SCIENCE OF SUCCESS

PSYCHOLOGICAL CHALLENGES

Amresh Shrivastava
MD, DPM, FRCPsych, FAPA,
Psychiatrist

Declaration

ll images have been taken from pixabay, royalty free, authorized for 'Free for commercial use, No attribution required' Pixabay (www. pixabay.com). We profoundly thank the company and the contributors of these images

Paperback ISBN 13: 978-93-90507-81-8
Paperback ISBN 10: 93-90507-81-2

Hardback ISBN 13: 978-93-90507-86-3
Hardback ISBN 10: 93-90507-86-3

Published by BUUKS Publishers, India

EDITORIAL SUPPORT

Ujwala Shrivastava
Siddhansh Shrivastava

ART CREDIT

Ajai Chavan

CONTRIBUTING AUTHORS

Dr Harneed Kaur MD

1. Adolescent mental health
2. Personal development

Dr Siddhansh Shrivastava MD

1. Brain structure and function
2. Stress and stress management

DISCLAIMER

The contents of this book are not a medical or legal document for any kind of evidence in any real-life situation. In this book every person's name and all kinds of identifiable information have been anonymised. The stories are edited for protection of privacy and confidentiality. This book is not intended as a suggestion, evidence or substitute for the medical advice of physicians. The reader should regularly consult a physician for matters relating to his or her health, particularly with respect to any symptoms that may require immediate attention, investigation, diagnosis and treatment. Contents of the book are neither any evidence nor support any legal positions that may arise in any situations pertaining to mental illnesses of an individual. The book is written for awareness, information and education in the field of mental health. It is not intended to form any opinion or pass any judgement or be pre-judgmental, be discriminatory, bring prejudice or cause any emotional or psychological trauma or damage about any patient or their families or caregivers. Any resemblance to demographic, history, social situations, illnesses, diagnosis, treatments, and consequences of illnesses or treatments discussed in the book is merely coincidental.

CAUTION

NOTICES

This book is about mental health and its role in accomplishing success in life. It discusses practice of spiritual sciences in dealing with psychological challenges, and accomplishing success in life.

TABLE OF CONTENTS

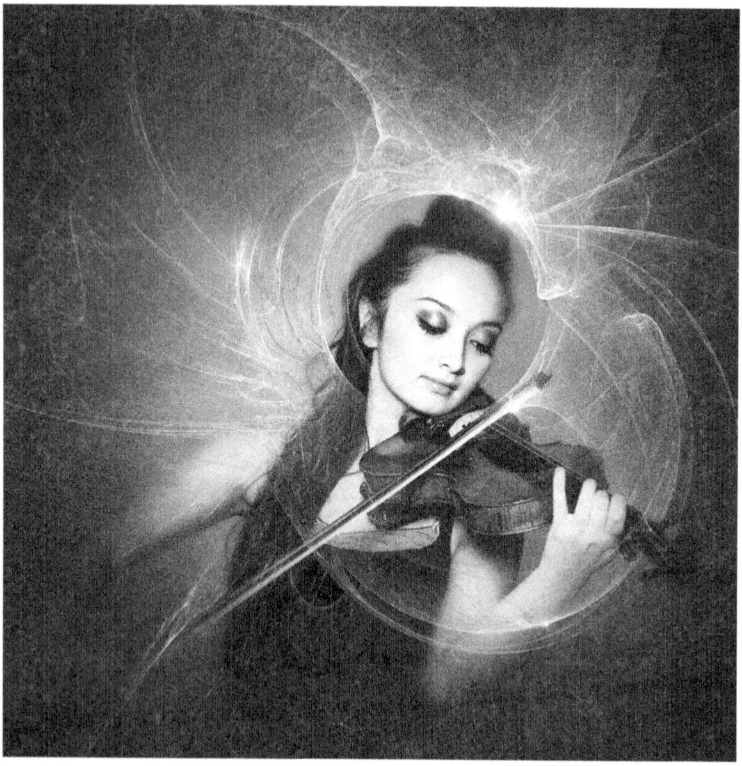

Success is not
for ever, but the
experience of success
is everlasting.

ACKNOWLEDGEMENTS

Writing a book for a new generation is far more challenging because one has to travel ahead of time to understand their demands and desires. They are several decades ahead of me. I have had to develop some unique methodologies to deal with this problem. I formed an informal group of discussants of students from different walks of life: medicine, science, art, literature and engineering. Most of the young minds who joined me to help are currently in universities and from my own family network.

Some of them discussed the issues with their friends as well and came up with unique suggestions; they also collected opinions from a few internet communities.

I remember hours of brainstorming with them to streamline the concept and content.

Mental health is not a very popular topic, but from their discussions I understood that the science of mental health makes great sense.

I am thankful to each one of them.

At several places they have contributed in writing as well, this book truly belongs to them. Thank you very much. I love you all.

Amishi Srivastava, Anirudh Shrivastava, Anshula Shrivastava, Divyansh Srivastava Lakshya Kaushal, Shivang Chavan, Shivank Srivastava, Shriansh Shrivastava, Siddhansh Shrivastava, Suryansh Kumar, Swati Shah Shrivastava, Ujwala Shrivastava and, Yash Srivastava.

The idea to write a book about basic information regarding mental health for students and young people struggling in their careers has been with me for quite a while. It gradually became much stronger as I worked with university students in India, UK and Canada. Interacting with them was quite insightful for understanding why they feel tense and depressed. It is very different in many aspects. I am thankful to each one of them who bestowed their trust in me, came up and spoke to me on matters that they would have never done with anyone else.

This book would have remained only an idea if not for the serious involvement of my wife Ujwala. She is the most deserving person to claim its credit. She took charge of editing this volume which has been a tiring job because the project has finally ended up with three different volumes: a comprehensive one for behavioural sciences, a shorter volume for students and the last one focusing on spirituality and mental health, which discusses the significance of spirituality in prevention of mental disorders.

One can write a book, but whether it will finally reach the right places or not, that is, in a book store can never be decided by the author. I would have seriously erred if I did not have ongoing support from Ajai Chavan who is a friend and a creative director in design; he has withstood my all-round nagging and has shared his ideas consistently through the process of putting this book together.

Siddhansh deserves a special mention for contributing, writing and reviewing the text of the book and bringing in contemporary thinking of medical students. I am particularly thankful to Dr Harneet Kaur for her collaboration.

I am grateful to Professors Nilesh Shah (Mumbai) and Nitin Gupta (Chandigarh) for reviewing the volume and providing their feedback. They assessed the contents and came up with valuable suggestions.

All images have been taken from pixabay, royalty free, authorized for 'Free for commercial use, No attribution required' Pixabay (www.pixabay.com). We profoundly thank the company and the contributors of these images

Last but not the least, I wish to thank my publishers, BUUKs publishers and their team specially Mr Prasad G.D and Sandra Sherin Naren Publishing Manager, who have made the book a reality and have produced a living example of knowledge translation. In addition, I would like to thank Miss Sonia Perumal, copyeditor for her contribution towards reviewing and proof reading the book. I have a firm conviction that knowledge transforms people; I am hopeful that readers of this book will be, at least, more careful in handling their life.

Thank you all.

PROLOGUE

His Excellency Ajay Bisaria
High Commissioner
High Commission of India
Ottawa, Canada

Science of success: Psychological Challenges
Author: Amresh Shrivastava

Suicide is a tragic way to end life and its prevention must remain a priority humane objective for society. Dr Srivastava has added valuable thought and research to the quest for a deeper understanding of suicide and related issues. His insights from science, religion and ancient learning moulded in a modern theoretical framework, would be a valuable addition to the thinking on this subject. Early intervention is critical to deal with complex mental disorders that drive people to end their lives. We, therefore, need every bit of expertise and research on this mental health issue to show us the light on prevention which can save valuable lives. In Canada, we have seen tragically high levels of suicide, particularly among young migrants from India going through difficult processes of adaptation to their new environment. Dr Srivastava has spent a lifetime in a stellar professional career spanning over 38 years, not just dealing with mental health issues but also in research and advocacy for preventing suicide. An integrative approach – that focuses on prevention and strengthening spiritual well-being through lessons from ancient Indian scriptures like the Bhagwad Gita and yogic sciences – is exactly what can provide us the way forward.

Dr Afzal Javed
President World Psychiatric Association

SCIENCE OF SUCCESS PSYCHOLOGICAL CHALLENGES
Book by Amresh Shrivastava MD, DPM, FRCPsych, FAPA, Psychiatrist

It is a great pleasure to write this note on the publication of a recent book, SCIENCE OF SUCCESS PSYCHOLOGICAL CHALLENGES, written by a well renowned psychiatrist, Amresh Shrivastava.

Dr. Srivastava's professional career spans over 38 years in mental health. He served in India, the United Kingdom and Canada in the fields of clinical academics, research, and education encompassing Government health services, private practice, universities, and professional organizations.

It is true that achievement and success can be described in several different ways. However, one dimension of success is the accomplishment of one's goals. The process, no doubt, is complex and besides other factors, mental health is one of its determinants. The importance of mental health is highlighted by the fact that despite excellent ability, many of us are still not successful, and many lose by just a margin. This is when we wonder whether the success is achievable with a little psychological support. It is therefore important to understand the role of mental health in success.

He has always been inspired by the complexities of mental health and its impact on day to day living along with understanding of its different dimensions. Dr Shrivastava's current book explains mental health and its role in accomplishing success in life & discusses practice of spiritual sciences in dealing with psychological challenges and accomplishing success in life.

A significant number of young people may suffer from a psychiatric ill-health or some problem arising due to stressful life situations. We thus need to gain better understanding of what changes are required, and what steps can be taken to preserve and promote mental health among these young individuals. This book certainly provides an account how to be successful and how to maintain success. It is hoped that this book will generate a lot of interest among public as well as for the mental health professionals in their practices.

I congratulate Dr Amresh Shrivastava for this work and hope we will continue getting further contributions from his clinical, academic, and professional expertise.

M.B.B.S; M.C.P.S; D.Psych. (Lond.); Board Cert.Psych. (U.K); M.Phil. (Edin.); F.R.C.Psych. (UK) F.R.C.P (Ireland)

President World Psychiatric Association
Consultant Psychiatrist & Honorary Professor Institute of Applied Health Research, University of Birmingham, UK, Honorary Associate Clinical Professor, Warwick Medical School, University of Warwick, UK,

Matra Raj Majmundar
President- International association of Yoga Therapy

A Story is one of the few mediums, if not the only one, through which one can impart complex concepts to a child or a scientist alike! Story creates a compelling urge to revisit its whole essence from time to time.

Through stories, Dr. Amresh Srivastav lays a strong foundation for readers. His stories are built by weaving universal principles of Ancient Scriptures and contemporary research. As a result, he is able to harness readers' inner awareness and offer bite-size doable practices. Dr. Srivastav gently nudges the readers to transition from self-doubt and self-inflicted mental negative barriers to, empathy, achievement, and self-freedom. Zapped of its power, self-doubts give way to a budding tiny voice. The voice gradually manifests itself in the birth of a seeker!

Thanks to stalwarts like Dr. Srivastav, growing understanding and admiration of holistic approaches - as a therapeutic methodology - is a novelty no more. The methodology is becoming a bridge between medical and healing community. Books like Science of Success have been a catalyst in bringing about such transformation. The transformation will foster an eco-system and bind forces of Healing Art and Science.

According to Dr. Srivastav, engagement in occupation and meaningful activity with purpose is an innate human need. Presence of these factors is necessary to achieve and maintain one's overall health and wellness.

Because mental health stressors are multifactorial, Dr Srivastava offers holistic multi solutions that are usable as daily tools. Not only that, he takes readers a step further - he exposes readers to ideas like Learned Optimism and Eustress (positive benefit of stress). This, in turn, brings changes in readers' mind-set. Result? -improved self-efficacy and desired performance in their chosen occupation! Talk about a domino effect!

How does Dr. Srivastava achieve such a feat? By convincingly demonstrating through his work that individuals, with mental health disorders or psychosocial differences, ***do and can,*** *improve functional outcomes – irrespective of their life roles – in their everyday lives.*

Dr. Srivastav dissects 'Success'! Being successful ***does not add anything to one's self-worth or attitude towards life.*** Instead, he argues, true success should be guided by one's belief system and wisdom – *for, Success is an experience that is only measured by what it means to each individual.*

Dr. Srivastav's focus on Early intervention is vital. Early Detection and development help in self-regulation, self-structuring, self-education and self-governance – to say the least. Reentry in family, community, and in one's occupation, can be achieved with the help of friends, family, community, society, educational institutions, and workplaces. Therefore, Dr. Srivastava suggests that availability of wellness programs and counseling services in schools, universities, and community centers must be accessible and made affordable right away.

Dr. Srivastav's armor is built with positivity and spirituality. Its ingredients include, but are not limited to, oneness, health and happiness, satisfaction, selflessness, trust, optimism, compassion, contentment, resiliency, self-witnessing, divinity, and loving-kindness!

Let us pause and ask ourselves - how can one enjoy utmost balance and optimal health? According to Dr. Srivastava, one should integrate (1) Ancient holistic Medicine - like Yogic practices Asana, Breathing-Pranayama, Relaxation, Mudras and Mindful Meditation; with (2) Ayurveda - based on individual's unique Personality- Prakriti. The integration will create a connection with agreeable natural elements and bio-fire blueprint. (3) Bhagvad Gita empowers people for culturing mind for detachment. All three enhance brain plasticity.

In light of the above, Individuals, Parents, Scientific Communities, Corporations, Military Leaders, Education Institutions, Hospitals, and Governments are more likely to embrace the findings of the 'Science of Success' to address intractable individual and social problems.

So, when all is said and done, a story merges into personal Sadhana to cultivate a sustainable lifestyle:

Din-charya by regular daily practice of Sage Patanjali's universal moral principles (Yama). To be a responsible Social Citizen through Self-purification and inner discipline (Niyama).

Matra Raj Majmundar OTR. C-IAYT AWC (Ayurvedic Counselor)
Certified - Mudra, Somatic Yoga Teacher and Peri Natal Educator.
Author-Yoga for Pregnancy, Birth and Vibrant Life.
President- International association of Yoga Therapy (Iayt.org)
The Y board member- Healthy Living and Youth Development.
Society for Art and Cultural Heritage of India (SACHI)- Past VP

Prof.Shailendra Singh, Ph.D., FNA Psy
Director,
Indian Institute of Management
Ranchi, India

All of us want success in life and work. But what is success in not clear to us. Some may think getting good grades in college is success. Another may think having good job and doing well in that is success. Still another may think being satisfied in personal and professional life is success. So, there is no universal definition of success. Success may be very subjective experience, measurement of which is also illusive. Thus, what make people a success is also debatable. The subject is so popular and also controversial that scholars from psychology, philosophy, management background, social scientists and many others have tried their hands to answer the question. Dr. Amresh Shrivastava , a medical professional and a trained psychiatrist has attempted to answer through his book titled, *Science of Success-Psychological Challenges.* Although, there are no easy answers to the question: what are the determinants of success? Hold on to your curiosity and read the book. You may find some interesting answers. I don't want to quell your exploration into the book and encourage you read the book and develop your own perspective from amongst multiple pathways to success.

The book touches on many psychological challenges people face in their lives during the journey of academic and professional careers. Read on. What Dr Shrivastava has narrated resembles with the story of many individuals struggling to make space for themselves in the world characterized by vulnerability, uncertainty, complexity and ambiguity. He goes on to provide perspectives on stress and its management, resilience, emotional intelligence, psychological challenges like feeling low, regulating moods, modifying behaviour, impulsivity, depression, anxiety, etc. He also tries to explain brain mechanism involved in these experiences.

Is personality related to success? How does it contribute to wellness? Can we transform our personalities? Can we change our destiny through life style interventions? Interested in knowing answers to these intriguing questions, you are invited to take dip into this book.

Once you have soaked the knowledge about personality, traits and their plasticity, you may develop a perspective that you can change your situation. Now you are ready to experience change, the book takes you to the spiritual retreat by showcasing the wisdom from Shrimad Bhagwat Geeta, Mahabharat, Yoga Sutra, Buddha, Gayatri Mantra, and the power of spirituality in healing, performance and success in very simple language.

The book is full of research-based recommendations and popular maxims of success. It also provides rich material on how to overcome psychological and mental challenges while progressing on the path of satisfaction and happiness. However, Dr. Shrivastava has put a disclaimer very clearly, that the book is not a substitute to psychotherapy. Please consult your doctor for treatment of problems.

The book is very timely addition to the literature of Success and Mental Health when the whole world is suffering under the grip of COVID-19 and anxiety, fear, depression, losses, bereavements etc. are on its peak. Readers may find some resolutions and gain perspectives on the challenging situation the world is facing.

Prof.Shailendra Singh, Ph.D., FNA Psy
Director,
Indian Institute of Management
Ranchi, India

PREFACE

Achievement and success can be described in several different ways, and no wonder there is no consensus definition. However, one aspect of success is the accomplishment of your goals. It is a process. The process is complex and besides other factors, mental health is one of its determinants. The importance of mental health is highlighted by the fact that despite excellent ability, many are still not successful, and many lose by just a margin. This is when we wonder whether the task was achievable with a little psychological support. Yes, it is, and thus it's important to understand the role of mental health in success. One always wonders where lies the difference that only a few can achieve what they desire? Predicting success would be the most rewarding job in this world. It is not possible so far. Achievement and success are too complex to predict. The main reason could be because we are unable to investigate and comprehend the process of success or define its pathways.

A significant number of people suffer from a psychiatric ill-health or some problem arising due to stressful life situations.

We need to gain better understanding of what changes are responsible, and what steps can be taken to preserve and promote mental health. We also need to find how advancement in mental health sciences can yield good social and psychological empowerment of students. However, in contemporary times, most young adults find it difficult to withstand the psychological, social and existential challenges. The problems of young students globally are the same, except for a few cultural differences and varying living socio-economic situations. They are struggling with issues like depression, suicidal thoughts, examination stress, addiction, etc. Their inability to cope with life stands out as the primary issue. Most of their problems seem to arise from challenges in personal life, like academic stress, unemployment or relationship problems, but at the same time, many seem to also be struggling with mental disorders without having much understanding of it. Academic life is getting harder due to various deficiencies, including the system of education, and it could be due to lack of good and sufficient number of teachers or other resources. Problems responsible could be enumerated but the list could be endless, and lack of required resources should speak for it all. But the main issue is explained a little better when we view the 'social conditions' and understand its intricate relation to mental health. It is very frustrating for students when they are faced with certain situations like lack of equal opportunities, inadequate funding for education, discrimination and so on, which makes them feel powerless since they do not have control over it. All these culminate into increased mental disorders. Poor mental health leads to poor educational attainment and poor academic progress resulting into further deterioration of mental health. There are still 58 million children out of school globally and around 100 million children who do not complete primary education. About one fourth of them have a mental disorder, and least to say that only a few of them have access to care.

The problem of student mental health is so compelling that this topic needs to be included in every student's academic curriculum. Knowledge translation is therapeutic; it is not merely a body of information but an effective tool to provide intervention.

I hope that students and other aspiring people will find it interesting, meaningful and stimulating.

This book is the third publication in series of mental health literature, authored by me and published by BUUKS publishers.

**All powers are within you,
You can do anything and
everything.**

Swami Vivekanand

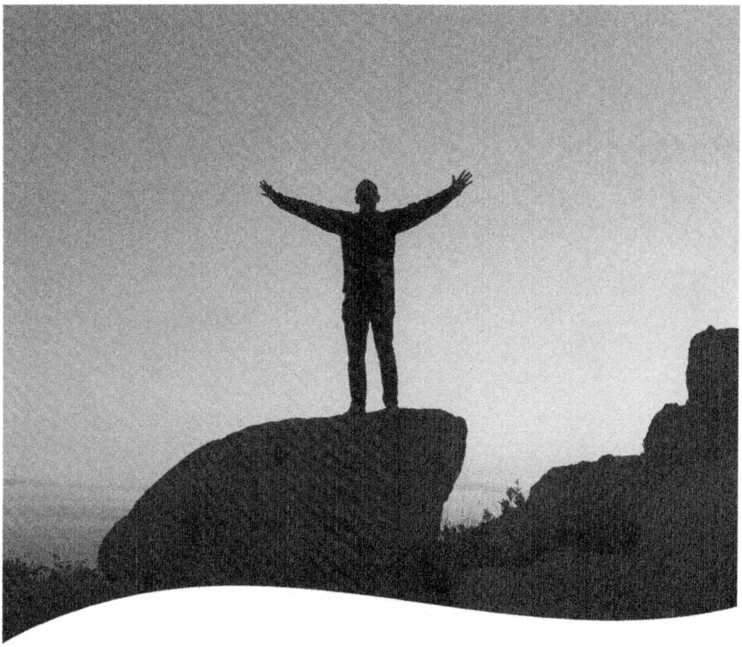

Those who have mental health problems also succeed

Around the world every 1 in 5 people
have a mental disorder.

At a global level, over 300 million people are estimated to suffer from depression, equivalent to 4.4% of the world's population.[1]

Student success starts with a positive mental health

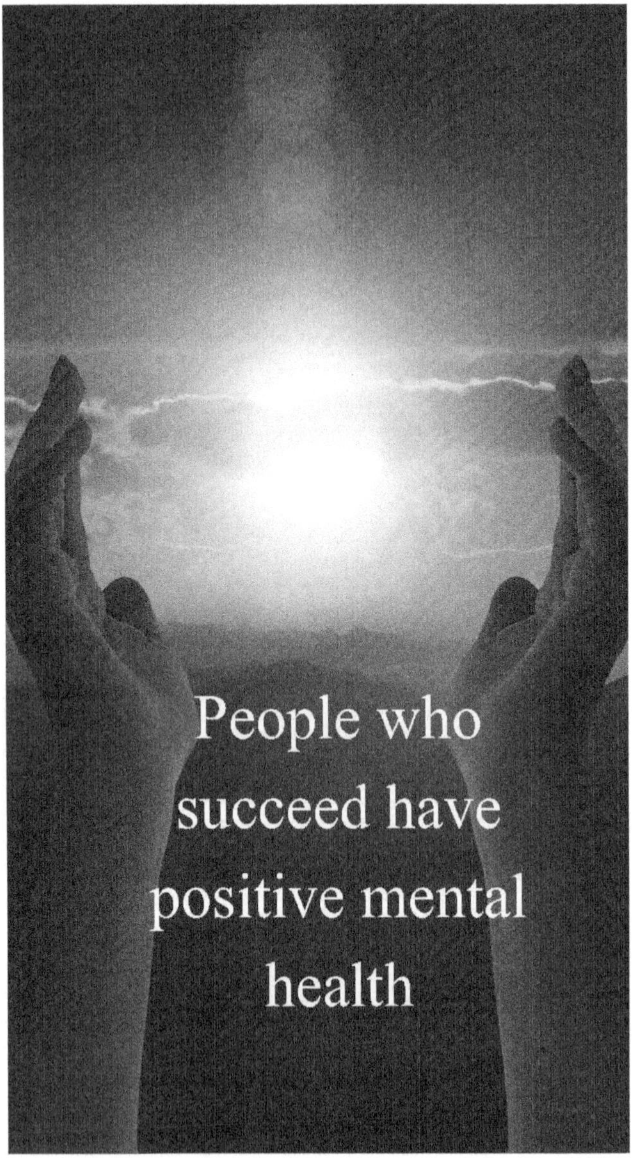
People who
succeed have
positive mental
health

SECTION 1

Everybody Wins

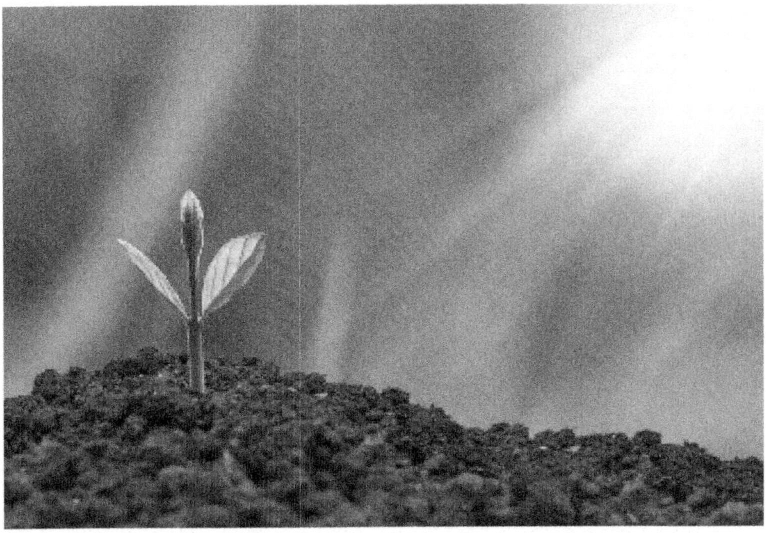

Success is a personal journey. It is an accomplishment which you cherish. If you are successful but unhappy, you will never treat this success with respect. Almost everyone who loses success either did not know the kind of success they aspired for, or they knew but chose to deceive themselves by setting wrong goals to achieve.

CHAPTER 1
SUSTAINING SUCCESS

1. SUCCESS UNLIMITED

Success is a dream and a cherished desire, but it holds a different meaning for everyone. Each one of us desire it for different reasons, but the psychological understanding remains the same. Success means to many, a matter of identity, their signature, their existence. Most people look at it as material achievement to be possessed or owned, and many people identify with it excessively. They want to be known as successful people.

Success is defined in many different ways. Several determinants have been discussed. For some it is a hard work, while others believe it is achieved with commitment and conviction.

As a result, it does not remain absolute; it becomes relative to something and especially something which others have. They want to match their success with that of others. This understanding is a road to frustration and guilt. Frustration because the sense of competitiveness is never-ending and guilt because what one loses while gaining a competitive success is always regretful.

Success is a credit only to those who are honestly aware of its true meaning.

It is neither a war to conquer nor a game to win.

Value of success is only the utmost when it works in your best interest.

The real definition is the one which can give you an insight to accomplish the kind of success that is good for your inner self.

Success is not time bound and definitely not short-lived, as for only today or tomorrow. It is more or less a continuous process. A success which comes with worries and without satisfaction or contentment is not 'the success'. If such a success gratifies you, that would mean you neither understood success nor have looked within yourself. An integral constituent of success is honesty. Your honesty to recognise and appreciate the need and nature of your success will be a true success for you.

Success is a personal journey. It is an accomplishment which you cherish. If you are successful but unhappy you will never treat this success with respect. Almost everyone who loses success either did not know the kind of success they aspired for, or they knew but chose to deceive themselves by setting wrong goals to achieve.

An individual's first test of honesty lies in making the choices for oneself. An honest choice is free from burden and obligations. You can own it. Thus, setting up goals for success with honesty will not leave you with pain, sorrow and regret, even if you do not accomplish it.

The challenges arise in knowing what is good for you.

The ability to know yourself is the best attribute that you need. Knowing your own mindset and the extension of your mental health is of prime importance while planning to succeed.

The very idea to succeed begins from a clear state of mind. A disturbed mind and defensive mindset plans with an ambivalence. The backdrop of ambivalence is a definite route to remain unsuccessful.

People hardly think about mind and mental health. It does not hit us that there is something like thought, emotion and memory which will determine whether you will be successful.

Not many are able to detect the psychological challenges interfering in the process of becoming successful. The mental health front of success and failure provides a unique perspective. A fresh look in deciding for a successful career or future with a prism of mental health gives clear imagery of success.

Awareness is an attribute which distinguishes a person from others on this planet. Humans have come a long way in millions of years, and in the process they have obtained increased brain mass and very fertile pre frontal cortex which gives us the power of understanding, insight, foresight, intellect, cognition and everything that determines 'sense of meaning and reasoning'.

What do we mean by knowing ourselves? It is about understanding body, mind and, spiritual values.

It is about looking into yourself with honesty. Being honest means knowing your mind, body and spiritual sense.

Success is a personal experience. What success means to someone depends upon his/her value system.

Success is not merely a gain or failure or even a loss.

Becoming successful does not add anything to your self-worth or your attitude towards life.

And becoming unsuccessful does not take away anything from you.

The fundamental questions which people face are

(1) How to become successful? and
(2) How to succeed again after becoming successful, or how to sustain the success?

Nobody wants to lose success.

Someone wants to become successful at any cost...

Life is not a war which you will have to win at any/all cost.

Thus, the consideration of cost in becoming successful is not appropriate.

Success is an experience; it is measured based upon what it means to you.

2. THE UNTOLD STORY - RAJAN - AN ASPIRING YOUNG MAN

It is difficult to be successful, but it is far more difficult to maintain success. Happiness of success is often lost for many. About half of the successful people develop significant psychological problems. Handling success has nothing to do with how educated you are, and it is not because of your intelligence, but it depends upon the basic value system which people possess. It depends upon understanding of success. It is a testimony of your belief in yourself. Many people are anxious to become successful, and they carry their anxiety with them even after becoming successful. Their psychological traits like fear, trust, faith and so on. interfere with their performance and decision making. Some people do not find a sense of fulfilment, and it is likely that they have chosen a wrong path. Their emotional and intellectual responses determine their involvement in the work they do. It can often go wrong. Only a few remain contented. They are the people of wisdom.

Rajan's course of life is perhaps the best way to understand the importance of mental health in the journey of life.

India was transforming rapidly, and young men in the society were aspiring and restless. They were questioning most things around them. The trend of globalisation had changed the common topic of discussion around in coffee shops or college street corners. Students had access to more money, and most of them enjoyed their independence and autonomy. It is much different than what was a few decades ago. Those days too, many bright students had decided to leave the country for further excellence. Then India was considered to be a place of limited opportunities, though not any more.

The environment now is encouraging and vibrant, full of hope and confidence. Students do not harbour a sense of self-doubt, anxiety or ambivalence; now it is a straight path, evident in their thoughts where their ambition and aspirations are the driving forces. Future of the young Indian generation is bright. I have reasons for my opinion; the last ten years have seen a large number of highly successful non-resident Indians in different countries as doctors, professors, CEOs, bankers, scientists, people in Silicon Valley and many more. In present times, I wonder what really is going through their minds, and what are the thoughts of today's graduates, do they still aspire to go abroad, or are the advances in this country inviting enough for the young to proceed and indulge in new start-ups or join the services right here. I hope whatever position they all reach, they will also be happy. There are very few people today who will say that their goal in life is to remain happy. Very few would keep happiness as a priority over achievement.

Immigrant Indians bear very great capacity to adjust in difficult, multicultural societies. They are known to be quite resilient. Rajan was one of them. He was 45 years old with a prestigious degree in business management. At the age of 25, he was offered admission in a US university with scholarship. A great opportunity and a golden chance to do another business degree and to go around the world. He immigrated and completed the course within the stipulated time frame and also took up another course in International law. It was an enviable situation and great qualification. He preferred to join a law firm as a financial manager. He told me that it was a difficult decision, but he did not want to look back.

Many people face difficulty of psychological nature. They are not abnormal. They may be at risk, or they may be vulnerable. Such people react very strongly to stress.

Significant number of people have several traits which are neither normal nor abnormal. When these traits become a symptom under stressful situations, a psychiatric disorder begins. Every psychiatric disorder starts with milder shades of abnormality in behaviour, personality, thoughts, mood or emotion. Though these problems present with some amount of limitation, they can cause severe dysfunction. This highlights several aspects of milder symptoms of mental health leading to significant disruption in the course of life.

When I received him in my office, I was surprised to hear the reason for his visit. He said that he was staying in the US for more than 20 years and now wanted to go back to India. He hoped to discuss this issue with me. It was interesting to see someone who was not ill. As a psychiatrist during most part of the day the talking and listening consists of stories of sadness, pain, depression, and trauma. It was refreshing. I thought to have the opportunity to learn newer things, but I knew it was not as simple as it was presented. I will have to determine if he was 'going away' from America or 'returning back' to India.

We had completed three sessions, within the following two weeks. I knew enough about him by now.

Rajan was an only son of a middle-class but educated family. His father was an accountant in a medical college, and mother was working in an insurance agency. They knew he was very bright and confident since childhood, unlike his father. Perhaps he was more like his grandfather because he reflected similar qualities. Since he was bright and hard-working, his parents invested all their energy and money to educate him. Rajan was brought up to be a respectful person with good moral values. He was also religious and believed in God. He would never fail to offer his prayers. He was a regular visitor to the local temple and was actively involved in the community. After his law degree in the USA, he joined a multinational organisation and started working with reasonable success, but soon after, his growth felt stagnating. He was neither promoted nor was his work acknowledged with any pay hike during the past five years. He worked hard, put in extra hours and as a result could not focus on his personal life. Somehow things were not in place. In every project he worked, the rewards acknowledged someone else in the team. This changed his attitude, and he started getting suspicious. On various occasions he expressed his doubts to his friend in India to confirm if he was wrong or prejudiced at the workplace. No one was in absolute agreement or could totally understand his issues. This was the beginning of his problems. His behaviour started changing, and he lost trust in people around him and his team. A team which was navigating his plans and projects was now discussing him in his absence. His secretary sensed his discomfort and offered that she would reconfirm his availability and willingness to attend before booking any meetings on his behalf. Colleagues were uncooperative, and it led to further isolation, within six months the team members were on divergent paths. He was fighting a lose-lose battle for nothing.

On arrival in USA, he married a Caucasian fellow student he had met at the university. Initially, for a few years he was able to manage the family well but after a while that too had failed. He was not able to spend time with his wife and two kids and now they were feeling neglected.

Rajan had not come to the country with any pre-fixed ideas, and he had no disregard for local culture, language or people. He projected as if he belonged to the country but was a very obstinate and obsessive person; extra careful about cleanliness, always organising his schedule, rearranging his belongings, his pen and paper, the computer mouse. The moment he would try to change the place even of a photo frame in his room he used to become anxious and after a few minutes, he would bring it back in its original position. He would go to a meeting and insist on sitting on a particular seat in a particular direction, and he believed that if he did not sit in a chair facing east or north-east, the decisions of the discussion will not be in his favour.

His work would not translate in any progress, despite all the hard work he put in. His networking was inefficient, and he was not able to socialise. He would spend time looking for ways to excuse himself from dinner meetings, and many times he returned from the venue and sent an apology. While in a crowd, he wondered if people were looking at him or trying to guess what was on his mind. He would then get anxious and leave. People perceived him as a loner which he was not. Was he a misfit? He often wondered how to have a job which will be a better fit.

He started getting bored and losing interest. During these five years, he had experienced a significant degree of emotional burnout. He started working mechanically; he did everything right except that he did not bother about how his efforts could translate into a profit for himself. His philosophy was that once he applied his mind to a project and did everything right, and it was not his problem how profitable it turned out to be. This nature did not help the organisation.

Along the same time, his marital life strained and his wife moved out of the house. His responsibilities increased as now he also had to look after the kids. He was now their sole caretaker. He took a break of three months and tried to cope with the home situation with his children. It was a kind of 'stress-leave'.

After a few months, he got another job and resigned from the present one.

He soon realised that he may have some limitations and thought it was apt to enrol in a course of personality development and effective communication even before he joined the new position. He prepared himself thoroughly, and collected information about every person in his team, his bosses and his clients. He attempted to learn things to help him function better in an organisation as a leader as well as a team member and tried to master several other skills which he felt he was missing.

He also visited a doctor to talk about his compulsive habits and stress. The doctor referred him to a counsellor with whom he spent about half a dozen sessions to prepare himself.

He improved significantly and was doing well in his new job, and his income improved. He even considered getting back together with his wife, and pocketed a couple of pay hikes. His opinion and guidance was of value now. But all was not that straightforward. Once his boss scheduled to come to his city, and a meeting was fixed between the two. Rajan had a golf meet with a business partner at the same time. His dilemma was not resolved, and he left the decision for the last moment.

On the very day, he chose to attend the golf meet and sent an apology to his boss. This behaviour was unexpected and unacceptable. It was documented in his confidential report, and he was called for a professional discussion. His organisation took it seriously, his performance was reviewed and to their surprise, they found several irregularities, he had missed out on a lot of meetings. Him assigning his jobs to the junior colleagues seemed to be a common practice, and they were happy to do so since it was adding to their work experience.

The report and feedback forced him to leave the organisation.

He chose to escape the humiliation with smoking and drinking. Stress was overpowering and only led to loss of good health. His elder son was eleven years old and the daughter was nine by then. He was keen on returning to India, but that option presented problems of where to leave the kids, and then there weren't any promising jobs or opportunities awaiting him in India.

Was he disappointed? Yes, of course. Were there options? Yes. Was he able to utilise those options? Absolutely not. Why? He was not in a right frame of mind.

Why was he in such a conflict? He came to me to talk about it.

He was drunk the night his wife walked out on him never to contact him again. But she was in contact with the kids and even chose their school bags and sports shoes. He did not care until he lost his job. In moments of despair, he missed her a lot. Loss of job was a loss of purpose. His knowledge was not enough to establish his own business of financial management. He was torn between the decisions and saw no options.

By now I had heard his story in five sessions without any comments. Only questions I asked were to collect additional information. He was keen on getting some answers from me, and he asked for my advice.

He wanted me to suggest a way out, 'That is not what is done in counselling or therapy', I said. He was now feeling better and thinking more clearly. He should decide, but it did not work, and he kept on insisting so I persisted with my reply.

As the sessions progressed, his ruminations and racing thoughts had increased.

Once he talked about his restlessness to his family doctor. This doctor prescribed some medication and explained that it is a symptom of a psychiatric disorder called obsessive-compulsive disorder. He said that the symptoms can appear with increased stress due to the heightened rumination of thoughts. Rajan did not follow the explanation and refused the medication.

Things were not getting any better and he had resorted to continuous use of alcohol. This was traumatic for the kids. They informed their mother who was scared for their well-being and safety. She arranged to get the kids under her care.

This event seemed to be quite an eye-opener, and he stopped drinking and decided to get things in order. He started spending time with his friends instead, but the anxiety was still building up. It was now clear that the therapy sessions with me were not working out or helping him.

His friends suggested that he should join some spiritual discourse groups, where he could meet new people, and a fresh insight may help him. They even gave him some information about a well-known Indian guru, whose groups he could attend.

Rajan appreciated the thought, since he saw no harm in taking up spiritual learning as this, he was sure, will at least not have any unpleasant side effects. Much was lost to stress, and he might as well take a break from the upheaval. His health was at its worst; weakness was increasing and the signs of depression were clearly indicated on his face. But he was against taking any medication.

His internet search led to a decision joining one of the Swami Chinmay Ananda's Ashram. Spiritual Camps, normally the week-long retreats, encouraged devotees to temporarily 'renounce' the world, briefly shelve daily problems and spend time in study, contemplation and introspection. It is an opportunity for total immersion in knowledge and devotion. He enjoyed the guidance as he got to learn many new things, but he was convinced that just doing a couple of courses was not going to get him anywhere. His friend in India advised that regular practice of yoga was a better option. Rajan was drained from trying out so many new things, which are known to show their effect if the practices were continued for a fair amount of time and brought in as a way of life.

He did not know, but his problem was fairly complex. He had a strong personality with number of adverse features. His ability to relate to trust was limited. The low-grade symptom of rumination of thought along with other symptoms were untreated. He got into a vicious cycle of psychological symptoms compromising his functioning and ability to connect with others. His significant drinking problems got him into trouble quite a few times. Any psychiatric disorders which are complicated with drugs and alcohol are hard to treat, and the response is poor. Also, the conditions which have some personality-related issues are also conditions for not a very good outcome.

It is almost a year now, and he is ritually practising yoga, both at home and attends guided classes at a nearby athletic club. His health is better now, though he has faced a lot of difficulties. He is still unemployed; during the tough times of economic recession, jobs are difficult.

It is not a matter of surprise that one has not shown good response to therapy with a qualified psychiatrist. Often clients are not honest and frank while discussing their problems thus evaluation does not necessarily become possible.

Culture influences our expectations about how person-to-person interactions will occur. Additionally, **culture** influences how we understand health and healing.[1]... **Cultural** ways of being are also present within **psychotherapy.**

Counsellors must incorporate culturally diverse clients' values and beliefs into the treatment process. **Cultural** belief systems like spirituality and family-centric issues may in themselves serve as therapeutic vehicles to promote healing[2] and self-awareness.

Throughout the year, Chinmaya Mission centres worldwide host spiritual camps or intensive residential courses for adults, children, youth or the whole family. Mission devotees also often choose to take a solitary retreat and stay at Mission ashrams.

Jnana Yajnas is a series of public discourses on a Vedantic scripture given by an Acharya of the Chinmaya Mission. It is for five to seven days. Jnana Yajnas are regularly organized by all Chinmaya Mission centres.

Spiritual Camps are week-long retreats organised by Chinmaya Mission in various ashrams and other locations all over the world.

'The evolutionary path is an uphill struggle, in ourselves, with us. Therefore, the seekers of spiritual life must have a few days of intense study and Bahasa [self-discipline] in a Camp consisting of similar hearts under the inspiring guidance of a Teacher, and that, too, in protected surroundings wherein the usual tussles of life will not reach him, nor the teasing temptations distract him. Such a spiritual holiday camp is a retreat.'[3]

- Swami Chinmay Ananda

3. MENTAL HEALTH AND MANAGING SUCCESS

Let us understand the case of Rajan, The mild degree of obsessive-compulsive tendencies did not interfere in several testing times, during Rajan's academic career. But when he started working, its consequences were apparent. People with obstinate nature are known to be careful and produce quality work, but due to mental exhaustion they are unable to get a high volume of work done, and therefore, their total output remains low. This limitation may also be referred to as a characteristic, possibly running in families. He had inherited and inculcated discipline and religiosity, but these strengths were not sufficient to deal with adversities. At the same time, he could make choices which are unconventional, for example, in his personal life, opting for an inter-religion marriage. No doubt Rajan was a virtuous man, but perhaps he could not transform his life in a manner as such people would normally do. His self-confidence and virtuous characters were not sufficient to save him from the consequences of the psychological stress in his life, and he succumbed to indulgence in smoking and drinking.

Though he is a careful and wise person, a history of longstanding failure makes him hostile. He was a man in a rush to achieve but he faced failure at every step in his job. He seemed to get the idea that things were not on a right path, but his intelligence was not sufficient enough to perceive the situation. He refused to acknowledge that his performance was declining. His inability to interact, form social relationships, review his style of functioning, identify his psychiatric or behavioural traits, be a good team player, conform to the prevailing style of functioning, change and over-value himself are some of the factors which he could have handled. But he was clearly not aware about it.

Did he need training for developing skills to cope with this limitation? No one goes for training for self-improvement before joining a job except for orientation about the nature of the job. There is an ongoing process of learning; if this particular feature is absent within you when your perception about yourself and others is incorrect, it results in situations of the kind Rajan had to face. In addition, he gradually became not only controlling but careless and complacent. He failed to realise his short-comings and finally made mistakes. The gravity of these mistakes cost him his job.

Success has several determinants. It depends on social and psychological characteristics, and not only on education and skills.[7, 8] Training and discourse can bring in a good change. Handling success has nothing to do with how educated you are, but it depends upon the basic value system which people possess. Everyone wants to succeed but everyone's definition of success is different. Some people relate success in a job of power which satisfies their need for control, some measure it with money earned which gives them the pleasure of money power, still, others want to remain content which gives them happiness they cherish and value. Success is a hard-earned treasure, many do not realise that it is too good to enjoy and too bad to envy.

Sustaining success and surviving in a job is a matter of cautious efforts. It is known that sustaining success is harder. Further psychiatric disorders or psychological challenges in day-to-day life are common. Often such problems are already a part of your personality since the beginning, but it accentuates when stress increases due to multiple demands and real-life challenges.

Whether it is employment, nature of work, cooperation by colleagues, rewards or lack of rewards or stresses arising from home situation or marriage, these are to be dealt with.

There is no single factor which can be held responsible. The responsible factors can be either external or internal. Both are constantly interplaying. External factors may be a reality, but these become more toxic due to internal factors.

Personality, ability to cope, psychiatric disorder, response to stress and nature of problem-solving are some of the predominant internal factors. External factors commonly include work environment, colleagues and lack of rewards.

Here is someone (Rajan) who is a motivated and a successful person, with no psychiatric history. He has a personality which reflects traits of obsessive behaviour, irritability, emotional rigidity and excessive confidence. He is conditioned to be appreciated all through his life due to his success in academic performance.

Overall, we can restrict this discussion to:

1. Personality traits or patterns
2. Psychiatric disorders or subclinical states
3. Coping ability and resilience

There is a significant overlap and inter-relationship between all three factors; none of the factors work in isolation. Most of the characteristics are part of behaviour, emotional response and cognitive abilities (e.g. intellectual ability). In other words, psychiatric disorder, personality factors and resilience are part of one's internal system. Some may change in intensity from time to time but most of them remain non-modifiable. However, the impact of these non-modifiable factors lead to limitations which can be minimised by treatment or training.

Experts in management psychology and organisational or behavioural sciences will provide a number of suggestions and tips about how to function successfully in a job. Their advice generally works when applied. They are indeed experts in this specialty.

Mental health professionals have multiple problems while handling such a case, for example determining the nature of the problem, finding the cause behind symptoms and having to not only deal with the symptoms but also their consequences, in a manner to make the best possible outcome possible. Their objective is to achieve a good quality of life and maintain the recovery.

Rajan clearly had undetected mental health problems which increased under stressful conditions. His coping was diminished and he developed a behaviour which caused so much damage to his health, occupation and family.

Are his problems modifiable? Yes, some of them are modifiable, their intensity and impact can be minimized.

Here are certain psychological features worth noting which are matter of concern in the present case: identification of traits of OCD, impulsivity, high need of appreciation, alcohol behaviour, life-style problems, skills for managing inter-personal relationship, marital relationship, management skills and effective conversation, conflict resolution, and skill for planning and execution of assignments.

Behavioural traits do not appear in a day or suddenly, these traits are a part of life, present in the personality but does not generally interfere unless there is any extraordinary or stressful situation. A problem which may be lying dormant may emerge in the form of psychiatric illness. Job is a significant stress. Before anyone joins in an employment, he or she should know about their own-self, strengths, weaknesses, blind spots, sore points, limitations, behaviours in relaxed time, and social and emotional support.

Origin of all behaviours is deep in genetics and experiences from environment and culture. All chronic or severe problems begin with milder symptoms. The opportunities to undertake corrective measures are often missed.

Those who think that their skills and academic qualifications alone shall give a successful and steady life are wrong. These qualities are not enough. You need emotional and social intelligence to prevent psychological problems. Awareness about this aspect of becoming successful is hardly discussed and therefore people may not be aware. Its indeed an important characteristics of personality and needs proper attention. Managing career needs several types of attributes. To become successful in a job demands great emotional strength and social skills, leadership style and collaborative strength; it demands emotional and social intelligence.

Periodic review and self-assessment, observing emotional states and following good lifestyle should generally be sufficient to avoid negative consequences. Managing mental health challenges, primarily addictions, marriage and stress are the main factors which help keep someone going irrespective of success or failure.

The story of Rajan is about 'sustaining the success'. He was a successful man, and his success did not help in having a healthy and fulfilling life.

He could not hold on to his success for long.

He lost success as well as many things which he thought he achieved because of this success, that is, his job, income, work, and health and family.

What was wrong ?

Vulnerability for psychological problems and inability to deal with the challenges in life

Rajan was perhaps vulnerable for developing psychological challenges, and he faced severe and challenging situations, as a result he developed problems.

What did he lack?

- Insight, understanding
- General knowledge of worldly affairs and life in general
- Principles of discipline, *dharma* and righteousness
- A sense of care and caution, self-care self-worth and confidence of his – being what he is.
- His respect, commitment for work/job and success

Precisely, he lacked –

1. The protective mechanism for mental health consequences
2. The ability to handle life and reduce the risks
3. The art of dealing with success
4. The principles of work and performance

He could not have done much for his vulnerability which is generally present since birth but was it possible to minimise the risk arising from these tendencies or susceptibilities so as to prevent the possibility of a mental disorder.

1. Inability to minimize the risk for psychological problems
2. Inability to deal with challenges in life

- o Inability to identify
- o Inability to learn
- o Inability to accept

1. Be aware of yourself, your strengths and your weaknesses.
2. Be aware of your values and your, meaning of life.
3. Be aware of knowledge and information in a general sense, like what is going on around us. No one can be ignorant.

He approached for treatment. He had some positive experiences and later on approached for lifestyle intervention and spiritual methods to deal with his problems.

What can he do now?

A few significant methods are helpful in deal with such complex situations in life, e.g. having full knowledge, developing abilities to change and being disciplined to comply with new learning, being honest with your own self, believing, practicing high ethical values and maintaining good physical health by life-style management. It is never too late to search and practice lessons for spiritualism that you believe in.

- In one of the clinical situations I am discussing why psychological problems develop and what role stress, risk factors and psychological challenges play.
- The second situation is discussed in section 3, where a young student develops a mental illness, receives treatment and recovers. He completes his studies and accomplishes whatever he wanted to.
- The difference in the two situation is in the manner they understood purpose of their lives. On one hand Suvarna, the young student could overcome all barriers and Rajan, a mid-career employee succumbs to the pressures, develops psychological problems but finally captures the lost ground.
- In both the situation what makes a difference in their life is the treatment of psychiatric disorders.

Rajan has a history of becoming successful in everything that he did, and his habit of succeeding has made him overconfident. He brings personal bias and callous conduct in his work ethics, gets easily stressed and fails to perform. He is quite impulsive, has difficulty in taking decisions and procrastinates while dealing with difficult situations. He did not develop a good rapport with his colleagues and doctors, to the extent that many of his colleagues isolated him and started taking advantage of him. He was not careful about social relations and interpersonal relationship. He drifted away in his marriage. This made his children lonely and frightened; they left him at one point of time. Finally, the worst thing which he could not deal with was the alcoholism. It took quite some time for him to trust someone and engage. He finally develops good connection with the place he received spiritual intervention.

Interventions from mental health or psychiatric intervention in form of medication, psychotherapy, social support, psychoanalysis, social engagement etc. have their limitation, no single treatment and most of the treatments in combination do not provide a response rate more than 60%. There is high rate of drop out and disengagement. Often people who non-comply develop serious problem.

These treatments are not designed to achieve what we are looking forward to bringing a positive change in overall life. Possibly a psychiatric intervention is only the first step and a good place to begin individual's transformation back to a 'healthy state'. We cannot say which treatment will work better or what are the treatments required. As modern science is evaluating several cultural, social and spiritual treatments I hope to have many people coming back to healthy state and a life with dignity and respect.

Further, psychiatric treatments are also not developed with objective of prevention of a psychiatric problem. We have limited knowledge about prevention. Overall we do not have a strategic intervention which can prevent an illness, there is no vaccine. Whenever methods for prevention be available, it cannot be a replacement for developing good character and resilient personality.

Good and happy human being will continue to be of prime and irrefutable significance.

4. PSYCHOLOGICAL HEALTH

Several reasons may make a student's life complex. Issues from their personal life back home, it could be differences with parents, and even matters like availability of funds for education. Diverse social and economic conditions always affect mental health. Thus, students suffer from both sets of problems, one which is a personal issue and the other could be an issue of global relevance.

Students' life represents an interface where psychological problems and problems of education are intertwined in a manner that one is inseparable from the other. If a student is in a crisis due to emotional reasons, school and education play a role. Since the students spend most time in school and its environment, facilities, culture, teachers, their behaviour, etc. influence their mind. Sometimes the impressions made in school can remain for life, particularly the negative experiences.

Suicide, depression, and alcoholism are not the only problems students face. They are pressured due to several other issues which never appear in the list of problems. e.g. 'lifestyle' constantly works on the minds of students. Much of the problems are local and cultural. Problems we see in universities and colleges in India are unique where student's problem is closely related to family's income, health condition, the distance of the school from home and lack of resources/teacher etc.

Research studies conducted provide reasonably good information. These studies have been conducted in communities by visiting people in particular areas. The major source of information about student's mental health comes from hospitals and clinics where these students are taken for treatment and this information is usually limited to the serious nature of problems. Minor problems are treated by counselors in the schools or by doctors in their clinics. Overall, a fairly good estimate becomes available about the mental health problems of the students. Studies show that about 25% of people in our society are likely to be affected; and about 10% are in the age range of 13 to 17 years have a mental disorder. Mental health issues have far-reaching consequences. It affects daily life activities, ability to learn and engage in gainful employment, the ability to develop social relations and thereby chances of leading a quality life.

The students go through a severe psychological turmoil which compromises their capacity to deal with changes, adversities, and stressors in their lives. They are in this age of 'transitioning' from one stage to another in biology and sexuality, they are trying to understand their own body, mind, and emotions. Their coping mechanism sometimes fall short of dealing with anxiety, depression, and academic failure. There are many areas in and around the student which could be the potential source of psychological problems and almost always remain at-risk. Why are students at higher risk? Sometimes students have a stress-related problem, but they also have sufficient mental strength to deal with such problems. Some other students may face similar problems but may not have sufficient mental strength or may not feel positive or motivated to help themselves.

Psychological Challenges:
Our first concern is as we know that students suffer from mental health problems. Let's see how common these are: e.g.,

- Some children are born with mental health problems like-intellectual disability, mathematical skills, writing reading, and language development, etc.
- The problems which are present since birth is more likely related to brain functioning.
- On the other hand, the problems which develop afterward during childhood or adolescence are generally minor.
- Only a small percentage of such students develop more serious or severe problems. Such problems can be like feeling anxious, depressed, inability to concentrate, or problems related to memory, loss of sleep or having poor appetite.

We can also look at the problems

1. **Arising from student's personal life**
2. **Arising from families and cultural contexts and**
3. **From school resources and environment.**

These problems often appear in form of complains in physical health. Health related symptoms are common as a presentation of mental pain. Emotional problems, emotional crisis, problems from inter-personal relationships, issues arising from attitude of people around the students are also very common.

Many times, these problems are left untreated or unattended.

It is not necessary that you have to always contact someone like a doctor or a counsellor. You can help yourself and sort out a lot of these difficulties. It is therefore important to know about mental health. If you know how to recognise the problems, what to do in that situation, you will not suffer but if such information is not known your problems can increase. This is exactly the purpose of this book; my objective is to inform you about mental health and its abnormalities. Similarly, I also want to tell you the merits and challenges of mental health, so that the quality of your life can be at its best.

Our mental health affects all areas of our life. It surely, therefore, influences our ability to work, to grasp, to apply our mind and all other mental faculties. Since education is related to mental faculties it is obvious that education and health, particularly mental health are intricately related. In fact problems of mental health become one of the toughest barriers for accomplishing objectives of education, which is one of the key characteristics to succeed. Our mental strength determines our conviction and confidence. Adverse mental health leads to tension, stress, depression and sometimes suicide, mental stress and mental disorders reduce the ability to function and do compromise mental well-being.

Problems like poor concentration, mood changes, addiction, anger, aggression, and many others are present commonly but may not be severe enough to require treatment or qualify for a diagnosis. When the difficulty increases and the symptoms start interfering with daily life's activities and ability to perform work or, are employed or cause harm to themselves or others e.g. not eating for days, becoming violent or talking about self-harm, then it may require appropriate treatment after a thorough assessment and achieving a diagnosis since these problems progress, changes in mood makes the person erratic and irritable, students start procrastinating, lose interest in doing daily activities, studies appear harder and harder, therefore they avoid academic work, consequently their attendance becomes poorer, they fall behind in examinations, lose their respect in a competitive peer group. Very slowly students often miss the opportunity to recognise it well in time. I will discuss this later in this book.

How a mental disorder develops is not precisely known. However, most researchers and experts agree on the current understanding that several factors combine uniquely leading to mental illness. There is a general understanding and consensus that mental disorders are multifactorial and no single factor can be responsible.

Mental Health is a dynamic state of internal equilibrium which enables individuals to use their abilities in harmony with universal values of society. There are few important components of mental health, which are maintained with the harmonious relationship between body and mind. Some of these characteristics are intellectual activity, cognitive functions and social skills. Ability to recognise, express and modulate one's emotions, ability to cope with adverse life situations forms the necessary features of mental health.

All psychiatric symptoms are neither a mental disorder nor do they necessarily develop into a mental disorder. Large number of people in society remain at risk for mental disorder however only a few of them develop an illness. Mental disorders present with both mental as well as physical symptoms. The symptom suggesting any psychological problem may have several correlates.

Most of these symptoms appear as changes in behaviour, mood, thought, inability to understand things surrounding them or changes in memory. These attributes are part of our psyche and represent normal traits of personality. The symptoms of mental disorders are often accentuation of these characteristics which becomes distressing. These symptoms may be present in low intensity and many people continue to live with it. These symptoms also do not interfere with daily life activity.

Typically, people begin with symptoms of withdrawing themselves from surrounding, friends or family members, remain reclusive, become excessively irritable or anxious, or sometimes developing episodes of rage or anger or they may present with abnormalities of mood.

Many people start forgetting normal events or if the problem has been existing since a long time they may be observed to have declined in their performance doing house-hold work or performance at work-place. Newer habits like excessive smoking or alcohol consumption or binging is not uncommon. The symptoms point out to the direction of developing a specific psychiatric disorder but it may change during the course e.g. a prodromal symptom of depression or mood is most likely to develop into an illness like major mood disorder but some such cases may develop into schizophrenia. We don't know any predictors and it is almost impossible to distinguish between those who may develop a mental disorder from who may not. Furthermore, it must be realised that a person who is at-risk remains under stress and functions poorly, they need help, and most importantly their sufferings need to be alleviated.[4]

The initiative to identify people at-risk for developing a mental disorder is one of the important developments in psychiatry. Current initiative is to identify people much before they develop any signs or symptoms. Several risk factors make people vulnerable to develop a mental disorder and therefore identification of specific risk factors is necessary. However it is difficult to find out specific risk factors because mental disorders are caused by a number of factors from social, psychological and cultural fields.

Childhood adversity, trauma and inability to deal with stress, coping ability of individuals, positive or negative environment, emotional health, and family dynamics tilt the balance in favour or otherwise, for mental disorder. Most important factor is the person himself and his ability to deal with environmental factors. High resilience is protective for mental health. Thus, any modality which can either minimise impact of environmental stress or enhance individual's capacity to deal, will be suitable for prevention of mental disorder much before the development of any symptoms.

Often it is difficult to describe or paint a picture of mental health when people enquire about it. It is a very common situation. Sometimes when I am introduced in social functions and confronted with this question, frankly, to be candid, my answers have been quite vague.

This applies to every aspect of our life. If we cannot clearly define a context, we can hardly think of dealing with it. Worse, still is the situation when we define it wrong.

The WHO definition of mental health may be correct from an academic point of view or from point of view of measuring mental illness but it is insufficient for people to exemplify mental health.

I firmly believe, the concept of mental health cannot be conceived without taking into consideration the fundamental attributes of a human being. A human being is identified with the characteristics and capacities which enable to live with contentment, satisfaction and the ability to have moral values.

Good mental health is not simply the absence of diagnosable mental health problems, although good mental health is likely to help protect against development of many such problems.

Good mental health is characterised by a person's ability to fulfil a number of key functions and activities, including:

- the ability to learn
- the ability to feel, express and manage a range of positive and negative emotions
- the ability to form and maintain good relationships with others
- the ability to cope with and manage change and uncertainty.

I will add two categories of attributes, the abilities and the characteristics e.g.

1. Abilities: the ability to tolerate, ability to contribute, ability to relate and ability to give.
2. Characteristics – compassion, honesty, volunteerism, forgiving, are some of the positive psychological characteristics which represent mental health much better.

I am aware that sometimes it can be said that the presence of such positive characteristics does not mean having normal mental health however 'positive' mental health is like normal mental health. Normal mental health and positive mental health are not mutually exclusive, there is an overlap.

One 50-year-old gentleman often missed most of the meetings which were scheduled for Monday mornings. He could not bring himself to office as he could not summon the energy to do so. This had been a pattern for several years. One of his colleagues suggested that it could be a psychological problem. He visited a counsellor and received treatment. It is a minor form of depression which is called 'Monday morning blue'. But by the time the issue was handled, many years had passed him by and much was lost in the growth of his career.

The brain is the most complex organ in the human body. Mental illness occurs when the brain, just like any other organ such as the heart, or the kidney, is not working the way it should. Mental illness is a collection of disorders such as depression, bipolar disorder, depression, and anxiety. The symptoms can range from loss of motivation and energy, changed sleep patterns, extreme mood swings, disturbances in thought or perception, or overwhelming obsessions or fears. Mental illness interferes with relationships and affects a person's ability to function on a day-to-day basis, often leading to social isolation.

Many people have mental health concerns from time to time. But a mental health concern becomes a mental illness when ongoing signs and symptoms cause frequent stress and affect your ability to function.

Mental health problems can have a wide range of causes.

These factors are biological, psychological, social, and environmental.[5]

Generally, mental disorder develops among vulnerable people. People who have mental disorders in their parents or other family members biologically related to them, are at a higher risk. The disease develops early in life. Besides family history, emotional experience, psychological stress and social conditions play an important role. A positive experience protects an individual while an adverse experience increases the risk.

The complex relationship between biological factors and social conditions also became much clearer when it was demonstrated that social factors may directly cause a detrimental effect on the brain. Several substances which connect brain cells and allow their normal functioning can increase or decrease. This cannot be generalised since for some psychiatric conditions; there are no brain changes. However, more research is being done to investigate this aspect. Progress in this area will ultimately unlock the secrets of the biology of major psychiatric illnesses and the mechanism of action of the drugs that are effective in treating them.[6] Similarly, it was observed that severe psychological stress also causes changes in the brain.

Genetic factors including a person's individual genetic make-up, may put them at higher risk for developing a mental illness. Factors can also include physical trauma, such as a brain injury, or the misuse of substances such as street drugs or alcohol. having a close family member with a mental illness can increase the risk. However, just because one family member has a mental illness doesn't mean that others will. Having a gene with links to a mental health disorder, such as depression or schizophrenia, does not mean that an illness will develop. Likewise, people without related genes or a family history of mental illness can still have mental health issues.

Certain genes may increase your risk of developing a mental illness, and your life situation may trigger it. Environmental factors that can negatively impact a person's mental health can include severe psychological trauma, such as war, or sexual abuse. Social factors such as where we live, whether we have strong support networks (close family and friends who make us feel safe and who we can rely on), and our work environment impact our mental well-being. The amount of stress people are under, and the duration of that stress can impact one's mental health, especially in situations where individuals are unable to change their circumstances.

Illicit drug use can trigger a manic episode (bipolar disorder) or an episode of psychosis. Negative childhood experiences such as abuse or neglect can increase the risk of some mental illnesses. Trauma and stress adulthood, traumatic life events or ongoing stress such as social isolation, domestic violence, relationship breakdown, financial or work problems can increase the risk of mental illness. Traumatic experiences such as living in a war zone can increase the risk of post-traumatic stress disorder (PTSD). Personality factors like some traits such as perfectionism or low self-esteem can increase the risk of depression or anxiety. Environmental exposures before birth inflammatory conditions, toxins, alcohol or drugs while in the womb can sometimes be linked to mental illness. Neurotransmitters are naturally occurring brain chemicals that carry signals to other parts of your brain and body. When the neural networks involving these chemicals are impaired, the function of nerve receptors and nerve systems change, leading to depression and other emotional disorders.

Main factors which increase the risk of developing a mental illness, include

- A history of mental illness in a blood relative, such as a parent or sibling
- Stressful life situations, such as financial problems, a loved one's death or a divorce
- An ongoing (chronic) medical condition, such as diabetes
- Brain damage as a result of a serious injury (traumatic brain injury), such as a violent blow to the head
- Traumatic experiences, such as military combat or assault
- Use of alcohol or recreational drugs
- A childhood history of abuse or neglect
- Few friends or few healthy relationships
- A previous mental illness

The effects of mental illness can be temporary or long lasting. You also can have more than one mental health disorder at the same time.

Symptoms

A mental illness can cause problems in your daily life, such as at school or work or in relationships. In most cases, symptoms can be managed with a combination of medications and talk therapy (psychotherapy).

Signs and symptoms of mental illness can vary, depending on the disorder, circumstances and other factors. Mental illness symptoms can affect emotions, thoughts and behaviours.

Examples of signs and symptoms include:

- Feeling sad or down
- Confused thinking or reduced ability to concentrate
- Excessive fears or worries, or extreme feelings of guilt
- Extreme mood changes of highs and lows
- Withdrawal from friends and activities
- Significant tiredness, low energy or problems sleeping
- Detachment from reality (delusions), paranoia or hallucinations
- Inability to cope with daily problems or stress
- Trouble understanding and relating to situations and to people
- Problems with alcohol or drug use
- Major changes in eating habits
- Sex drive changes
- Excessive anger, hostility or violence
- Suicidal thinking

Sometimes symptoms of a mental health disorder appear as physical problems, such as stomach pain, back pain, headaches, or other unexplained aches and pains.

Complications

Mental illness is a leading cause of disability. Untreated mental illness can cause severe emotional, behavioural and physical health problems. Complications sometimes linked to mental illness include:

- Unhappiness and decreased enjoyment of life
- Family conflicts
- Relationship difficulties
- Social isolation
- Problems with tobacco, alcohol and other drugs
- Missed work or school, or other problems related to work or school
- Legal and financial problems
- Poverty and homelessness

- Self-harm and harm to others, including suicide or homicide
- Weakened immune system, so your body has a hard time resisting infections
- Heart disease and other medical conditions

There is no physical test or scan that reliably indicates whether a person has developed a mental illness.

However, people should look out for the following as possible signs of a mental health disorder:

- withdrawing from friends, family, and colleagues
- avoiding activities that they would normally enjoy
- sleeping too much or too little
- eating too much or too little
- feeling hopeless
- having consistently low energy
- using mood-altering substances, including alcohol and nicotine, more frequently
- displaying negative emotions
- being confused
- being unable to complete daily tasks, such as getting to work or cooking a meal
- having persistent thoughts or memories that reappear regularly
- thinking of causing physical harm to themselves or others
- hearing voices
- experiencing delusions

'All mental processes are brain processes, and therefore all disorders of mental functioning are biological diseases,' he says.[7] 'The brain is the organ of the mind. Where else could [mental illness] be if not in the brain?'[8]

Preventive strategies thus involve method to:

1. Preserve brain maturation
2. Reduce risk for mental disorder (biological, social as well as psychological)
3. Improve protective factors
4. Self-development and Promotion of mental health
5. Develop positive mental health

There are several means to achieve this. This topic is currently being investigated all over the world to find best possible methods for prevention.

However, all possible methods will be helpful depending upon the state of personality and positivity. Growth and development in early childhood is the key objective for this purpose.

Prevalence of mental disorders in patients with chronic physical diseases is about 40–50%. The overall current mental health morbidity was 10.6% of which 10% prevalence was accounted for by Common Mental Disorders (CMDs), which include depression, anxiety, and substance abuse.[9] Literature highlights that child and adolescent age groups are severely affected, and suicide is emerging as a major concern with 1% population reported having high suicide risk.[10] Despite efforts to provide care, a huge treatment gap exists for all types of psychiatric disorders. Mental illness results in the poor quality of life decreased productivity, and lower earning potential.[11]

It is important to note that those who develop a mental disorder are not the ones having an only stress-related problem they are particularly at risk or vulnerable due to a number of reasons, high vulnerability increases their risk for developing a mental disorder.

Timely attention to the group of people suffering from stressful conditions and mental ill-health will reduce psychiatric problems among people with mental illness, minimise the possibility of developing a medical disorder, improve quality of life, minimise the burden of psychiatric disability, reduce the prevalence of mental disorder or delay the onset of mental disorder, besides improving their quality of life and level of satisfaction, when this is done for children and adolescents its helpful for robust personality development.

Mental disorders develop due to a number of causes. The determinants of mental health include not only factors related to actions by individuals, such as behaviours and lifestyles, coping skills, and good interpersonal relationships, but also social and environmental factors like income, social status, education, employment, housing and working conditions, access to appropriate health services, and good physical health. Fostering of these individual, social and environmental qualities and the avoidance of the converse are the objectives of mental health promotion and prevention of mental disorders.[12]

Most of the symptoms of mental disorders reflect in changes in sleep pattern, emotion, mood, concentration, energy level, feeling of pleasure, anxiety, aggression, violence, problems related to memory, sometime loss of control on self, abnormal thoughts and problems related to perception and interpretation of changes in vision, hearing, etc. Mental illness takes many forms, including eating disorders, which influence eating behaviour and are accompanied by negative thoughts about body shape and weight. Although suicide is not itself considered a mental illness, it is often the result of some underlying mental illness.

A vast majority of individuals with mental illness continue to function in their daily lives and can lead a good quality life. But some people may become so sick that they may need hospitalisation to ensure their safety.

Some disorders can be severe. These are also called major mental disorder like psychosis, schizophrenia, major depression, bipolar disorder or alcoholism and addiction, majority of the patient recover well when treated early. Most of the mental disorders are treatable with fairly good outcome.

IMPORTANT FACTORS INVOLVED IN DEVELOPMENT OF MENTAL ILL-HEALTH

- *Some people are highly susceptible to mental disorders*
- *This is determined by our genetic make-up as well as by early life experiences*
- *It is affected by use of drugs and alcohol*
- *Stress refers to challenges faced in our lives*
- *It is affected by our coping mechanism, social support and involvement in meaningful activities*
- *There is biological vulnerability among people who develop mental disorders e.g. presence of any physical disorder*
- *Genetic factors because the illnesses run in family*
- *Vulnerability is also influenced by birth complication, prenatal nutrition, stress, birth complication, early experience in childhood*
- *Similarly some people are more vulnerable to develop drug, alcohol problem as well as a mental disorder.*

I recollect an incident worth mentioning here. A young scientist, with no known mental health issues, traced the phone number of a clinician who was also a professor of psychiatry in a medical college and called her. He gave his name and other details and said that he wanted to inform her of his decision about killing himself, before he acted upon it. The doctor was at the dinner table and found it very difficult not to hear him out. While she could develop any plan for helping him during this crisis, she decided to engage him in conversation. He did not agree to go visit any other doctor or hospital or even speak to any friend or relative. He instead tried justifying life and death philosophically, saying that he believed that the soul never dies, so it was perfectly fine if he kills himself. It was quite a stressful situation. It took her two hours to get through his mental state when he promised to see her once and finally came to the hospital and decided to 'defer' the decision of committing suicide.

Psychological Characteristics

Psychological symptoms	Level of satisfaction
Productivity	Quality of life
Educational achievement	General well-being
Social functioning	Emotional intelligence
Social intelligence	Ability to learn

You have to grow from the inside out. None can teach you, none can make you spiritual. There is no other teacher but your own soul.

Swami Vivekanand

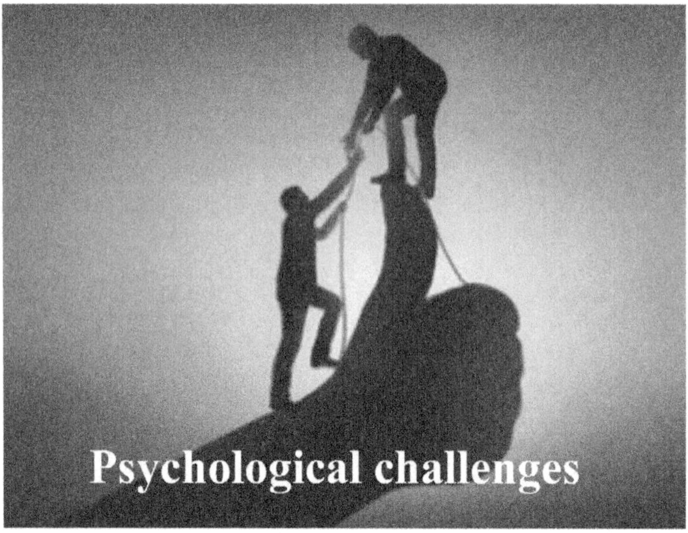

Inability to change

Compliance in daily life

Modifying behaviour traits

Decision making

Hopelessness,

Regulating the mood

Emotional conflict

Stress in children

Obesity and smoking

Alcohol and drug abuse

NATURE OF MENTAL HEALTH PROBLEMS SEEN AFTER BECOMING SUCCESSFUL

- Psychological stress and deterioration in physical health
- Problem in behaviour - increased risk behaviour, smoking, addiction and lack of self-care, change in behaviour leads to several problems e.g. anxiety, aggression or depression, social and legal difficulties
- Family related difficulties, relationship / interpersonal and marital difficulties
- Increase in vulnerability for mental illness
- A full-blown psychiatric disorder

Mental health problems seen among successful people

Psychological Stress

Deterioration in physical health

Risk behaviour' - smoking, addiction etc

Psychological symptoms e.g. anxiety, aggression,

social or legal problems

Challenges in family relationship

Increased vulnerability for mental disorder

Psychiatric disorders

Relapse of pre-existing psychiatric conditions

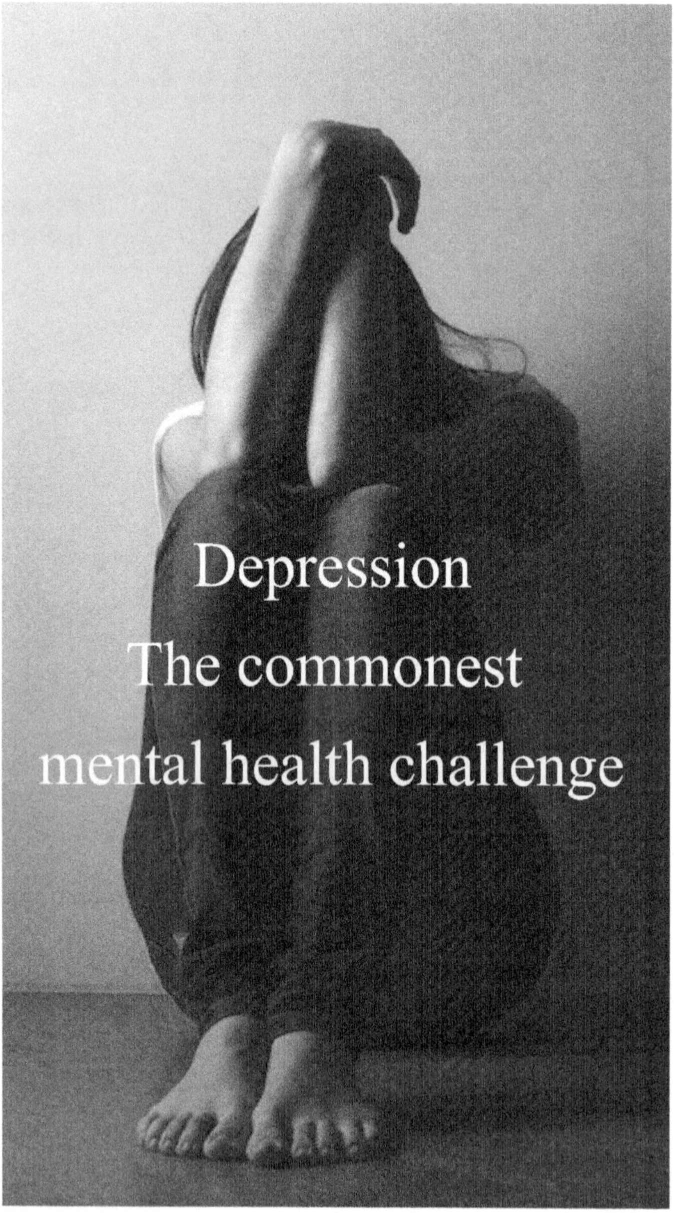
Depression
The commonest
mental health challenge

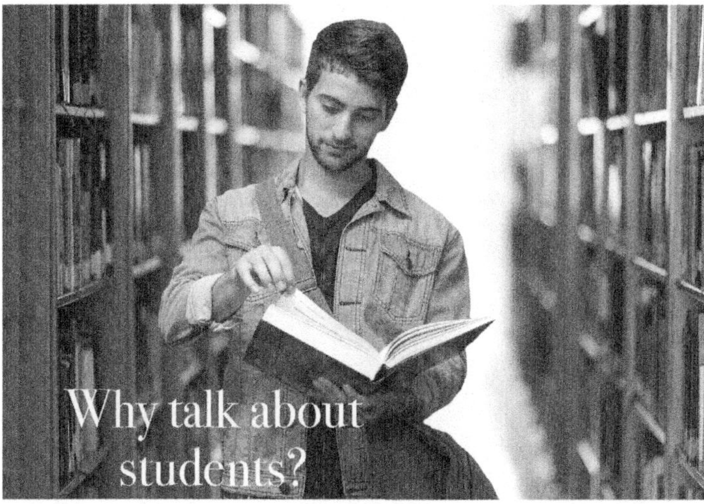

Sever Psychological Stress

At least one mental disorder (in life-time) 35%

At least one mental disorder in previous 12 months 31%

symptoms typically appear in early or middle adolescence

50% mental disorders begin at 14 years and

75% between age 17 ad 21 years

CHAPTER 2
PSYCHOLOGICAL CHALLENGES

5. INABILITY TO CHANGE

The resistant behaviour leads to unhappiness and unsafe life.

Behaviour is not exclusively a psychological feature. It takes place in a social environment; therefore, some types of behaviors are specific to a social situation. Also, behaviour of people is known to change while in a group. When the behaviour pattern coexists with other psychological traits, the problems and the consequences increase many folds. Conditions like anxiety, restlessness, irritability, impulsivity, etc. commonly complicate the behaviour. Further, symptoms like anger, mood changes, stress, difficulty in social relations, tendency for alcohol and drug abuse, make resistant behaviour far more severe.

Resistant behaviour is not a mental illness; however, it is undoubtedly a high-risk factor for mental as well as physical illness. Due to these complications, people with resistant and complex behaviour have a shorter life span. Their main psychological difficulty remains poor level of satisfaction, feeling frequent episodes of depression, suffering guilt and hopelessness. This further increases the consequences of the behaviour pattern. Resistant behaviour appears to be a spiritual health issue and modification of such behaviour can be best addressed by spiritual intervention and not only by counselling and behaviour modification.

Behaviour becomes resistant because the abnormal pattern is deep rooted in personality when the personality is developing. At this stage subtle symptoms of mental ill-health start appearing due to which the mood remains unstable which may lead to complications.

Study of behaviour needs a multidisciplinary approach. It includes psychology, sociology and behavioral sciences which provide good insight of the causes and consequences of behaviour. It takes shape early in life. One can say that people are born with behaviour pattern, with about 50% being the genetic causes and 50% shapes up with environmental influences. However, no specific gene has been isolated. Environmental experiences play a crucial role. They are known to arise from emotional attachment with mother. Poor physical bonding with mother during the first year after birth is known to be associated with violent behaviour in the future. Other environmental factors are stress, trauma, abuse which play an equally important role, leading to difficulty in behaviour.

Generally, families fail to pay sufficient attention to such behaviour, or whenever they are even able to identify these flaws, they are unable to help because of the nature of the resistant behaviour. It is difficult to identify resistant behaviour, but it is important that the problem be addressed by proper investigation and treatment since it could be a serious risk to life. Good treatments are available nowadays.

6. COMPLIANCE IN DAILY LIFE

Outcome of an intervention whether advised by a doctor or any health care worker, depends upon your ability to understand, believe and comply. Most of the treatments or suggestions fail because of difference in opinion, disbelief or bias. If you are not open to suggestion or you have problems following the advice, it will always be hard to be beneficiary of the treatments. More than 80% patients who are given medications for psychiatric disorders discontinue much before the stipulated time period. Majority of them have stopped it within 3 to 4 weeks,

There are many reasons for it e.g. social and cultural belief, attitude towards the medication, adverse effects, ability to understand i.e. cognitive functions, psychological bias or social consequences or stigma are some of the causes for the non-compliance. People often fail to remember the consequence of such behaviour.

People who non-comply take a chance and put their life at risk, i.e. risk for diminishing the gains made during the treatment, risk for future episode of illness, risk for adverse outcome of a relapse i.e. suicide, self-harm, violence or complications in family or work-related matters.

They also do not realise that the response to the same or better treatment regimens may not give the quality of recovery which was obtained in previous treatment. Most important aspect is to remember that life with an illness becomes harder day by day, every day with an active illness is adding up to toxic state. The effect of non-compliance on quality of life, well-being, participation in social roles, happiness and enjoyment is insurmountable. Non-compliance make the problem chronic and irreversible,

Thus, when you take responsibility of correcting yourself, it's in fact a huge responsibility. One may decide to have supervision or support and not take the entire responsibility to implement a treatment regime, this responsibility may be gradually transferred to you by your support worker or a family member, when you are able to take over with full responsibility. Your inability to take care about yourself is by no means demeaning or insulting or a reflection of 'bad' or 'poor'. It should not convey the meaning that you cannot do it but it always done in your best interest in order to minimise the chances or error.

The same applies to any treatment or 'attempt to change' yourself. When you decide to be a responsible person for 'self-care', it implies that you are going to comply with an intervention 'prescribed' by yourself. Same principles apply to medical treatment, social discipline, managing risk behaviour, personal development and any other life-style intervention.

The social and psychological intervention have the same principles of effect and side effect that applies to a medication or any procedure that is performed by your doctor or therapist or dentist. Non-compliance is the worst enemy for personal growth and development.

Compliance is a discipline, it is an intellectual attribute.

It reflects in social and emotional intelligence, social behaviour, ability to perform, success and failure. Compliance is one psychological characteristic common to all walks of life. It is also determine by certain biological factors, specific brain circuits which may explain the behaviour of non-compliance.

Compliance is a matter of brain and behaviour. It is an outcome of your ability to understand and act as you like, Others ability to influence you, your tendencies to be over-compliant or defiant.

It does not mean that there are fixed structure and rigid functions which cannot be optimised or changed. The therapy of behaviour modification is based upon the principle that may aspect of our behaviour can be changed by changing thought processor cognitive re structuring.

Our actions and responses are influenced by our thinking and judgement and at the same time there are other factors which influence us and change the course of our actions e.g. social situations, similarly on many occasions opinion and advise given by others also influences our judgement and responses. It depends upon a ability of other person to influence you and also on your ability to get influenced. Thus compliance is determined by multiple factors, the best one can do is to recognise and assess the possibility of good or poor compliance and take a decision of working alone or in a supervised manner.

It is truly an ability to change opinion and behaviour – a popular concept in behavioural science which has enormous influence of mental health

Self-help is the first step towards prevention of psychiatric disorders. Self-help can offer effective intervention. It is not an alternative for professional help by doctors, psychologist or social workers. It is rather complementary and necessary part of treatment for mental health related problems as well as mental disorders. The objective for self-help is clearly defined:

- To arrest progression of symptoms and the illness
- To treat the symptoms and its consequences on the person, others in all walks of life
- To ensure safety, i.e. suicide prevention, prevention of violence, and prevention of physical deterioration
- Develop a crisis plan to deal with any emergency situation
- Improve level of education and awareness about mental health

It is important to have full information about the health condition while planning for self-care. Mostly people do not give much thought about it. One may be committing similar mistake by not knowing what needs to be done just in the same way as; wrong dieting or unscientific manner of physical exercise or unsupervised yoga therapy for a patient of heart disease can be counterproductive

Some of these are: assess and Identify the strength, weakness and limitation of the individual e.g. nature of illness, medications, ongoing problem of addiction.

The risk benefit of compliance to an advise also depends upon resilience and ability to deal with adverse situations. Resiliencies an individual's characteristic which allows people adaptor adverse or challenging or traumatic situations. Its purpose is to protect our inner self from external threat and generally refers to characteristics of: Adaptability, Optimism, Satisfaction, Contentment.

Thus personal development by whatever modality is serious manner and it must be properly planned for prevention of psychological challenges, some of the important methods for psychological intervention which result in positive characteristics are given below:

1. Enhance stress threshold
2. Coping mechanism
3. Personality development
4. Identifying personality traits for optimising its functioning
5. Identification and treatment of mental illness
6. Volunteerism
7. Social engagement
8. Building resilience
9. Treatment of minor psychiatric clinical factors
10. Personal development
11. Self-esteem, self-confidence
12. Lifestyle intervention
13. Exercise
14. Group discourse
15. Prayers
16. Spiritual intervention

7. HARD TASK - MODIFYING BEHAVIOUR

He is 65 years old now, obese and retired. Since early adolescence he was a rigid and strong-minded person. He was never amenable to any suggestions. All was well, until 42 when he had to undergo four-vessel coronary bypass surgery. Even then, his difficult behaviour was the reason for not complying with doctor's advice. He tried to make lifestyle changes, but obviously he did not succeed. The resistance was so severe that he could not keep up with diet and exercise programmes. At the age of 50 he developed diabetes, which remained uncontrolled and as a result he frequently went through hypoglycemic episodes. Diabetes continued to get worse. By the time he was 63 years old he had undergone another angioplasty for 2 more vessels, he was managed on multiple medications and insulin, however, nothing changed in his lifestyle. Subsequently it was found that he had severe depression. This was missed and remained untreated. Even after the treatment for depression, the improvement in symptoms was relatively mild. He started showing some change, and the good part was that he was no more in denial. Now he could entertain a frank discussion about the resistant nature of his behaviour. He is retired at 64 due to health reasons and resting at home in an almost dysfunctional state. He does not have any engagement, this again made him further lethargic, depression increased and all attempts to change the behaviour became useless. It's the worst possible health condition that can be seen due to problems of 'inability to change'. Later I came to know that he had a strong family history of similar type of behaviour.

People are identified by their behaviour, personality and character. Mothers and grandmothers were able to predict the conduct of a child, by taking into account the present behaviour of a child, during the early days of life. While behaviour of a person is fairly predictable, it is also related with severe problems. Some people have behaviour which is not malleable to change. They have a fixed behaviour pattern, which is not in their best interest, but they are not able to change. These inabilities lead to severe health problems. Such people develop adverse habits like smoking, eating excessively, indulging in alcohol etc. Despite realising and making all possible efforts they find themselves unable to bring substantial change, and as a result end up leading an unhealthy lifestyle.

Behaviour which is resistant to change is a severe problem. E.g. inability to live a proper lifestyle, leading to increased risk for cardiovascular diseases.[13] Resistant behaviour is a critical public health issue, number of people with type II diabetes is expected to rise from 366 million in 2016 to 552 million in 2030,[14] whereas 17 million people died due to cardiovascular diseases in 2008, and some 23 million are expected to do so in 2030.[15] This disorder is a problem arising from lifestyle management which demands several changes in behaviour.

8. PERSISTENT BEHAVIOURAL TRAITS

Personality traits are significantly related to academic achievement. This position is based upon the observation that what an individual can do is the reflection of cognitive ability,[16] whereas, what an individual will do is a reflection of personality traits. Educators and researchers have worked on academic achievement problems for years. It is reported that besides cognitive abilities, non-cognitive factors which are known as personality traits are responsible for academic achievement.[17] Several personality traits are related to academic achievement. There is support for the idea of evaluating personality traits as predictors of academic achievement based on several works that have done on personality.[18]

Cognitive and non-cognitive factors are both responsible for academic achievement. The role and impact of cognitive ability in relation to academic success is well documented, and a strong correlation between grades and cognitive ability was found the relationship between personality and academic achievement.[19] Predictors of academic achievement often lay on a continuum with cognitive measures, intelligence and mental abilities.[20] Trying to predict academic achievement have yielded different results, they have consistently pointed out the role of cognitive abilities and personality characteristics in academic achievement.

The mental health aspect of achievement is closely related to individuals' psychological characteristics as personality as well. One of the interesting parts if this is the minor traits or 'typology' or 'psychological feature in an individua's personality. Personality is everyone's unique feature, the way of thinking, feeling and behaving, it includes one's behaviour and the way they solve their problems, how well they can connect with others, how they become comfortable with themselves, their ability to regulate their mood, ability to identify. Though these traits are milder they may cause significant dysfunction. As we know everybody has a typical personality it is a characteristic which identifies the person. More often than not, these traits become the identifying features, e.g. some people may be very obsessive, or very restless, or may suffer from frequent bouts of anger, or be very suspicious. We also know that these traits are often associated with brain related changes and level of functioning. Some of the key constructs included in the reviewed studies include *adaptability, attitude, affect, anxiety, belief, basic skills, classroom behaviors, control strategies, cooperation, curiosity, discipline, effort, elaboration strategies, emotion, engagement, extracurricular activity, habit, help-seeking, homework, independence, etc.*[21] Personality traits reflect people's characteristic patterns of thoughts, feelings, and behaviors. Personality traits imply consistency and stability—someone who scores high on a specific trait like Extraversion is expected to be sociable in different situations and over time. Thus, trait psychology rests on the idea that people differ from one another in terms of where they stand on a set of basic trait dimensions that persist over time and across situations. Mental health status can be assessed by symptoms reflecting functions of mind. Generally, mood state, thought, behaviour, and cognitive functions give us a fairly good idea of the presence of mental ill-health. We find 3-4 types of abnormalities, some people have frank psychiatric symptoms, which qualify for psychiatric disorders, those who have milder symptoms, will turn to become a disorder in future. There is a third group of population where they suffer from one or two behavioral traits, sometimes these are precursors of related psychiatric diagnosis. These traits may remain as such for life and accentuate during times of stress. Often people refer to them as 'personality traits'.

9. A STATE OF HOPELESSNESS, WHY?

When we realise that someone is feeling hopeless, we wonder, why? What is important to know is, whether it is a normal function or an abnormal state, whether this state of mind can do any harm, what might happen if it does not disappear.

Conditions which lead to hopelessness include problems related to memory, thinking, brain injury, stress, hormonal problems like hypothyroidism besides any physical problem of persistent pain.

Hope is closely related to thought process. If someone is getting excessive thoughts the mood will change, if someone starts feeling low, the thought process changes if the mood is normal the mathematical or intellectual characteristics are much brighter.

Emotions not only influence our thinking, intelligence and ability to perceive, they also affect our internal body system.

Sometime diseases of brain e.g. any neurological condition like epilepsy, there is also the symptoms of hopelessness present. It can be present in association with or may appear prior to other symptoms in several conditions, e.g. people who are developing dementia or forgetfulness sometimes present with ideas of hopelessness. These ideas are not taken seriously and after sometime problems related to memory functions appear. It may present secondary to endocrine related problems e.g. in diseases related to thyroid hormone. Many times people do not speak about it and its detected only when someone starts a conversation. Occasionally people will find such ideas serious or abnormal, to consult someone for help.

Some people by nature may feel hopeless, some may have always been feeling joyful and happy and suddenly or gradually their emotions change it. This may happen because of stress, social situation, a physical illness or a mental illness.

Emotion is most important feature of mind. It represents not only how you are feeling but also about how you can regulate several other features of mind. Mood is indicator of state of mind. Several features coordinate with each other to represent mood state at a particular moment. Hopelessness is an emotion which is typically characterised by a lack of hope, optimism, and passion. It's important to recognise when you or someone around you is feeling hopeless. There is sometimes very thin boundary between ideas of hopelessness and depression. Though hopelessness is a part of depression, but every condition of hopelessness does not progress to a state of clinical depression. In some situations of hopelessness one should discuss with a doctor if the ideas of hopelessness are persistent all the time and are increasing or if there are any severe stressful factors associated with it. Many times hopelessness may be present due to number of physical conditions, e.g. illnesses related to hormones like thyroid, or as psychological reaction secondary to major illness e.g. heart attack.

One should not be surprised if these ideas persist for long, neither increase nor decrease by any significant degree. Many people have a typical personality which is of a 'depressive nature' and they live with ideas of hopelessness for lifetime. An individual who feels hopeless may often have no expectation of future improvement or success.

Most times hopelessness are related to life events. Negative life events can change the cognitive style. Mechanism of the risk due to hopelessness is related to cognitive abilities. Negative cognitive style leads to hopelessness. Hopelessness has been suggested as a central dimension of depression[22] as well as a marker of anxiety and a predictor of clinical depression.[23] Specific relevance for hopelessness lies in predicting improvement of various health conditions. Though hopelessness is a cardinal feature of depression and suicide, every one feeling hopeless is not depressed. Feeling of sadness and despair may begin slowly and increase at a slow pace but finally take over most time of the day. It is associated with several other symptoms, most commonly it is accompanied by crying spells, feeling easily tearful, feeling worthless, feel as though the time is not passing by at all. Generally it indicates mood disorder but it may also be the initial features of many other psychiatric or medical conditions.

Several studies indicate that hopelessness is a stronger predictor of suicide.[24] A sense of hopelessness is characterised by a sense of futility and negative expectations about the future and one's personal goals. Hopelessness seems to lead to more negative evaluations of new situations and less effective coping strategies. While hopelessness is often a major symptom of depression, it may play a distinct and larger role in the development of cardiovascular disease. Sometimes these ideas may increase, prolong or develop into other symptoms like sleeplessness, loss of appetite, severe depression or ideas of suicide. If ideas of suicide are present along with hopelessness one must always approach the hospital or one's doctor and seek proper psychiatric intervention. Self-help in presence of suicidal ideas has limited merit. Ideas of hopelessness are closely linked to Impulsivity. In fact Hopelessness, impulsivity and depression, together form very high risk for suicide attempt.

When the symptoms of hopelessness persist for long, it is deep-rooted in the personality, thus it becomes part of your life. Such feeling of low mood, irritability, getting easily worked up, inability to enjoy, lack of pleasure, instability of emotions etc. maybe be present since long. These are certainly distressing. It is 'normal' and many people have it, presence or absence of these psychological traits make people different and therefore it is difficult to take it out or get rid of these. The best possible way is to:

1. identify and be sure that these are your shades of life,
2. it is wrong to consider these as negative or bad, limitations or a roadblock to your career or personal satisfaction.
3. this is not a mental disability,
4. identify the symptoms which bother you most and try to change the symptoms or change your style of dealing with symptoms.

There are millions of people and each one is different, the expectation to fit everyone in the jacket is impossible, there will have to be space for flexibility, if that's not given, there will be significant non-compliance e.g. in every field where there will be people who are unable to comply – many will not be able to attend work on time, sleep on time, or follow the instruction given to them.

You may not be able to do much for the aspect of your life which is regulated by others, but you certainly have the options of regulating and optimising your own life, depending upon your psychological needs. The low symptoms cannot be suppressed, if these symptoms interfere too much with daily life i.e. if you are getting distressed, it is important to establish communication, discuss and find answers with anyone you like. You may seek professional help, but we must realise that professional help is not personal. There is a delicate and smart balance between what is required and what is permitted to be done by a professional. Beyond doubt, the decision is always left to the person seeking help.

5. Respect yourself: no one will respect your problems if you do not recognise that these are not a stigma or shame or guilt.
6. Be quiet when you feel hopeless or talk if it helps you but do not isolate yourself.

10. SUBTHRESHOLD DEPRESSION

Some people are vulnerable for a psychiatric disorder. Many of them develop minor symptoms which are not severe enough to qualify for a diagnosis, however these symptoms are also distressing and lead to some degree of functional loss. Such conditions are known as subthreshold disorders or subclinical conditions. In general these are quite significant because:

1. Large number of people suffer from this disorder.
2. Significant number of people with such problems develop frank and full-blown depression in years to come, however, about 10 to 20% of such cases develop a full-blown depressive disorder during two to three-year follow-up.[25] Rest live with low degree of symptoms.
3. People with subthreshold symptoms remain unidentified. Relatives and friends often wonder but do not get any answers as to why the person sometimes behaves distressed and appears ill.
4. On many occasions physicians decide to treat such conditions. The decision to do this is entirely dependent upon the risk which the patient carries.
5. This condition is treatable.
6. In most people its cause is not known. Probably, it has started with some traumatic event in the childhood.

Besides the frank and diagnosable depressions, there are two other conditions which hit our people hard. One in which they are suffering from a condition in which they do not have all the symptoms which can qualify for a depressive disorder however the single or insufficient symptoms are no less incapacitating-then subthreshold depression. Subthreshold depression is far more prevalent than clinically diagnosable depression.

The second group of patients who pose serious problem but suffer, are those, who have mild and low potency symptoms since a long period of time where the depressive tendencies are integrated within their personalities, such conditions had invariably started during adolescence when personality was growing, and this depressive feature has become part of their life. It also interferes with proper growth of their personality in terms of adequate coping abilities, ability to work to be enterprising and innovative, frustration tolerance. They have low anger threshold, become easily anxious and respond poorly to social stress and conditions. They remain vulnerable to developing several psychiatric conditions and physical illnesses.

There is another group of people who are at a higher risk of developing a frank disorder, they may have hereditary factors or may have parents who have suffered from similar disease. They may have developed some symptoms, at times the intensity of such symptoms might increase.

Risk factors for developing this problem are lower social support, recurrent short episodes of depressive symptomatology, remitted and current anxiety disorder, remitted substance use disorder, suicide thoughts, a chronic physical disorder and diminished mental and physical functioning.[26]

11. IMPULSIVITY

Generally, everybody has a particular type of behaviour, and we seldom think that this behaviour can become a problem for managing day to day life. If you look around, you will easily find people who display unprovoked anger, or suddenly become aggressive. We wonder what exactly happens. People with this kind of behaviour find it difficult to adjust in family and job situations because they themselves fail to understand why they behave as they do, suddenly and without any provocation. This problem neither reduces nor ceases. Sometimes, it becomes matter of great concern and people turn to seek help. Nobody is worried when such anger or aggressiveness occurs in adolescence, since it is quite common and everyone is aware that they will eventually outgrow this problem. Those people in whom this problem persists find it very challenging to function.

Most people have acted sometimes in their life on an impulse or at the spur of the moment. It's not only due to the way one thinks, feels or gets angry, but such impulses originate from deeper structures of the brain and various brain chemicals pave the way for such behaviour, which becomes abnormal for a short time. Several psychological factors also contribute to impulsivity.

The terms 'impulsivity' and 'disorders of impulse control' have customarily been used interchangeably. Yet there have been contrasting definitions in the literature. 'Impulsivity' has been defined as a decreased sensitivity to negative consequences, rapid unplanned reactions to stimuli (without adequate processing of information), and lack of regard for long-term consequences. 'Disorders of impulse control' have been characterised as repeated failures to resist an impulse or perform an act that is harmful, with a preceding subjective sense of increasing tension (or arousal) and an experience of pleasure or gratification, i.e. catharsis, while committing the act.[27]

Behavioural impulse is a type of normal impulse which generates movements of the body. This movement is under the control of brain mechanism. It's different in nature, than just acting quickly. Seldom it is a positive feature of our life. It is the tendency to respond prematurely or in an unduly risky fashion, which is becoming an increasingly important construct for mental health.[28]

It's not seen in adolescents alone; many adults and even older adults exhibit the features of impulsiveness. Impulsivity is an uncontrollable urge. People find it difficult to contain it, by the time they think something might happen, the act has already taken place, even if it was not provoked.

Sometimes it can be prolonged too, and that's a more serious condition. It truly is a neurobehavioral process (a process which involves mechanism which determines the behaviour). If the severity of the impulsivity is such that it can interfere with the smooth functioning of life or it causes social or personal consequences, it is considered as abnormal.

The impulsive behaviour which does not affect the day to day functioning or poses a risk to anyone or self, is not a clinical problem. However, it's common to find people with impulsivity getting into trouble with the law, fights with people in the family or outside home or in school. It also represents a specific type of personality. It is associated with mental disorders, head injury or brain diseases, alcoholism and drug addiction. It can be perceived as a risk factor for an impending episode of violence and suicide.

Many reasons are cited for impulsivity, significant ones are:

- Poor mother-child bond,
- Separation from parents, especially the mother,
- Child abuse,
- Sex abuse,
- History of violence amongst parents,
- Emotional trauma,
- Brain damage at birth,
- Weak physical growth in early years of life and
- Physical disorders,
- Personality development contributes to health and management of impulsive behaviour.

Unfortunately, it's not only limited to these conditions, but it is closely associated with suicide, attempted suicide, alcohol or substance abuse, mood disorder, attention deficit disorder, or several neurological disorders. It is one of the essential features of attention deficit disorder. It is very challenging for parents to cope with impulsive behaviour.

Some of the types of impulsivity may become a psychological problem. That's because there are consequences of such behaviour which are often harmful.

Such behaviour is called 'impulse control disorder' which is characterised by the features like:

- Acting on the spur of the moment (motor activation) remains the key feature, which is associated with several mental disorders,
- Acting without thinking,
- Not focusing on the task at hand (inattentiveness), and not planning and thinking carefully,
- Decreased sensitivity to negative consequences of behaviour,
- Unplanned reaction to stimuli before processing the information thoroughly,

- No regard for long-term consequences of a behaviour,
- Fast reaction without thinking and conscious judgment.

'Disorders of impulse control' have been characterised as 'repeated failures to resist an impulse' or 'perform a harmful act'.[11, 21]

The consequences are usually harmful, with subsequent feelings of regret or guilt. Low level of serotonin (a chemical substance) is found in the brain among people who have impulse control problem, which makes such individuals highly vulnerable to depression, suicide as well as other mood disorder.

Purpose of discussing it here is to highlight that impulses are normal in everyone but if impulses are such that you want to control and you cannot resist it, it may be a clinical problem demanding adequate assessment and treatment.

One of the major impacts of this condition is inability to focus and poor concentration which leads to poor academic progress.

12. FACTORS AFFECTING MENTAL HEALTH

Risk factors	Protective factors
Academic failure	Ability to cope with stress
Attention deficit	Ability to face adversity
Caring for chronic illness	Adaptability
Child abuse neglect	Autonomy
Chronic insomnia	Early cognitive stimulation
Chronic pain	Exercise
Early pregnancy	Feeling of mastery and control
Elder abuse	Good parenting
Emotional immaturity	Literacy
Excessive substance abuse	Positive attachment
Exposure to violence	Early bonding
Family conflict	Positive parent-child interaction
Loneliness	Problem-solving skills
Low birth weight	Social behaviour
Low social class	Self-esteem
Medical illness	Skill for life
Neurochemical imbalance	Conflict management skills
Parental mental illness	Social and emotional growth
Parental substance abuse	Stress management
Perinatal complications	Social support
Personal loss-bereavement	
Poor work skill	
Stressful life events	
Substance use during pregnancy	

13. FEELING LOW

Hope hardly dies.

Hope of the rising sun

Hope is like rising sun...it sets in every evening
Only to rise again the next day.
Is there anybody who has not felt 'low'?
I doubt.
But if I ask how many people 'live with feeling low'?

It's not rare, in fact it may be common. Don't be surprised its felt by people who are young as well as those who are elderly.

Few neurons in middle of the brain protected by hard skull regulated all our feelings, hope, aspiration, pleasure or happiness.

We are born with it. Newborns may not speak but they feel it and experience the joy. Hope keeps us moving forward all the time.

People who suffer from depression obviously suffer from hopelessness but if we consider those who do not have any psychiatric problems like depression, we find that about 10% adolescent,15% college students, 10% adults and 20% to 30% elderly people experience emotions of hopelessness.[29, 30]

Hopelessness: Hopelessness is an emotion characterised by a lack of hope, optimism, and passion. An individual who feels hopeless may often have no expectation of future improvement or success. Hopelessness is common and it can become a matter of concern in some conditions.

Hopelessness is truly a reflection of mood. The state of hopelessness may be a permanent trait, it may be existing for a long time or it may have come up recently due to any stress or other problem. Hope is the emotional driver of life; lack of hope may be called hopelessness. But it is much more than loss of hope.

Hopelessness is not an abnormal emotion in in normal circumstances, it's a precursor of depression. There is hardly any situation in which people may be depressed but not hopeless, however it is not necessary that an emotion of hopelessness will grow into depression.

There are several emotions which appear similar to depression but ideally those may be different e.g. sorrow, sadness, despondency, dejection, pain and many more. We can include all these under the rubric of hopelessness for the sake of our discussion.

It is expression of emotion which is very specific to an abnormal state of mind. You may feel hopeless in response to some event or it can appear on its own. Most often we find that hopelessness is present since long time but remained unnoticed because it did not interfere with daily life routine.

Many times depression responds to a treatment but hopelessness persists.

It has its specific biological feature.

It is important to understand it in relation to depression because both the conditions present as an abnormality in the emotion. It appears that depression may be a severe form of hopelessness but that's not true. Hopelessness is an independent psychological characteristic representing a form of emotion. If the hopelessness is of recent origin and in response to stressful factors, it is likely to be cleared off soon, but sometimes it has persisted for long. In such conditions, it has remained unidentified and consequently it has not been treated. Long standing feeling of hopelessness is sometimes embedded in the personality. It exists as a trait of personality, generally these emotions arise during childhood, most likely response to adverse emotional experience.

Hopelessness is an important co-existing symptom. It is a part of dependence symptom clusters and also increases during craving for alcohol. Sometimes, the brain is affected due to addictive substances and mood changes appear. Hopelessness has been related to the onset and prognosis of mental and physical health outcomes including the development of depression, suicidal ideation hypertension,[67] subclinical atherosclerosis, adaptation following acute cardiac events[33] and progression of carotid atherosclerosis, including breast and haematological cancers,[70, 71] although the evidence is not consistent.

The psychological features do not work in isolation, its closely related to several other brain functions which lead to significant change in our ability to withstand stress which leads to change in stress hormone, heart rate and blood pressure.

55-year-old gentleman came to meet me; He was working on this ship and had fairly decent life. He came because of vague psychological symptoms; He was not clear what these symptoms were, but he knew that something was not right.

When I asked him what brought him here, he said he wanted to feel happy. It was quite simple I thought it may be one of the common diagnosis like depression. While discussing the details, he insisted that he did not have depression, but he was also not feeling happy. The symptoms were always there since he was 30. He had met few psychiatrists in the past but there was no change in the health condition.

His expression of not feeling happy was unique. He described that nothing would make him happy. Good company, friends, festival, just nothing. He did not present any other feature which could have suggested the possibility of depression.

He had lived with these feeling for a long period now. I explained that this problem is not only arising from psychological factors but there is a specific place in the brain and emotions are regulated from that particular place. Generally, it responds to medications but training his mind to control negative thoughts and ideas were necessary. I arranged for a psychological therapy called cognitive behaviour therapy, in which the thought and mood processes are restructured by training the thought pattern.

Hopelessness has a specific centre of origin in the brain. A recent research highlighted that the place where hopelessness 'resides' is the Neural circuitry in the midline regions of the brain, along the cleft between the brain's two hemispheres.[72]

It is also said that some people are of a negative mindset and they 'learn' to feel hopeless from their environment.

There are significant changes taking place in the brain. These studies show changes in neurotransmitter, memory, intelligence, and change in brain areas.

In modern brain scans like positron emission tomography (PET), the findings provide an initial glimpse into the cerebral neurobiology of the psychological dimensions of states of hopefulness. The psychological states involved the participation of brain areas that deal with the functions of cognition, language, perception, vision, audition, and emotions.[31]

Consequences of emotional abuse leads to several problems. Detachment with mothers, changes in personality, social isolation, psychiatric disorders and several other psychological and social consequences are common amongst children who are abused.

Psychological abuse is often combined with other forms of abuse.[8] The present state of research indicates that depressed and helpless people have trouble learning.

The obvious question arises about how to help deal with it. In most situations it is self-help. Many times reaching out to anyone who is trustworthy is of great value. The proper management is to understand it. Though these methods are effective, it is very difficult to take initiative to change your mood. It appears hard and a task in itself.

The best possible course is to do activities which are of your interest. Any activity like connecting with people, reading or attending discussion groups is helpful. One must avoid drugs and alcohol. Alcohol is known to make your mood sad and it is thus counterproductive. The advice that small amount will not hurt is not true. If the state of mood is deteriorating you must seek help from your doctor.

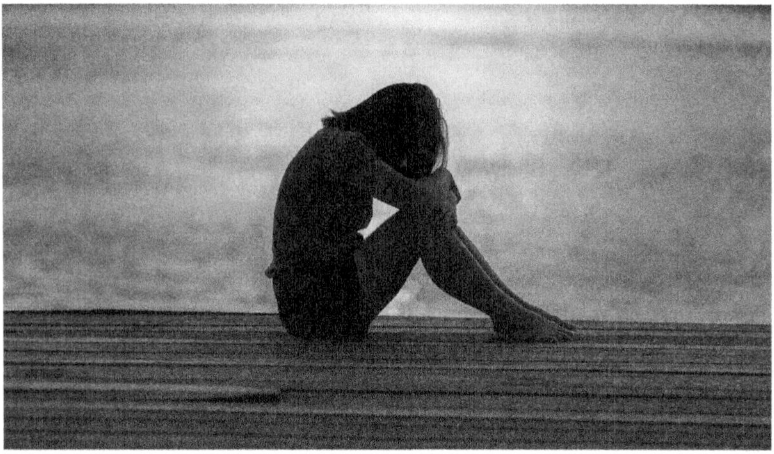

The abnormality of mood can present in various ways. The mood can change all of a sudden, or it may be going down slowly towards a depressive feeling. It may only occur for a few days, or the changes in mood like feeling low or high can become a regular phenomenon oc- curring at a fixed interval.

14. REGULATING THE MOOD

Mood is an emotional state which affects us all the time.

Nobody has a flat state of mood. The mood is variable throughout the day, during the week and season. The control mechanism of mood present within the brain is highly sensitive. It varies due to change in environment, social cues, and psychological condition. The fluctuation in severity and duration of mood is also variable. Mood can be affected by the level of noise, seasons or weather. Abnormality of mood is also commonly seen in stressful conditions as well in psychiatric diseases and amongst people who are highly vulnerable to develop depression. Normal mood always has two different poles or endpoints, which is referred to as 'bipolarity of mood'. Presence of bipolarity is perfectly normal, and it should not be mistaken with bipolar disorder.[32]

Mood may change in its intensity and appear high and low or become extreme. When this happens, it affects our lives. Most common abnormality due to mood dysregulation is the mood disorder.

Mood is not the same as emotion. Mood tends to be far longer lasting, it goes on for hours and days, while emotion last for short time, it could even be only a few minutes. Emotion is specific for a particular situation or a person or cues in the surrounding while mood is much more diffused. Mood is a general feeling not a reaction to anything, it is also not as intense as emotion. You may find emotions creating strong reactions around you, e.g. the emotions of terror or exhilaration. However the two are closely linked.

Mood originates from the part of the brain-called prefrontal cortex influences mood. It is also connected with the middle part of the brain called 'limbic system'.[33]

Some people seem to experience a positive mood when they have an emotional state which is not stirred-up, have had a good night's sleep, and feel relaxed. Mood state is also related to memory, mental ability and intellectual abilities. Some mood states have a severe effect on our ability to remember, recall or to perform any intellectual task.[33]

Low mood often seen in clinical depression is also related to several other features; e.g. loss of energy, irritability, forgetfulness, easy distractibility and suicidal ideation, difficulty in concentration, disturbed sleep and appetite.

Mood disorders are a group of mental illnesses that affect how you feel and think about self, other people and life in general. There are a few different types of mood disorders: depression, dysthymic disorder and bipolar disorder.

The abnormality of mood can present in various ways. The mood can change all of a sudden, or it may be going down slowly towards a depressive feeling. It may only occur for a few days, or the changes in mood like feeling low or high can become a regular phenomenon occurring at a fixed interval. Such changes may also appear due to other mental or physical problems, e.g. it may appear after a heart attack or viral fever, and it may appear prior to a psychiatric or physical illness, e.g. mood changes may be the first symptom to start with several neurological disorders. Very often, mood changes also take place before suicidal ideas appear. The emotion of depression precedes almost all incidents of suicide.

Mood changes are an integral part of one's personality and character, and in such cases, whenever there is any change in personality, there will be changes in emotion.

Wide fluctuation in the range of emotionality is typical for people who may develop mania, especially amongst grown-ups and sometimes even during childhood.

If someone is feeling rhythm of low and high mood, it is perfectly normal because that is the very nature of mood which is a cyclic feature, it goes up and down.[34]

Mood state is also related to memory, mental ability and intellectual abilities. Some mood states have a severe effect on our ability to remember, recall or to perform any intellectual task.[35]

Low mood often seen in clinical depression is related to several other features; e.g. loss of energy, irritability, forgetfulness, easy distractibility and suicidal ideation, difficulty in concentration, disturbed sleep and appetite.

Mood disorders are a group of mental illnesses that affect how you feel and think about yourself, other people and life in general. There are a few different types of mood disorders: depression, dysthymic disorder and bipolar disorder.

The abnormality of mood can present in various ways. The mood can change all of a sudden, or it may be going down slowly towards a depressive feeling. It may only occur for a few days, or the changes in mood like feeling low or high can become a regular phenomenon occurring at a fixed interval. Such changes may also appear due to other mental or physical problems, e.g. it may appear after a heart attack or viral fever, and it may appear prior to a psychiatric or physical illness, e.g. mood changes may be the first symptom to start with several neurological disorders. Very often, mood changes also take place before suicidal ideas appear. The emotion of depression precedes almost all incidents of suicide.

- Mood fluctuations are normal state in everyone.
- Mood states may develop into depression in response to potential stress.
- Depression, mania or bipolar disorders are abnormalities of mood.
- Disorders of mood are closely associated with suicide.
- Treatments are very effective for mood disorders.

Mental disorders are common in India.

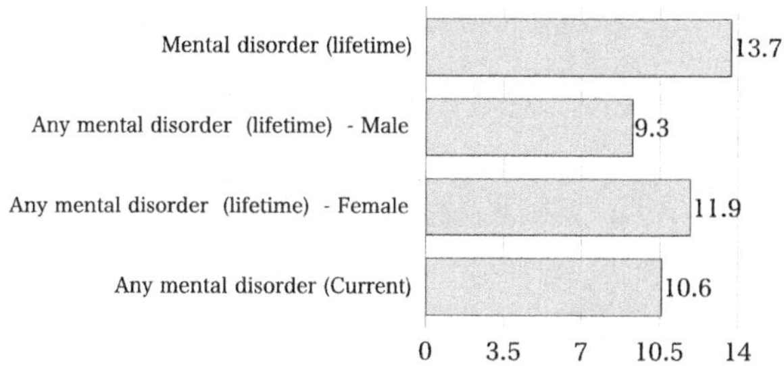

Source: National Mental Health Survey, National Institute of Mental Health and Neurosciences (NIMHANS) Bangalore, Government of India, 2016

True guidance is like a small torch in a dark forest, it doesn't show everything once. But gives enough light for the next step to be safe.

Swami Vivekanand

'Mental health is essential to students' academic success as well as their ability to participate fully and meaningfully throughout all aspects of their lives and throughout their lifespan.'

Mental health issues affect academic performance.

Students who experience mild or moderate symptoms of depression or anxiety also demonstrate more academic difficulties and achieve poorly in examination.

Students who receive treatment for depression report substantial gains in academic performance.

Many students prematurely end their education due to psychiatric disorders.

Mental disorder among adolescents

At least one 1 in 8 adolescents are at a higher risk for developing a mental disorder.

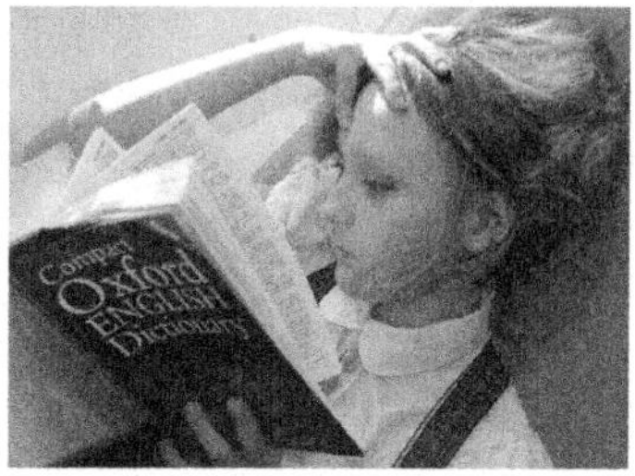

Thapar, A., Collishaw, S., Pine, D. S., & Thapar, A. K. (2012). Depression in adolescence. *Lancet (London, England)*, *379*(9820), 1056–1067.

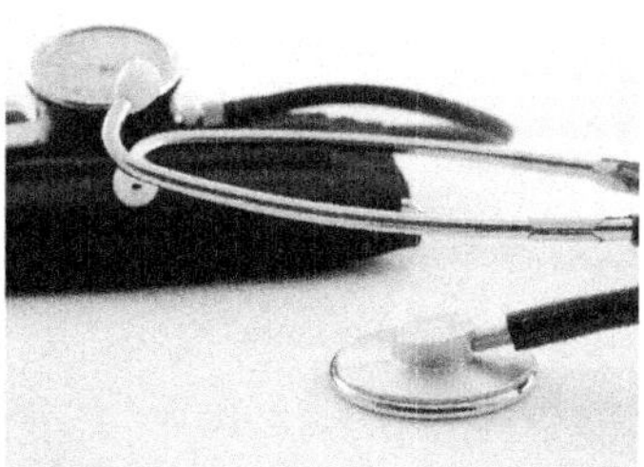

About 80% medical students in India experienced 'burn out'.

Farrell SM, Kar A, Valsraj K, Mukherjee S, Kunheri B, Molodynski A, George S. Wellbeing and burnout in medical students in India; a large scale survey. Int Rev Psychiatry. 2019 Nov-Dec;31(7-8):555-562.

Like a fire in a piece of flint, knowledge exists in the mind.

Suggestion is the friction which brings it out

Swami Vivekanand

EMOTIONAL CONFLICT

Dialogue and communication are the best ways to resolve conflict.
Conflict spares no one. However, if you have the strength to face consequences then you are in a better position.

We live in a society with strong opinions and a value system which is, of course, welcome, but it often contradicts with a young student's biological, emotional and social needs. Recently we are seeing a welcome change where parents are more supportive in dealing with their children. They sometimes make their life easy by removing barriers and welcoming their children's partners into their home while they are still in a live-in relationship and not yet married. Having said this it is also important to know that such an arrangement can also put a different kind of pressure of adjustment within the family, many times, especially since you are not married. This kind of disturbance may also build up some pressure on the student's mind.

Conflict gives rise to stress, it needs to be resolved, everyone finds his way to solve or resolve conflicts. The conflict can be in which you are directly involved, and it can also be of eh type in which you're personally not involved i.e., the outcome of conflict may not directly affect you, you may have a situation for which you are competent to solve it, or you may face a situation in which you lack skills to solve the problem, Conflict resolution is closely related to decision making but both are not the same. there are always 3 options 1- to resolve it one way or the other 2- postpose it for tomorrow 3- leave it for hoping for an automatic solution of leaving it to God. The existence of conflict produced psychological and physical symptoms which shows up as stress, such stress brings symptoms in the person and people close to them, one should remember not resolving conflict is like 'resolving it the way you don't want it to be resolved' that means handing over the outcome to your worst possible fear. Leaving it to God also means you can do without it and you do not care if it is not resolved in your favour. From mental health, perspective conflict is a health risk for both physical and mental illness, it can kickstart any such problem, make the existing problem worse or slows down or delays the recovery in health-related matters. Anxiety increases, the tendency of avoidance stein people become frightened of dealing with similar situations if the stress of conflict continues, Stress can change given behaviour. Negative psychological effects lead to low confidence, low mood, ad risk for a psychiatric disorder. One should consider the psychological state, bearing stress of conflict for a normal individual and people with a psychological disorder is different, it is far more stressful for people with serious physical disorders one can avoid the conflict in which it affects you, but you cannot avoid if it directly does not affect you. You may not be able to avoid the conflict, but you can certainly avoid the psychological and health consequences arising from the stress of the conflict. The best way to help you is to deal with it without delay either by yourself or with your trusted people or in a suitable scenario let someone else do it for you and be ready to accept the outcome, the mere presence of a problem in form of conflict means it is not in your favour, but it can be in your favour. It is easy to solve if the conflict is between two positive options and it is easy to decide if the conflict is between two negative options however if it is between two divergent choices, it is much more complex. One should consider the impact of the outcome and the suffering in the process of deciding. Thus, the best to avoid it is to deal with it.

HOW TO MANAGE PERSONAL CONFLICTS?

The most important question we face is how to resolve a conflict? Most conflicts are best resolved through opening lines of communication. Inner conflict is best resolved by drawing on your inward resources. The best possible resolution comes by using the certain basic and important resource in one's character e.g., logic, intelligence, strategy, resilience, foresight, firmness. Further personality factors like risk-taking ability and experience of the past should be taken into consideration. What you should do is to

- Identify the conflict
- Assess or evaluate the merit or consequences of it
- Analyse each option
- Execute the plan of decision

Identification means full knowledge of the nature and stakeholders of conflict-generating forces. Assessment involves the study of potential consequences. Analysis means considering the possibilities of various methods for reaching its logical conclusion and finally, execution means employing the best possible method and concluding the chain of the process. The relevance of these details draws a lesson that it is an art, and everyone should learn to resolve the conflict based on the method and consequences as stated above. To summarise, it's recommended that:

- Do not delay resolving a conflict
- Prevent complication by using your understanding
- Be logical and deal with intelligence
- Identify stressors
- Accept the outcome
- Learn from experience.

There is no magic pill for the treatment of the behavioural problem, but it is heartening to know that about half of the adolescents grow out of such problems fully, and the other half persist with a minor or major psychiatric problem that can be treated with some success. Professional help is necessary.

It is helpful if parents can observe the behaviour of their child from an early age and do a proper intervention. It's difficult to define the term 'proper' but it means respectful treatment relating to them and open lines of communications. Adolescents need to be heard. On many occasions, their fears are genuine, but they are denied the opportunity to express them. Traditions, excessive control, the presence of stress, an unpleasant family environment, etc. contribute to the occurrence of such episodes. When a crisis erupts, it is important to ensure the safety of everybody concerned. Due to misunderstandings, there are high incidents of tragic happenings like consuming an overdose of sleeping pills or trying to run away from the house or attempt suicide. It is also important to remember that the difficulty arises more because of the consequences and complications related to adolescence rather than from the crisis itself. If the crisis is not attended to and the behaviour continues, they are conveying a clear signal to be understood and the attempt should be made. At the same time, the treatment of anxiety is also important.

In our society, treatment for behavioural problems is not easily available and it is also not the mindset of people to approach mental health professionals for what they call 'day-to-day' difficulties.

The best answer is to remain vigilant, identify early and intervene on a priority basis by talking and educating, children and their parents. We must provide an answer to emotional problems. Finally for severe cases no doubt a psychiatric intervention would be necessary. Dialogue with parents about handling adolescents can, however, go a long way to provide answers.

15. DECISION MAKING

A COMPLEX NEUROBEHAVIORAL PROCESS THIS INVOLVES

A brain function: Decision making is not only about 'personal choice' like in selecting a career or a partner or making a bid in the stock market or a casino. It's much more.

Characteristics of the person who is making the decision (emotional regulation, anxiety, executive function, i.e., brain ability for planning and execution, memory and recollection of the experience, personality characteristics, intelligence, ability to see the question from an overall perspective and long term outcomes- insight and foresight) the situation in which the decision is to be made (social support, threats or stress factors in the environment, presence of friends or adversaries)

The main outcome involved in decision making, how important is the question for the person who is making the decision, and what is the implication of this decision on others, the time duration involved for making the decision.

Factors that limit the ability to make good decisions include missing or incomplete information, urgent deadlines, and limited physical or emotional resources. When making a decision, we form opinions and choose actions via mental processes which are influenced by biases, reason, emotions, and memories.

Decision making is the cognitive process that results in the selection of a course of action or belief from several possibilities.

Heuristics are simple rules of thumb that people often use to form judgments and make decisions; they are good for most situations but can sometimes lead to errors in judgment.

The anchoring effect happens when a person must choose a number, but the number is influenced, or "anchored," by the person having just heard a different number.

The framing effect occurs when the way a decision is framed (i.e., positive or negative) affects the decision-making process.

Some decisions are 'conditioned responses' that means the choices you have made at various times in the past and the outcome has not been adverse in a given situation where the quick answer is required one usually goes by this 'Response'.

However, there are steps to ensure that people make consistently excellent choices, including gathering as much information as possible, considering all the possible alternatives, as well as their attendant benefits and costs, and taking the time to sleep on weightier decisions.

One must allow time for an in-depth study before taking a decision. Emotional overtones may adversely affect the decision; however, there is hardly any situation which is free from the emotional component because emotions are a part of the system. Therefore, one needs the skill to optimize intelligence, past experience, and psychological overtones involved in specific decision making. Every individual has characteristics which affect their decision making.

Several features in an individual affect their decision making, e.g., need for easy and early gratification, high sense of urgency, presence of excessive anxiety, competitiveness, foresight-ability to sense what may happen, resilience – the ability to adapt to any new and challenging situation.

MENTAL HEALTH AFFECTS DECISION MAKING:
Those suffering from depression or dementia or early memory lapses either due to any metabolic or hormone problem or severe anxiety state, often make mistakes while making decisions.

It is not clear if decision making has a set pattern or it varies at different times in an individual.

When you practice methods to remain calm, it means maintaining the functioning of a brain in a state so relaxed that it will not allow adverse factors to interfere, an internal atmosphere which can provide a clear state of free will, analytical capacity, and judgments which are free from personal biases.

The complexity of decision-making is, therefore, a process which involves brain functions. It requires a brain-mind behavior, previous learning, intellectual capacity, and resilience. The simple act of decision making means you apply your free will, weigh benefits, and assess the cost of making a choice. Factors like personal biases, unconscious desire, or irrational thinking, adversely affect the process of making choices. While making the best possible choice which is relatively 'risk-free', one should try to resist using previous experience without considering the studied outcome of current challenges. Know your limitations or the characteristics of your personality and practice how to overcome factors which interfere with it adversely, e.g., need for urgency or undue anxiety. Maintain your motivation while solving the problem. Avoid quick decision making. The best thing you can do to remain 'risk-free' is to pause before decision-making and allow emotional turmoil to settle.

A brain function: Decision making is not only about 'personal choice' like in selecting a career or a partner or making a bid in the stock market or a casino. It's much more.

If someone has taken a particular decision in the past in a given situation, will he again make a similar decision if those circumstances again came up? Generally, there is a pattern. System of 'reward' in the brain decides this factor to a certain state if the previous decision has been positively rewarding you are more likely to take the similar decision, in such a situation your current perception of choice comes in conflict with the experience. It is this situation which makes people unique. Your ability to take every decision and deal with every question as a new question for problem-solving, you are more likely to be correct. You do not win in the gamble only because you won in the past with a similar technique. A successful person will view every problem as a new and nascent problem. It is the most straightforward argument to say that "I did so...because it always worked with me," it is more helpful if you say that .."I did so because, in my opinion, it was the best possible thing to do."

Another set of situations which influence the decision making is the surrounding involved in the decision making, i.e., any person or any situation, the context of 'social cognition,' i.e., how you interpret the social stimuli which influences your choice, everyone has different capacity of perceiving and reading another person and surrounding space. Social cognition is a unique characteristic which adds to one's personality.

16. MENTAL HEALTH AND DECISION MAKING

Those suffering from depression or dementia or early memory lapses either due to any metabolic or hormone problem or severe anxiety state, often make mistakes while making decisions.

It is not clear if decision making has a set pattern or it varies at different times in an individual.

When you practice methods to remain calm, it means maintaining the functioning of a brain in a state so relaxed that it will not allow adverse factors to interfere, an internal atmosphere which can provide a clear state of free will, analytical capacity, and judgments which are free from personal biases.

The complexity of decision-making is, therefore, a process which involves brain functions. It requires a brain-mind behaviour, previous learning, intellectual capacity, and resilience. The simple act of decision making means you apply your free will, weigh benefits, and assess the cost of making a choice. Factors like personal biases, unconscious desire, or irrational thinking, adversely affect the process of making choices. While making the best possible choice which is relatively 'risk-free', one should try to resist using previous experience without considering the studied outcome of current challenges. Know your limitations or the characteristics of your personality and practice how to overcome factors which interfere with it adversely, e.g. need for urgency or undue anxiety. Maintain your motivation while solving the problem. Avoid quick decision making. The best thing you can do to remain 'risk-free' is to pause before decision-making and allow emotional turmoil to settle.

STRESS OF DECISION MAKING

One of the most important mental activity faced by everyone, not just the students is about making a decision. It's not that decision making is of significance only in making a career choice or marriage, decision making is involved at every step irrespective of the nature of question involved. If you are deciding to attend a class or not to attend, the logistics for making a decision is same. whether will have long-term or short-term reward or punishment depend upon how you make a decision. this psychological task is not only complex, but it has the potential to make life stressful. There is nothing like a big decision or small decision, easy decision or difficult decision. A question which is difficult for you may be difficult for others. Level of distress that you will feel depends upon how strongly you associate yourself or identify with the question.

Though it may be difficult to change the behavioral pattern that you have developed for problem solving or decision making yet it is worth understanding the process. The objective of making a decision is not that you to yourself with guilt or remorse, it also not to bring you in a situation where you start feeling unduly responsible. Sometimes, you may be taking decision on behalf of others and may start feeling more responsible than what you should be. Thus, decision making is a cognitive process, but it has huge emotional overlay.

It is also important to know how and when not to make a decision.

Characteristics of the person who is making the decision (emotional regulation, anxiety, executive function, i.e., brain ability for planning and execution, memory and recollection of the experience, personality characteristics, intelligence, ability to see the question from an overall perspective and long-term outcomes insight and foresight) the situation in which the decision is to be made (social support, threats or stress factors in the environment, presence of friends or adversaries).

The main outcome involved in decision making, how important is the question for the person who is making the decision, and what is the implication of this decision on others, the time duration involved for making the decision.

Factors that limit the ability to make good decisions include missing or incomplete information, urgent deadlines, and limited physical or emotional resources. When making a decision, we form opinions and choose actions via mental processes which are influenced by biases, reason, emotions, and memories.

Decision making is the cognitive process that results in the selection of a course of action or belief from several possibilities.

Some decisions are 'conditioned responses' that means the choices you have made at various times in the past and the outcome has not been adverse in a given situation where the quick answer has required one usually goes by this 'response'.

However, there are steps to ensure that people make consistently excellent choices, including gathering as much information as possible, considering all the possible alternatives, as well as their attendant benefits and costs, and taking the time to sleep on weightier decisions.

One must allow time for an in-depth study before taking a decision. Emotional overtones may adversely affect the decision; however, there is hardly any situation which is free from the emotional component because emotions are part of the system. Emotions are created when the brain interprets what's going on around us through our memories, thoughts and beliefs. This triggers how we feel and behave. All our decisions are influenced by this process in some way. Different emotions affect decisions in different ways. If you're feeling sad, you might be more willing to settle for things that are not in your favor, such as not putting yourself forward for promotion, or remaining in an unhealthy relationship. But sadness can also make you more generous – research shows that unhappy people are more likely to be in favor of increasing benefits to welfare recipients than angry people, who are lacking in empathy.[36]

Therefore, one needs the skill to optimise intelligence, past experience, and psychological overtones involved in specific decision making. Every individual has characteristics which affect their decision making.

Several features in an individual affect their decision making, e.g. need for easy and early gratification, high sense of urgency, presence of excessive anxiety, competitiveness, foresight ability to sense what may happen, resilience – the ability to adapt to any new and challenging situation.

17. DECISION MAKING AND BRAIN FUNCTION

Decision making is not only about 'personal choice' like in selecting a career or a partner or making a bid in the stock market or a casino. It's much more.

If someone has taken a particular decision in the past in a given situation, will he again make a similar decision if those circumstances again came up? Generally, there is a pattern. System of 'reward' in the brain decides this factor to a certain state if the previous decision has been positively rewarding you are more likely to take the similar decision; in such a situation your current perception of choice comes in conflict with the experience. It is this situation which makes people unique. Your ability to take every decision and deal with every question as a new question for problem-solving, you are more likely to be correct. You do not win in the gamble only because you won in the past with a similar technique. A successful person will view every problem as a new and nascent problem. It is the most straightforward argument to say that; 'I did so…because it always worked with me,' it is more helpful if you say that 'I did so because, in my opinion, it was the best possible thing to do.'

Another set of situations which influence the decision making is the surrounding involved in the decision making,[37] i.e., any person or any situation, the context of 'social cognition', i.e., how you interpret the social stimuli which influences your choice, everyone has different capacity of perceiving and reading another person and surrounding space. Social cognition is a unique characteristic which adds to one's personality.

CHAPTER 3
RESTORING PSYCHOLOGICAL HEALTH

18. IDENTIFICATION OF MENTAL DISORDERS

Mental illness involves changes in thinking, mood or behaviour, or a combination of these issues. Symptoms include significant distress, inability to function as needed over an extended period. These symptoms can be mild or severe, depending on the type of mental illness the individual is suffering from, family, patient's environment.

Though identification of mental disorders is important, even more important is to have the ability to identify the symptoms which are not very obvious. Besides this we also need to have the capacity to recognise the social, psychological factors or any trauma which may be interfering in our daily life, and thus resultantly is interfering in the pathway to success; symptoms like sleeplessness, loss of appetite, excessive thinking, mood variation, restlessness, aggression are some conditions which are not psychiatric disorders per se, but they are widely prevalent and have great significance because they cause some amount of distress. These are important, however small, because they are known to keep the affected person preoccupied and one is not able to focus on several other important things in life.

There are three groups of factors which interfere in one's daily life and also in the functioning and preparedness for good success or while preparing for any test or competitive sports or any kind of activity, and these are the symptoms of mental disorders which are present but also fail to amount to a mental disorder, the factors to which we are unable to adjust or cope. Most symptoms of mental disorder are problems related to mental health which are initially not very obviously seen. They are mild, may appear very gradually and progress slowly. Once these symptoms start, they persist for fairly long period of time. Very few conditions are self-limiting or disappear on their own.

This is one of the great problems while understanding mental illness, by the time you approach anyone in the family, a friend or a doctor, it becomes clear that the symptoms have been existing for a very long time. e.g. difficulty about sleep, may have 2 or 3 types of abnormalities 1st: Problem while getting into sleep, remain restless in bed before sleep, 2nd sleep being interrupted in the middle of the night and thereafter you can't fall asleep again, and 3rd: is waking up very much early in the morning, before 5 am, or so. This is not about the early risers, who have a different biological rhythm, and start the day early.

By the time the complaint is made one should realise that a good amount of period has passed by and the person has at least suffered for more than 6 months. People want to observe if the symptom of sleeplessness will go away on its own. A 6 month or 1-year long persistence of the symptoms has already tired the person out, and even led to difficulty in concentration. Thus, it is important that the symptom is recognised at an early stage. It does not necessarily mean that it can be categorised as 'sleep disorders', those are different things. Sometimes there are many other conditions related to sleep which will generally be missed and worsen if not reported in time. E.g. Restless leg syndrome (jerks in legs), or sleep walking.

Similarly, other symptoms of mood, emotion, behaviour, thinking, etc. also begin slowly and it is important to watch out if these symptoms are interfering with daily life activities, then one must seek medical opinion.

Mental health is as important as physical health, and they both directly affect each other. People with physical health problems often experience anxiety or depression, which affects their recovery. Similarly, mental health factors can increase the risk of developing physical problems, such as diabetes, heart disease, weight gain, or loss.

Adult mental health disorders begin during adolescence. This seems a simple enough statement that suggests we cannot understand mental illness affecting adults unless we appreciate what goes on during the preceding period of life. If true, childhood and adolescence, divided by the biological gateway of puberty, would-be crucial epochs in terms of understanding causes and mechanisms of adult illness. This would frame attempts at early intervention and both primary and secondary prevention. The seeds of many conditions manifesting in this period are sown earlier in life, could be even during childhood. Family members are often the primary caregivers in cases of mental disorders. The extent of the burden of mental disorders on family members is difficult to assess and quantify and is consequently often ignored. However, it does have a significant impact on the family's quality of life. In addition to the health and social costs, those suffering from mental illnesses are also victims of human rights violations, stigma, and discrimination, both inside and outside psychiatric institutions.

FEW COMMON SYMPTOMS TO IDENTIFY MENTAL HEALTH PROBLEM AND MENTAL DISORDER

Interest or pleasure

Feeling down or depressed

Trouble falling asleep

Feeling tired

Feeling loos of energy

Poor appetite

Feeling bad about self

Trouble concentrating

Moving or speaking very slowly

Thoughts that one would better be dead

Worry

Being afraid

Thinking unusual

Feeling that someone may be looking at him

Any abnormal behaviour

Feeling insecure

Speaks unusual thoughts or world

No more trust others

Remains suspicious

Feeling nervous, anxious, or on edge

Not being able to stop or control worrying

Worrying too much about different things

Trouble relaxing

Being so restless that it is hard to sit still

Becoming easily annoyed or irritable

Feeling afraid

More social or outgoing than usual

You were much more interested in sex than usual

You did things that were unusual for you

Spending money got you or your family into trouble

Have you heard unusual sounds like banging, clicking, hissing, clapping or ringing in your ears? Field is required.

Do things that you see appear different from the way they usually do?

Have you had experiences with telepathy, psychic forces, or fortune telling?
Have you felt that you are not in control of your own ideas or thoughts?
Do you have difficulty getting your point across?
Do you have strong feelings or beliefs about being unusually gifted or talented in some way?
Do you feel that other people are watching you or talking about you?
Do you sometimes get strange feelings on or just beneath your skin, like bugs crawling?
Do you sometimes feel suddenly distracted by distant sounds that you are not normally aware of?
Have you had the sense that some person or force is around you, although you couldn't see anyone?
Do you worry at times that something may be wrong with your mind?
Have you ever felt that you don't exist?
Have you been confused at times whether something you experienced was real or imaginary?
Do you hold beliefs that other people would find unusual or bizarre? Field is required?
Do you feel that parts of your body have changed in some way, or that parts of your body are working differently? Field is required?
Are your thoughts sometimes so strong that you can almost hear them? Field is required?
Do you find yourself feeling mistrustful or suspicious of other people? Field is required?
Have you seen unusual things like flashes, flames, blinding light, or geometric figures? Field is required?
Have you seen things that other people can't see or don't seem to see? Field is required?
Do people sometimes find it hard to understand what you are saying? Field is required?
Top of Form
How afraid are you of gaining 3 pounds?
When was the last time you went on a diet?
Compared to other things in your life, how important is your weight to you?
Do you ever feel fat?
Exercised excessively?

Are you currently in treatment for an eating disorder?
Did you have nightmares about the event(s) or thought about the event(s) when you did not want to?
Did you try hard not to think about the event(s) or went out of your way to avoid situations that reminded you of the event(s) ?
Have been constantly on guard, watchful, or easily startled?
Did you feel numb or detached from people, activities, or your surroundings?
Did you feel guilty or unable to stop blaming yourself or others for the event(s) or any problems the event(s) may have caused? Top of Form
Do you take unnecessary risks?
Do you feel hurt frequently?
Do you seem to be having less fun?
Do you act younger than children your age?
Do not listen to rules?
Do not show feeling?
Do not understand other people's feelings or
Tease others?
Blame others for your troubles?
Take things that do not belong to you?
Refuse to share?
Do you have any emotional or behavioural problems for which you need help?
Have you ever felt that you ought to cut down on your drinking or drug use?
Have people annoyed you by criticising your drinking or drug use?
Have you ever felt bad or guilty about your drinking or drug use?
Have you ever had a drink or used drugs first thing in the morning to steady your nerves or to get rid of a hangover?
What substance or addiction are you concerned about?
Alcohol
Marijuana
Cocaine/crack
Heroin
Prescription opioids

19. WARNING SIGNS FOR A MENTAL HEALTH PROBLEM

If several of the following are occurring, it may useful to follow up with a mental health professional.[40]

Sleep or appetite changes — Dramatic sleep and appetite changes or decline in personal care

Mood changes — Rapid or dramatic shifts in emotions or depressed feelings

Withdrawal — Recent social withdrawal and loss of interest in activities previously enjoyed

Drop in functioning — An unusual drop in functioning, at school, work or social activities, such as quitting sports, failing in school or difficulty performing familiar tasks

Problems thinking — Problems with concentration, memory or logical thought and speech that are hard to explain

Increased sensitivity — Heightened sensitivity to sights, sounds, smells or touch; avoidance of over-stimulating situations

Apathy — Loss of initiative or desire to participate in any activity

Feeling disconnected — A vague feeling of being disconnected from oneself or one's surroundings; a sense of unreality

Illogical thinking — Unusual or exaggerated beliefs about personal powers to understand meanings or influence events; illogical or 'magical' thinking typical of childhood in an adult

Nervousness — Fear or suspiciousness of others or a strong nervous feeling

Unusual behaviour – Odd, uncharacteristic, peculiar behaviour

20. MENTAL HEALTH SCREENING

A mental health screening is used to help diagnose mental disorders. Your primary care provider may use a mental health screening to see if you need to go to a mental health provider. A mental health provider is a health care professional that specialises in diagnosing and treating mental health problems. If you are already seeing a mental health provider, you may get a mental health screening to help guide your treatment.

- Common signs may include:
- Excessive worrying or fear
- Extreme sadness
- Major changes in personality, eating habits, and/or sleeping patterns
- Dramatic mood swings
- Anger, frustration, or irritability
- Fatigue and lack of energy
- Confused thinking and trouble concentrating
- Feelings of guilt or worthlessness
- Avoidance of social activities

21. MANAGING STRESS

We always hear the term stressed out. Students may complain of examination stress, adults of financial strain, the stress in relationships, and even in day to day life.

'Stress' is a word that has multiple meanings and holds different connotations in different situations. 'Stress of life' is perhaps the most popular use of the word, as it relates to the world we live in, and it points out the challenges we face and how we react to them.

The word 'stress' became more popular in the mid-nineteenth century and made its way into our daily vocabulary: today, we might be hard-pressed to find a word that can provide the same meaning. The concept of stress itself was introduced to what is considered 'modern medicine' in the 1930s, by a European scientist Hans Selye.[41,42] He was the first to take serious note of the changes brought about in a person facing an adverse situation. He was also the first one to notice the impact of what we nowadays call 'stressors' (or 'stressful events') on the general health of people. He named the set of effects observed as 'General Adaptation Syndrome', and defined it as a non-specific response of the body to any demand.

The study of stress is now a scientific discipline that holds a lot of potentials. One that concerns us here is the link between stress and illness, particularly mental illness. There have been numerous studies and theories published which offer a comprehensive view of stress and its relation to health. The concept of stress is not new; it has existed ever since the age of 'Vedic sciences'. It was described in the Vedas as a 'disequilibrium' between different biochemical constituents of the human body.[43] This has been a clear and undisputed concept of health in the medical sciences of Indian civilisation from the time human beings began to exist. Although a detailed discussion on this aspect is out of the scope of this book, it is reasonable at this point to briefly mention two important theories which should help us understand stress, and how to deal with it.

THE CONCEPT OF STRESS

The first question people ask about stress is 'what is stress all about?' It is a common term which people use but seldom understand because it remains ill-defined. Almost every factor we know has been implicated as stress, it may be cultural, social, economic, academic, personal, or work-related.

(Contributed by Siddhansh Shrivastava, MD)

It becomes important to answer some of the critical questions like:

Which factors constitute stress
What are the factors which can become potentially stressful?
Why does a situation become stressful?
To answer these questions, we need to know the concept of stress:

The idea of stress can be explained as follows:

1. The structural or physical human body does not contain or limit the mind. Though the mind is an integral part of life, it has no boundaries. Mind and body work together to maintain all functions of life.

2. There is another concept of equal importance. According to Ayurveda medicine, there is a biochemical energy system constituted by three elements, [*Doshas viz. vāta, pitta, and kapha*]: they control the health of both, body and mind. Disequilibrium of these elements will result in disease.[44] If we translate these concepts into the way we understand medicine today, we get the statement that the psychological, physiological, and biological systems maintain the equilibrium between the mind and brain. It becomes much clearer to understand when we expand the concept of mind and body to 'mind-brain-and-body' and still further to 'mind-brain-and-behaviour.' In this framework, any event (such as an abnormality, fear, threat, emotion or thinking) is likely to either disturb the biochemical or the mental mechanism. This idea gives rise to the concept of 'stress'.[45]

Several medicinal and yogic practices have been recommended for, first, dealing with a disease (intervention and treatment), and second, keeping life healthy and free from disease (preventive medicine). Mind and body work in conjunction. The way they are interrelated allows people to fight threats or dangers that they may find in their everyday life in a manner that does not affect their normal functioning.

Proper functioning of body and mind determine positivity, a sense of well-being, productivity, involvement, learning, and interpersonal relationships. However, when something goes wrong, abnormal situations arise. Such unusual conditions can disturb our emotions, alter the regular functioning of our body, elevate our heart rate, blood pressure, glucose levels, etc. The body adjusts to these factors to counteract the damage done by the trauma. Stress, at a reasonable level, is thus the body's way to protect itself from adversity.

Even though it is hard to define stress, we all intuitively understand what 'being stressed out' means. It is used in everyday language to express the pressure that life exerts on us and how it makes us feel, especially when we think we are struggling to cope with the events we are facing. However, the extent of information that the general public has on stress may not be accurate enough. One of the limitations is everyday use. Thus, grasping scientific facts about stress is difficult. Notwithstanding, we can notice when something is not right with us; even in cultures where people are not allowed to express their feelings freely or clearly, and where people fail to recognise when they feel stress, even they feel that something is out of line when they face specific life events.[46]

Words like 'anxiety' or 'burnout' have been associated with stress, but they don't mean the same thing. 'Anxiety' can be described as an internal feeling triggered by stress.[47] It may be expressed in several dimensions, such as behavioural (difficulty sleeping, avoidance, shaking, stuttering). It may also be present as an internal factor (a feeling of dread, fear, sense of unreality, feeling overwhelmed, feeling tense, etc.), or a physiological factor (rapid heartbeat, sweating, clammy hands, dry mouth, to name a few). Stress has a deep-seated role in our mind as well as our body. When a response to stress or an anxious state is dragged on for a long period, it impacts the physical and psychological health. The most evident effect of this impact is cardiovascular disorders, peptic ulcers, gastroesophageal reflux disease, loss of sleep and other sleep disturbances, weight loss or gain. The public widely recognises all these as standard manifestations of stress. Many different complications arise from stress, some of which are typical to chronic stress, and some are mostly related to immediate stress. Over-stress, or repetitive patterns of stress, can also create psychological effects among people: some of them are workaholic or indulging on binge eating or shopping, are mild in severity and socially acceptable to a certain degree, but some others can develop into toxic personalities, counter-productive behaviours and so on.

WHY PEOPLE FEEL 'BURNOUT'?

'Burnout' can be understood as an outcome of prolonged stress. It occurs when we feel we can no longer cope with the problems we face and feel like giving up.

Arch Hart, a psychologist, differentiated 'stress' from 'burnout' in a straightforward and applicable way, inspiring new ideas on what stress should and should not be.[48] For example, stress heightens and over stimulates emotions, whereas in a burnout the emotion is blunted; exhaustion in stress affects the levels of physical energy, whereas, in burnout, exhaustion affects the drive and motivation. Where stress produces disintegration (loss of strength), burnout produces demoralisation. Where stress invokes a sense of urgency and hyperactivity, burnout invokes a sense of helplessness and hopelessness. Where stress produces panic, anxiety or phobic disorders, burnout produces paranoia, depersonalisation and detachment disorders.[49] These comparisons constitute some of the root components involved in psychotherapy, pointing at the fact that scientific work in the field of stress holds a lot of potential for use in today's world.

When understanding stress as a protective system that helps us react in the face of danger, challenge or difficulty, it goes without saying that Stress is a temporary facilitator helping us cope with the situation at hand. Therefore, a prolonged state of stress is not desirable, and will slowly impact upon health. Some studies label such an extreme amount of pressure placed on the body as an 'allostatic load'.[50]

Many mechanisms in the body are inbuilt to cope with stress. An imbalance in such mechanisms, especially with hormonal involvement, over time, leads to illnesses—heart conditions, obesity-related diseases, and higher incidence of diabetes increase mortality in men with competitive jobs. Moreover, there are many physical, psychological and social consequences of stress worth mentioning; the burnout syndrome, depression, insomnia, an earlier onset of conditions normally expected in old age, kidney diseases, liver conditions, lowered immunity causing infections, addictive personality, and social impacts such as divorce, debilitating effects of depression-like low productivity, sexual inadequacy, gambling, trauma, suicide, and crime. In pregnant women, stress is particularly damaging, as it affects the maturation of the brain of the unborn.

Stress is an everyday issue and all around us. A proper understanding of stress involves the mind, body, environment, and social factors. It represents how stressors affect our mind and body.[51] It is interesting to notice that these stressors can be real-life problems or imagined possibilities of danger. Thus, a worker may feel stressed when he is notified that his boss is considering to fire him from his job, and he does not have a backup plan or any savings. But he can feel equally stressed when he hears the rumour that one person is going to be fired, even though there is a low-to-none possibility that he is the one; the physical and emotional impact of stress is the same in both the real and the imaginary case.

Of course, people can face stressful situations (of both kinds) in positive ways: not every stressor will impact negatively on the long-term life of people. The key notions of having in mind when facing a stressful situation are, first, the fact that we all are more than able to manage it positively: there is no problem that we cannot cope with. Successful management of stress should consider all the factors that can lead to stress-induced issues. First, we must manage to reduce the causes of stress, trying to solve the problem that is causing it. The consequences of the problem must be addressed too. Second, our mental mechanism to solve the problem must be addressed, starting from being certain of our capacity of solving the problem effectively. We can take care of the physical effects we may experience by consulting a physician when we feel the situation is negatively affecting us.

The social dimension of stressful situations can be managed too: letting our loved ones know that we are stressed can be a great tool. Speaking about our problems may help us look at them from another perspective. Relatives who are familiar with our situation may be more understanding when we are in a bad mood or irritable. Social situations often trigger stress. But stress itself also disrupts the social life of the person suffering from it. Thus, the consequences of stress are not only physiological or physical but also bring about unfavourable changes in the social setting. In turn, adverse social situations created by stress can contribute to the strengthening of the feeling of stress itself. A woman may be under stress due to a chronic disease, and because of this, her mood may change. Her typical way of dealing with her everyday life and emotions may be altered, and this may have an impact on her relationships in her workplace or with her family. Her interests reduce, her interaction with the people in her workplace become negative, causing an adverse work environment and an unwelcoming family climate.

Stress that is triggered by a problem in the workplace often reflects in the behaviour of the affected person at home. The stress caused by a mood change in a family member affects the emotions and behaviour of the other people in the household. Thus, poorly managed stress may affect not just an individual but an entire family. For this reason, it is important to notice when a family member or a relative is on the verge of experiencing stress or is unable to cope well with it. Many situations may trigger anxiety and be on the lookout for potential stressors may help people to cope better.[37,38] Financial trouble or work-related instability, social changes (divorce, children leaving home, or additions to the family), moving houses or cities, illness of a relative or a loved one, or strains in a marriage, are some of the stressors that are considered to be potentially serious. Stress has a negative impact not only on our physical health but social wellbeing as well. Stress is part of our lives. It instigates our ability to deal with adversities, the outcome may be favourable or not. With information, effort, practice and sometimes medication, it can be minimised. Once a positive response appears, it sets a chain reaction of positivity.

Finally, stress cannot be managed on the illness-or-disease model. Managing stress is the art of maintaining the equilibrium in the mind-body and brain mechanisms. Its responses are 'learned-responses' which can be changes achieved by the practice of keeping harmony in mind and body.[52]

HOW TO RECOGNISE STRESS AND WHAT ARE THE SIGNS OF STRESS?

We cannot do away with stress. Even if you are calm and cool-headed by nature, there are bound to be incidents in your life which cause stress. Recognising and overcoming stress can help us in our lives.

Stress generally affects all areas of life. Although, people usually, discuss only symptoms which are related to body and mind, there are always social, economic and personal consequences in a person who is facing problems-related to stress, we may see:

Changes in physiology, i.e. in several systems of the body, e.g. heart rate, blood pressure, muscle tightness or twitching.

Changes in psychological symptoms, i.e. changes in mood, thoughts or behaviour, thus the children or adolescents may complain of feeling anxious, fearful, panic-stricken or depressed or with poor concentration. Stress may also manifest it self in the form of physical problems like body ache, acidity etc. Stress can arise suddenly, i.e. a response of the body to a sudden change, i.e. you receive a piece of bad news or get exposed to a traumatic situation, in such situations most often people will complain about internal symptoms; the mental symptoms appear after some time. If the stress persists, i.e. long-standing stress, it leads to a chronic anxiety state. It has a complex presentation of several changes in the body and mental mechanism. People do come up with symptoms of depression or various body-related symptoms which are popularly called psychosomatic symptoms, such as tension headaches and heartburn.

The stress response also depends upon cultures. People living in societies which are more communicative and psychological minded can express that they feel stressed whereas societies like in India, people develop various body symptoms, e.g. a headache or pain in the back as a response to stress. It is important to understand the cultural differences because mental mechanism is guided by social factors which include traditions and practices. As society is changing this trend is changing. People often express that they feel 'stressed'. It is very difficult to pinpoint the cause of stress exactly. One thing is certain that there is no single cause, It depends upon an individual's nature, i.e. everyone has a particular threshold (stress threshold); everyone remains comfortable as long as the stress is below this level. If this threshold is crossed, then problems appear.[53] The stressful factor in case of students can arise from academic or non-academic aspects; it can be the curriculum, lack of support, failure in examination, parental pressure, or non-academic, like adverse home situation or a childhood adverse event of a flashback of any traumatic memory or a social conflict. In most of the conditions, many factors work together to cause symptoms of stress.

22. BUILDING RESILIENCE

Resilience is the characteristic which allows adaptation to adverse circumstances.

- Resilience is a neurobiological condition.
- It has characteristics of adaptation, optimism, satisfaction and contentment.
- Resilience can determine outcome of a psychiatric intervention.

Resilience has been broadly defined as a dynamic process, wherein individuals display positive adaptation despite experiences of significant adversity or trauma.[54] Resilience is often conceptualised as existing along a continuum with vulnerability, and implies a resistance to psychopathology, though not total invulnerability to the development of psychiatric disorder. Resilience is seen as more than simple recovery from insult, rather it can be defined as positive growth or adaptation following periods of homeostatic disruption.[55,56] The first theory about the resilience relies on the characters that related to positive outcomes in exposure to difficulties of life.[57] The current theories believe that resilience is a multidimensional construct comprised of constitutional variables such as temperament and personality accompanied with specific skills for example problem-solving skills.

Resilience[58] is the capacity people have to adapt swiftly and successfully to stressful/traumatic events while not reverting to the original state. Resilience is described as an evolving process influenced by a variety of biological, social, and environmental factor[59] is the growing evidence supports the notion that resilience is involved in the development of positive psychological traits.[60] Various studies have illustrated the critical role of resilience on the individuals' capacity to form a healthy response while enduring trauma, and this has been noted across all ages. Human beings have the capacity to protect themselves and deal with the adverse events or stimulus, which can challenge their psychobiological homeostasis. Here resilience contributes as a defence mechanism and a protective factor.

Resilience is extremely valuable in life. It is resilience which helps us get up when we're knocked down. It can help us in times of failure, grief and dealing with unexpected adversities. This quality helps us ward off psychological problems.

Resilience is an individual's characteristic which allows them to adapt to a new or adverse, challenging or traumatic situations. Its' purpose is to protect our inner self from external threat and generally refers to characteristics of:

- Adaptability
- Optimism
- Satisfaction
- Contentment

It is a psychological concept which is a derivative of brain mechanism. Resilience can help protect you from various mental health conditions, such as depression and anxiety. Resilience can also help offset factors that increase the risk of mental health conditions, such as being bullied or previous trauma. If you have an existing mental health condition, being resilient can improve your ability to cope.

23. RESILIENCE CAN BE IMPROVED

Get connected, make your day meaningful, learn from experience, remain hopeful, take care of yourself.

You can overcome defects in your personality and cultivate positive traits. To some extent it is the presence of a positive person around you and to alarge extent it depends how the positive person treats you, the quality of interaction, encouragement, faith and generating confidence. This may change the situation and transform the personality. Human beings have immense capacity to learn as well as to unlearn, when personality transformation is taking place, not only do some qualities have to be learned, but certain characteristic have to be re learned. Personality structure has dual features. The major part of it is constructed before the age of sixteen or seventeen. Some of the transformations continue to take place lifelong, certain other features can be changed by making a conscious effort. That is exactly what psychologists and psychotherapists do when they are treating a condition or illness. By using specific treatment, theytrytocorrectthefeaturesofpersonalitywhichareinterferinginthefunctioning of one's life. So everyone should keep the hope for change alive.

There is strong argument which claims that response to trauma develops through resilience, and although some neurobiological changes correlate with resilience and trauma, it is unclear whether the nature and degree of response to trauma is dependent on the extent of neurological changes alone. The level of resilience protection and modification also depends on other complex factors that shape the influence that resilience has on individuals experiencing trauma.

There are multiple factors influencing the 'strength' of resilience which are not yet determined. I believe that there are underlying cognitive features, which are strongly related to resilience, and may play a significant role in determining how appropriate and sufficient a response is, or how well the symptoms are minimised in a specific patient's case. Resilience is the human capacity to adapt swiftly and successfully to a stressful or traumatic event and manage to revert back to a positive state. Therefore, resilience creates a potential preventative measure for mental illness, and has a critical effect on health status of individuals.

24. BIOLOGY OF RESILIENCE

The neuroscience of resilience is beginning to uncover the circuits and molecules that protect against stress-related neuropsychiatric diseases. Glucocorticoids (GCs) are important regulators of basal and stress-related homeostasis that influence a wide array of genes in almost every organ and tissue. Changes in neuroplasticity, HPA (Hypothalamic-pituitary-adrenal axis) axis response to stress, neurotransmissions of dopamine, serotonin, and norepinephrine play an important role in maintaining homeostasis of resilience plasticity. The main neurochemical substance in this process is glucocorticoid. Neurochemical changes suggest that, cortisol-related sustained, enhancement of amygdala and hippocampus may lead to loss of functional connectivity. Research of gene environmental integration offers a host of significant findings, which support the concept of resilience being an independent paradigm. Such findings help establish the idea that genetic and environmental factors (i.e., early life stress, and chronic stress during adulthood) can produce a situation of enhanced vulnerability and a reduced resilience of the brain, which in turn leads to unsuccessful aging of the brain. Individuals possess the capacity to learn to be resilient by developing protective mechanisms that prevent them from the maladaptive effects of stress. It is not clear whether resilience is a modifiable or non-modifiable factor. Studies report that resilience is affected.

25. ADDICTION

Addiction is related to compulsive seeking of a substance or drug which is difficult to wean off or even reduce. It becomes a way of life.

People with addiction (severe substance use disorder) have an intense focus on using certain substances, such as alcohol or drugs, to the point that it takes over their life. They keep using even when they know it will cause problems. People with a substance use disorder have distorted thinking, behaviour and body functions. Addiction is widely prevalent among high school and university students. Students at a vulnerable age are swayed by peer pressure.

People can develop an addiction to Alcohol; Marijuana, PCP, LSD and other hallucinogens, Inhalants, such as, paint thinners and glue, Opioid painkillers, such as codeine and oxycodone, heroin, sedatives, hypnotics and anxiolytics (medicines for anxiety such as tranquillizers), Cocaine, Methamphetamine and other stimulants, Tobacco.

Sleeping pills addiction is becoming an issue. The medications prescribed for control of anxiety, commonly called benzodiazepines, are one of the most prevalent addiction which remains grossly hidden for years. When the person develops withdrawal symptoms like shaking or fits, due to non-availability, that is when others come to know of the problem. Sometimes simple medicines like cough syrup can also be abused. Memory impairment is almost always associated with such addiction.

Facts

Addiction is a common problem in all societies and cultures.

Problems related to addiction are rapidly increasing.

Due to increase in social stress family and economic factors

Alcoholism continues to be a challenge in adolescents, adults as well as elderlies, further, alcoholism in females needs special attention for treatment and prevention.

Every year worldwide alcohol is cause of death for 1 in every 20 cases, and about 300 million people throughout the world have an alcohol use disorder.

Vulnerability to develop abuse and dependence also depends upon genetic factors, socio-economic and cultural causes.

Prevention is understood as an activity designed to avoid substance abuse and reduce its health and social consequences. Prevention can modify the trend, generate, reinforce or help diminish the rising trend.

Demand reduction is done through special programmes with an objective to modify factors which make individuals vulnerable for substance abuse.

There are several subgroups in addictive behaviour and each one has their specific problem from prevention point of view. For example,

1. People suffering from addiction as well as mental disorder.
2. Someone who has developed a recent addiction problem but has no other mental disorder.
3. A person who is at a high risk because of either addiction or a mental disorder in one of the parents.
4. Teenager or a student who is at risk.
5. Person suffering from a mental disorder who remains at risk for developing addiction also.

People with addictive disorders may be aware of their problem, but are unable to stop it even if they want to. Addiction may cause health problems as well as problems at work and with family members and friends. The misuse of drugs and alcohol is the leading cause of preventable illnesses and premature death.

Many times mental health disorders are the root cause of addiction.[62] More than 50% of people with substance use disorders also have a mental health problem at some point during their lifetimes.[63] When people have mental health problems, even limited substance use can worsen it. Some people may inherit a vulnerability to the addictive properties of drugs.[64]

Much of the battle to deal with this problem is fought by the individual with the help of the family and therefore the strategy should be tailor made considering the nature and degree of addiction, presence of other psychiatric and medical illnesses, resources with the family, and social and economic conditions. These strategies are developed based upon the principles like:

1. To set an achievable goal depending upon the prevailing conditions.
2. Early identification of addictive problem.
3. Increasing awareness and level of education.
4. Recognising that the most common barrier for treatment is 'denial' and denial should be considered as a symptom.
5. Treatment of comorbid conditions is necessary to achieve successful prevention.

6. It is important to deal with psychological stress, precipitating factors and stressors arising from family and workplace.
7. Encouraging involvement of the family.
8. Psychosocial development of children of parents

26. PREVENTING ALCOHOLISM

Prevention of mental disorder as well as substance abuse goes hand in hand. Many people who are at risk for addiction are also likely to develop a mental as well as a physical disorder. Multiple factors are responsible for addiction and thus preventive approach is multipronged. The strategy for prevention involves harm reduction as well as supply reduction and much of these strategies are developed and implemented by governments and policy planners.

Earlier primary prevention, which is the intervention before onset of symptoms, was considered as the only true form of prevention. It is now recognised that effective prevention is required before and after symptoms become apparent, since substance abuse disorders are chronic and relapsing.[65] [R] Further, the personal and financial cost is largely due to episodes that follow the first onset. Thus, relapse prevention is also an authentic preventive strategy. Series of risk and protective factors have been identified which affect the likelihood of abuse. The preventive strategies are designed depending upon varying degree of vulnerability to substance abuse, e.g. abuse dependence, continuous use etc.[66] Suitable interventions for prevention target high-risk individuals who are identified with detectable signs or symptoms. In this regard early intervention strategy is most effective. The approach of reducing the harm. This type of prevention is a measure to reduce health and social consequences. The risk factors are seen in different domains, e.g.

- At individual level [some mental disorders or a drug seeking personality]
- In the family [living with a depressed or substance dependent parent]
- At school [poor academic performance]
- Among peers [friends using substances][67]

The protective factors can also be found in different domains, e.g. high self-esteem at the individual level, living with parents who are able to meet children's emotional demands in the family, complying to school discipline at school level, peers with low tolerance of drug use and a strong social network.[68] Presence of a protective factor does not mean absence of a risk factor. Both risk and protective factors have their own contribution in prevention of addiction.[69]

The important type of interventions involve identifying the vulnerable group, which is generally achieved through screening of the high risk population. After identifying the at-risk candidate, it is important to engage them, through groups or individual programmes in order to deal with denial, provide support and intervention in crisis situations. When necessary, treatment for psychiatric or medical conditions is absolutely important.

One of the comprehensive strategies depends upon the fact that addiction is an illness arising from social, psychiatric, medical and spiritual dimensions. Effective treatment to deal with all five domains provides a comprehensive approach. The social treatment consists of dealing with psychosocial and family situations, including issues like, trauma, marital discord, and alike. Presence of psychiatric illness requires appropriate psychiatric intervention. Similarly, medical morbidity, e.g. either directly due to addiction, hepatitis due to alcoholism, also needs a medical intervention. There is strong evidence to suggest increased recovery and quality of life by providing spiritual intervention on both short and long term basis.

27. OBSESSION

Obsessional character is a normal shade of human personality and people with such personalities are more likely to develop this disorder. They have a low degree of symptoms which are hidden, when unmasked these traits become abnormal and present a full blown illness.

There are many people whom you will observe washing their hands at very frequent intervals or checking the light switches almost every five minutes. We may dismiss them as finicky, little realising that their actions are a result of a mental disorder related to anxiety.

A young woman educated up to 6th standard, coming from a middle socio-economic status was admitted in a psychiatric ward with complaints of fear of contamination. She insisted that her clothes and hands are soiled with faeces. She was repeatedly washing her hands, going to the toilet to check her clothes, not able to do any household work and experienced a disturbed sleep. All these complaints were going on for more than 2 to 3 years. But her distress had markedly increased since the last 15-20 days. She had obsessions that everything around her was dirty. She felt a compulsion for checking her body and washing her hands repeatedly and becoming anxious whenever she tried to resist these feelings and attempted to stop the repeated actions.

This disorder is known as Obsessive compulsive disorder or OCD.

She was treated with medications and talking therapy to change this peculiar behaviour. This treatment is known as behaviour therapy; more precisely known as cognitive behaviour therapy.

Obsessive-compulsive disorder is an incapacitating mental illness. It has two clinical components; obsessions and compulsions. People may experience either obsessions, or compulsions, or both.

OCD traits include preoccupation and insistence on details, rules, lists, order and organisation; perfectionism that interferes with completing tasks; excessive doubt and exercising caution; excessive conscientiousness, as well as rigidity and stubbornness.

People with traits of obsession in their personality have very high need for perfectionism in all walks of their life. In majority of these individuals the traits persist and do not cause much difficulty. Everyone recognises them as people with great perfection or 'orderliness', in some of them it increases and starts causing anxiety, their behaviour changes and new behaviour patterns remain focussed on their nature of 'perfectionism' or persisting with particular type of action. It sometime gets complicated and people suffer a great deal of anxiety.

I remember two students who were sharing a room in the hostel. They used to get supply of a milk bottle every morning. To save some money they were taking one bottle and sharing before leaving for their classes. They had decided to keep the bottle outside the room on alternate days. One of them was very obsessive, he used to keep the bottle of right side, often he would ask if the other friend did so or not. It was working out but gradually his behaviour stated changing. He started remaining unsure if the bottle was kept on the right side of the door, he started leaving the class and to come back and physically check if the bottle was indeed kept on the right side or not, though he always found it to be. He did not have any reason to believe that it might not have been kept on right side but that's the way his personality was and it changed to a significant degree.

Such behaviours may continue to become severe and start interfering in life, and it may acquire a dimension which is called Obsessive compulsive personality disorder.

It originates from dysfunctional beliefs thought to be established in early adolescence[70].

These rigid beliefs can cause inner cognitive dysfunctions,[71] leading them to push their beliefs onto others, creating difficulties in social interactions. Inflexible cognitions such as 'my way is the correct way', 'I must own the truth' and 'all is not well unless it's done this way' are deeply ingrained, so that they are resistant to acknowledging alternatives to their ways of thinking. In Obsessive compulsive personality disorder (OPCD), inadequacies are only recognised in others and the external environment and patients do not harbour ego dystonia or question themselves.

On the surface, people with OCPD can appear confident, warm, organised and high-achieving; their meticulous standards can benefit them in certain professions. However, as with any personality disorder, overexpressed traits will cause dysfunction and OCPD frequently occurs with psychiatric comorbidities.

People with an obsessional personality are often imprisoned in their own cage of fixation and therefore they cannot compromise. They are unable to change their views and may jeopardise relationships or their own personal or professional development as a result. They are willing to lose anything as they cannot break through the wall of obsessiveness.

People with OCPD present with few characteristic features. They find it hard to express their feelings. They have difficulty forming and maintaining close relationships with others. They're hardworking, but their obsession with perfection can make them inefficient; They often feel righteous, indignant, and angry; They often face social isolation; The anxiety and depression that occurs with OCPD is often confused with an anxiety disorder called obsessive-compulsive disorder (OCD). However, they aren't the same.[72] The exact cause of OCPD is unknown. Like many aspects of OCPD, the causes have yet to be determined. OCPD may be caused by a combination of genetics and childhood experiences.

Obsessions are unwanted and repetitive thoughts, urges, or images that don't go away. They cause a lot of anxiety. For example, someone might worry about making people he or she loves, sick by bringing in germs. Obsessions can focus on anything. These obsessive thoughts can be uncomfortable. Obsessions aren't thoughts that a person would normally focus on, and they are not about a person's character. They are symptoms of an illness. Compulsions are actions meant to reduce anxiety caused by obsessions. Compulsions may be behaviours like washing, cleaning, or ordering things in a certain way. Other actions are not obvious to others. For example, some people may count things or repeat phrases in their mind. Some people describe it as a feeling that they have to do something until it feels 'right.' It's important to understand that compulsions are a way to cope with obsessions. Someone who experiences OCD may experience distress if they can't fulfil the compulsion. People who experience OCD usually know that obsessions and compulsions don't make sense, but they still feel these are beyond their control. Obsessions and compulsions can also change over time. This is a specific disorder with a central abnormality in the brain which leads to abnormal production or thoughts. These thoughts get trapped in abnormal neuronal pathways.

People show a lot of improvement when treated in the early stages of the disease and if treatment is continued for some time as required. It's a disorder of young people, generally begins between age group of 14 to 18 years and therefore it interferes with growth and development on psychological, social and academic characteristics. Students who suffer find it difficult to do their studies properly. Most people who are victims of this disease fail to receive timely treatment mostly due to lack of awareness.

A negative mind will never give you a positive life...

Common obsessions in the decreasing order are:

Doubts – obsessions about whether or not some action was performed. E.g. did I lock the gate? Did I turn off the gas? Have I locked the car?

Obsessive thinking – One thought leads to another and results in the formation of a chain of thoughts which results in day dreaming and delay in important works.

Fear – Internal cringe from a specific stimulus such as dirt, contamination, sex resulting in compulsive behaviour.

Impulses-Urges to commit any obscene act or say something offensive in public.

Images appearance of violent, horrific, sexual or any other unsettling images in mind.

Common themes of obsessions include contamination, doubts, symmetry, aggression and sexual.

What can you do to treat OCD?

OCD can make normal life of the patient and his or her family members go haywire increasing their distress. Cleanliness and being orderly is good but when it becomes an obsession then it is necessary that the patient receives the right treatment.

If you find yourself suffering with OCD and it is disrupting normal life then you can seek professional help.

Do not be ashamed to talk about it.

If any near and dear one is suffering from OCD, do talk to him.

Do not confuse perfection and orderliness for OCD.

If we have fever we know that we are ill and we rush to the doctor. Similarly, we should be alert for any signs of mental illness. Everyone should consult a psychiatrist if they sense trouble.

28. CANNABIS

Cannabis is a drug that comes from Indian hemp plants such as *Cannabis sativa* and *Cannabis Indica.* Cannabis is now the world's most popular recreational drug.

Cannabis is a depressant drug for central nervous system. Depressant drugs do not necessarily make you feel depressed. Instead, they slow down the activity of the central nervous system and the messages going between the brain and the body. When large doses of cannabis are taken, it may also produce hallucinogenic effects. Different forms of psychoactive cannabis are: marijuana, hashish and hash oil. Cannabis has a neurotoxic effect on the adolescent brain and highlights the importance of prevention and policy efforts targeting adolescents.

There are three main types:

Marijuana is the most common and least potent form of cannabis. Marijuana is the dried leaves and flowers of the plant.

Hashish ('hash') is dried cannabis resin, usually in the form of a small block. The concentration of THC in hashish is higher than in marijuana, producing stronger effects.

Hash oil is a thick, oily liquid, golden brown to black in colour, which is extracted from cannabis. Everyone's response to cannabis differs and can vary from one time to the next. Hash oil is the strongest form of cannabis.

It can affect your mental health and Short-term health effects:

Adolescents are initiating cannabis use at younger ages, and more adolescents are using cannabis daily.

The flowers and leaves of the cannabis plant cause distinct effects on the mind, including feeling high (euphoria), a sense of well-being, relaxation, heightened sensory experiences: sight, taste, smell, sound. While cannabis may make you feel relaxed and happy, your body and brain may also experience effects that are: negative, unwanted, unpleasant. Some of the short-term effects on your brain can include confusion, sleepiness, fatigue, impaired ability to remember, concentrate, pay attention, react quickly, anxiety, fear or panic.

Overall cannabis abuse is common in the community. It has a biological mechanism which increases the risk for a mental disorder.[73]

Cannabis contains hundreds of chemical substances known as cannabinoids. The main active chemical in cannabis is THC (delta-9 tetrahydrocannabinol), is responsible for the way your brain and body respond to cannabis, including the high and intoxication. THC has some therapeutic effects but it also has harmful effects. Harmful effects may be greater when the strength of THC is higher. The potency (concentration or strength) of THC in cannabis is often shown as a percentage of THC by weight (or by volume of an oil). THC potency in dried cannabis has increased from an average of 3% in the 1980s to around 15% today. Some strains can have an average as high as 30% THC. Cannabis that contains very low amounts of THC in its flowers and leaves (less than 0.3%) is classified as hemp. Cannabidiol (CBD) is another cannabinoid. Unlike THC, CBD does not produce a high or intoxication. There is some evidence that CBD may block or lower some of the effects of THC on the mind.[74]

How does it affect the brain?

The THC binds to a part of nerve cells known as the CB1 receptor, similar to the way a key fits into a lock. These receptors are present on many different nerve cells, spread widely throughout the brain. THC is much more effective at binding to the CB1 receptors and affecting the nerve cells than the natural endocannabinoids.

Cannabis use is associated with neuropsychological decline broadly across domains of functioning, even after stopping use of cannabis for years. Cannabis uses show cognitive problems. Impairment of cognition is people who start cannabis use during adolescence. More persistent use is associated with greater decline. Further, cessation of cannabis use may not fully restore neuropsychological functioning among people who start using it during adolescence. Cannabis can cause drowsiness, slow reaction times, lower the ability to pay attention and impair coordination. Using cannabis and then driving or operating equipment can result in an accident, serious injuries or death[75]

The risk is falls and other accidents. This is because THC can affect your: coordination, reaction time, ability to pay attention, decision-making abilities, ability to judge distance. Combining cannabis with other psychoactive substances, especially ones with sedative effects such as opioids and benzodiazepines, can increase the effects of the drugs. Mixing cannabis with alcohol increases the level of impairment and leads to an even greater risk of accident. About 80% of subjects with severe mental disorder use marijuana.

Despite popular myth, driving after using cannabis is not safer than driving after drinking alcohol. Cannabis impairs you differently than alcohol but it still impairs. Performance becomes even worse if drivers combine drugs, such as cannabis, with alcohol. The long-term effects of cannabis on your brain can include increased risk for problems with memory, concentration, intelligence (IQ), ability to think and make decisions. It can make it harder to learn and remember things. Cannabis can impair your thinking, concentration, memory and decision-making, and can impact your ability to perform well on the job or at school.

Using cannabis frequently (daily or almost daily) and over a long time (several months or years) can: Hurt your lungs and make it harder to breathe, if smoked: Cannabis smoke contains many of the same harmful chemicals found in tobacco smoke. Frequent use of THC over a long time increases the risk of cannabis dependence, also called: addiction; cannabis use disorder; problematic cannabis use. It is also associated with an increased risk of developing or worsening the disorders related to anxiety and depression.[76]

In some people, cannabis use increases the risk of developing mental illnesses such as psychosis or schizophrenia, especially those who: start using cannabis at a young age, use cannabis frequently (daily or almost every day), have a personal or family history of psychosis and/or schizophrenia. Frequent cannabis use has also been associated with an increased risk of suicide, depression, anxiety disorders. Stopping or reducing cannabis use can improve your mental health.

Short-term effects on body can also include: decreased blood pressure, which can cause people to faint, increased heart rate, which can be dangerous for people with heart conditions and can lead to an increased risk of heart attack. Though cannabis can cause euphoria (a high) it can also cause anxiety or panic. In some cases, cannabis can trigger a psychotic episode (not knowing what is real, experiencing paranoia, having disorganised thoughts and, in some cases, hallucinating).

THC produced perceptual alterations and spatial memory impairments; however, the results of several reviews regarding the connection between cannabis and cognition remain inconclusive. Cognitive dysfunction associated with long-term or heavy cannabis use is similar in many respects to some types of schizophrenia. There is ample evidence that cannabis use has a heritable component, yet the genes underlying cannabis use disorders are yet to be recognised.[77]

The relationship between cannabis and psychotic disorder is complicated. Cannabis also leads to psychological dependence, anxiety, depression and dysphoria. Individuals using marijuana are at high risk for schizophrenia and psychosis.

29. POOR COPING MECHANISM

The word 'cope' is derived from the Latin word *colpus* meaning 'to alter' and, as defined in the Webster's Dictionary, is usually used in the psychological paradigm to denote 'dealing with and attempting to overcome problems and difficulties'.[78]

Coping or ability to cope is the most internal resource or strength everybody has. It is one such psychological characteristic which allows us to survive throughout all our good and bad times. Then it could be our day to day difficulties or minor stressors or catastrophic situations in our lives, the ability to cope allows us to sail through. It is therefore important to know more about it. We hardly pay attention to it or close our eyes and assess our capacity. Yoga and meditation or just focussing on our inner strength, should help us in many ways by providing strength to our coping mechanism.

Coping skills are abilities or talents employed to effectively respond to adversity. These skills are applied all the time, some with conscious thought, some without. It is a response to physical, cognitive, and psychological stressors.[79]

Every one has coping abilities even if the levels could be in different. Some may successfully cope with most difficult situations while some may cope with difficulty. If we fail to cope to an adverse situation and succumb to any out-side pressure, the result is an unfortunate outcome. Coping being very plastic in nature, it can increase with no limits, except the limits that you decide for yourself. It can be practiced; unique methods can be used to enhance it.

We generally possess an adequate level of coping. it remains healthy without any adverse consequences. Ability to coping remains maintained throughout our lives.

The best possible method to increase this ability – is very personal; what will make my coping mechanism better may not be the best method for someone else. There are many factors which determine the coping ability.

We are born with this ability and several factors like how we are trained, what kind of environment we grow in, what have been our childhood experiences, presence of motivating folks around us, moral and ethical values are taught to us and our belief systems of 'self' contribute in construction of a system which determines our coping ability. Our belief in the *truth, dharma, righteousness, ability to do everything for others,* all these factors should be considered while dealing with our coping ability.

Coping strategies typically involve a conscious and direct approach to problems.

Having a good coping mechanism is many times referred to having a good level of self-confidence, self-esteem, social support, inner strength, mental strength, strong will power and a robust personality. Positive coping strategies increase long-term resilience and wellbeing. In contrast, negative coping strategies usually only produce a helpful distraction in the short-term. Coping skills and abilities can be enhanced by practice of psychosocial methods. Every human being faces problems many times their life. It could be a difficulty in preparing for an exam, or problem in relationships. It is the coping ability which helps people sail through difficult times. Coping is our ability to successfully deal and solve personal and interpersonal problems.

There are two main challenges are:

1. To cope with adverse situations and
2. To enhance the capacity for a state of readiness for future or anticipated stress.

Optimism is the core characteristics which allows coping, thus the strategies which build 'optimism' facilitate 'coping'. People who have negative thought process, or hopelessness or persistent sadness are known to lack optimism and therefore their ability to cope also remains poor. Further, optimism is one of the feature or characteristic of resilience therefore all measures which enhance resilience e.g. life-style, yoga, physical exercise ultimately increase individuals coping ability. Almost all psychological interventions also enhance coping ability to allow individuals to deal with adverse situations.

Depression among Indian University Students

1. With the increasing recognition of child mental health issues and the use of more psychotropic medications, the number of young adults with mental health problems entering college has significantly increased.[4]
2. About 15.6% of the students who were either suffering from severe or extremely severe depression required immediate mental health support Students who reported positive views about the university academic environment and living arrangements had lower level of depression compared to their counterparts.

4. Pedrelli, P., Nyer, M., Yeung, A., Zulauf, C., & Wilens, T. (2015). College Students: Mental Health Problems and Treatment Considerations. Academic psychiatry : the journal of the American Association of Directors of Psychiatric Residency Training and the Association for Academic Psychiatry, 39(5), 503–511. https://doi.org/10.1007/s40596-014-0205-9
5. Deb S, Banu PR, Thomas S, Vardhan RV, Rao PT, Khawaja N. Depression among Indian university students and its association with perceived university academic environment, living arrangements and personal

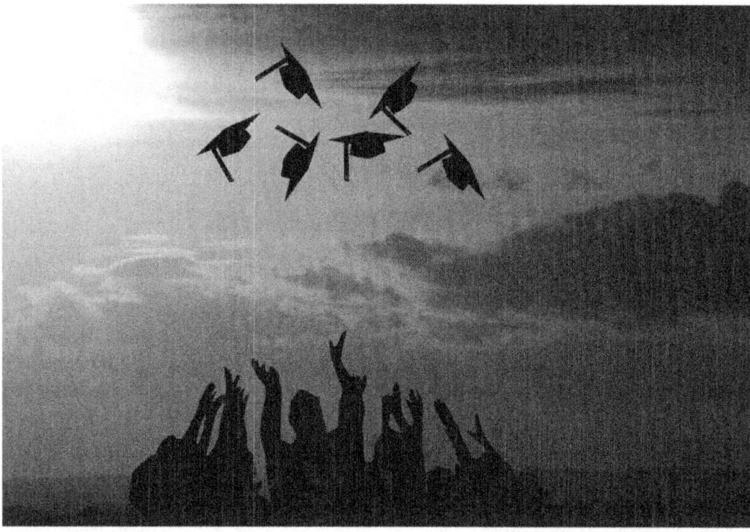

Success has several determinants. It depends on social and psychological characteristics, and not only on education and skills.Training and discourse can bring in a good change. Handling success has nothing to do with how educated you are, but it depends upon the basic value system which people possess. Everyone wants to succeed but everyone's definition of success is different.

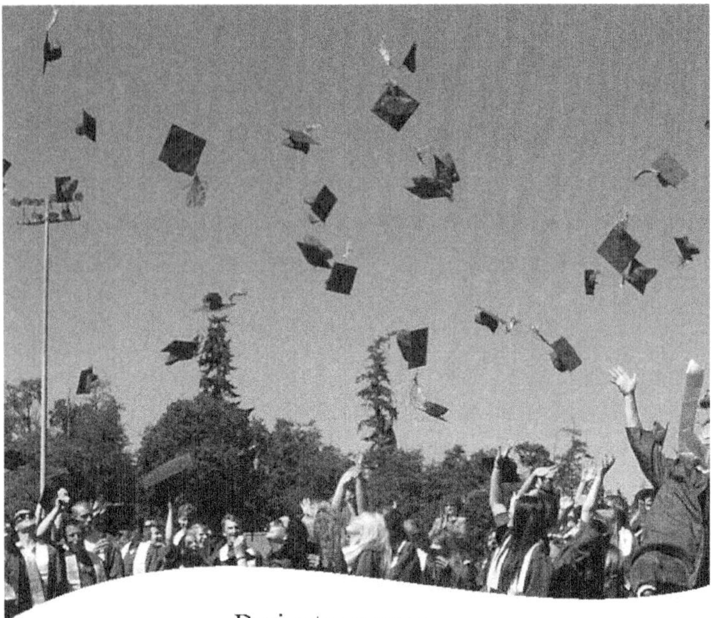

Determinants of success

- Desire to success
- Mindset and ambition
- Grit and personality
- Psychological health
- High educational attainment
- Intelligence but not necessarily
- Emotional and social intelligence
- 'X-factor'
- Stress tolerance
- Cognitive ability
- Healthy Competitiveness
- Brain mechanism

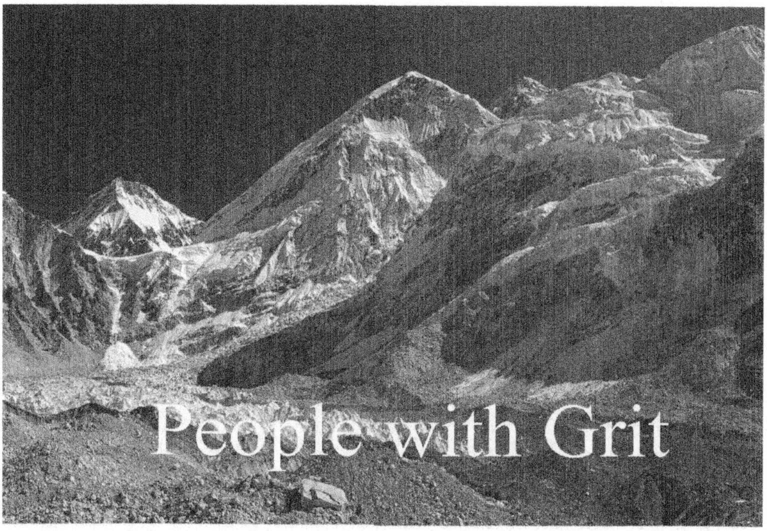

Conscientious

High need for achievement

Social and emotional

intelligence. They are

Visionary for long-term.

Grit is not tied to

intelligence

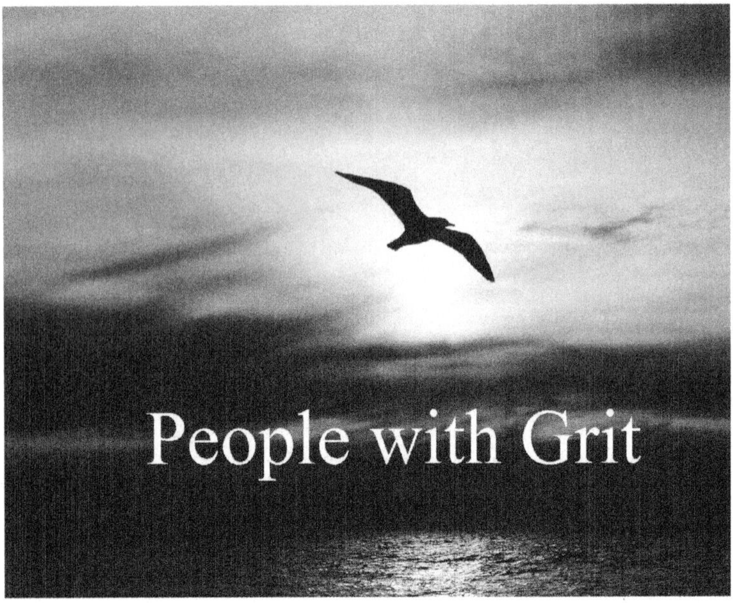

Maintain high determination

Confidence,

Intellectual talent,

Educational attainment,

Academic performance

Optimism and

Resilience

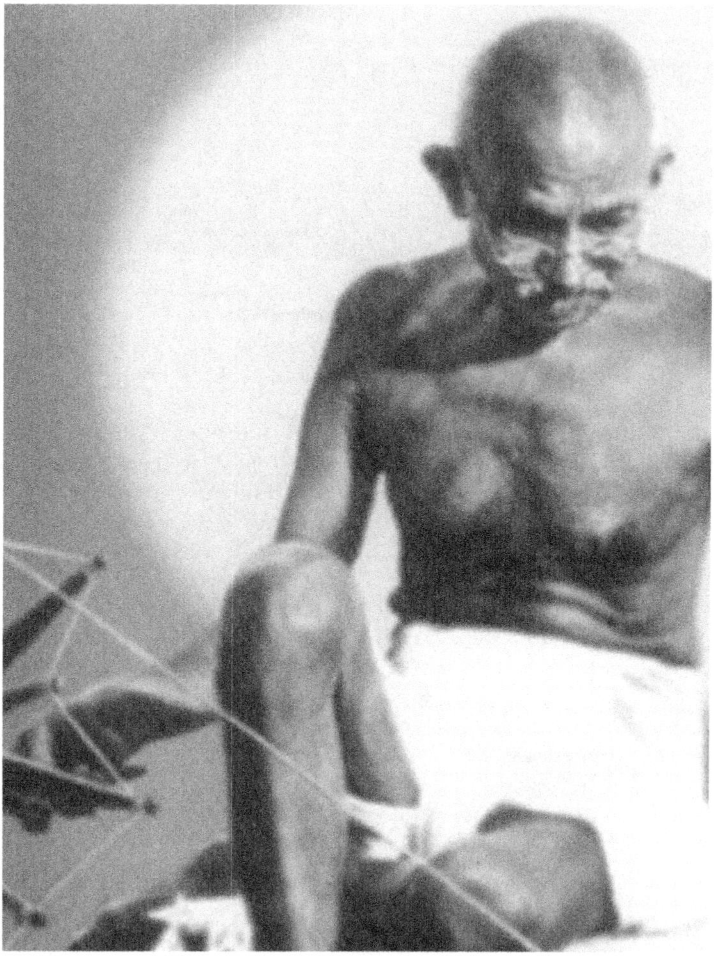

Grit

A predictor for "perseverance and passion for long-term goals"

Perseverance and tenacity

Father of the Nation: M.K.Gandhi

CHAPTER 4
SCIENCE OF SUCCESS

30. ACHIEVEMENT AND SUCCESS - A MENTAL HEALTH DIMENSION

Success is a psychobiological process and Mental health related factors are involved in the process of success and achievement.

Mental health issues are common and interfere in almost all areas of life. Mental health abnormalities, symptoms as well as mental disorders adversely affect performance, learning and quality of life. Most of these abnormalities are treatable conditions.

'Success' personifies a person whether in the family or at workplace.

When I recap the problems of young students who approach a psychiatrist or a counsellor or mental health professional, I find a pattern in their presentation. Most of these are related to:

- Psychiatric symptoms without any particular cause or a history of psychiatric problems.
- Presence of behavioral traits which are distressing and likely to progress to a disease state.
- As a result of pressure of exams or competitions.
- Psychiatric symptoms due to unsuccessful treatment

Psychiatric conditions appear to be related to stress due to the fear of failure.

It is found that the candidates who do not succeed are at high risk for developing a psychological problem. Individuals with a pre-existing condition who achieve less than they have expected may also experience accentuated symptoms.

Success and achievement is (Though) one of the most important aspects in our lives it is not well researched from mental health perspective.

Success is psychologically driven, which is most addictive, and it keeps people moving forward in life. We may try to avoid thinking about it, but it won't come naturally to us.[80, 81]

Success is an objective achievement but with a subjective perception, one may succeed and feel that he has not achieved enough, or one may fail but see a ray of hope that an attempt was not bad, therefore it has lot to do with expectation, ambition and perception.

Parents and teachers provide a fairly good account of what the students may be going through but since they themselves have limited awareness and knowledge about mental health, they cannot exactly point out the nature of problem. It is very difficult to make a correct estimate of how many students may be suffering from psychological issues because people do not report it, they are always frightened about problems related to the mind and they feel that the people they interact with will pass judgement or may start disliking them.

There are several observations which establish firm relationship between mental health and chances of success. Patients suffering from a psychiatric disorder perform poorly. Several psychological attributes are involved in it, e.g. cognition, mood regulation, decision making, and these are complex neuro-behabitual aspects of mind-and brain. Many people succeed but they are unable to sustain their success, and significant number of them develop psychiatric disorders. Mental health conditions are treatable, and treatment shall benefit the candidates.

Mental health characteristics can enhance the psychological attributes and facilitate ability to perform and cope with adverse situations as well.

Overall, there is a relationship between mental health, stress, and success or achievement. It remains unknown if the relationship is causal, meaning that stress or fear of failure may lead to a psychiatric problem or a psychiatric problem may lead to a sense of failure and in some cases an actual illness may develop. In fact, both are true.

There is another perspective into the game of success and failure. This is about happiness or satisfaction. One may succeed but not feel satisfied. Such success is meaningless. It is merely achievement, a true success is one where you achieve and feel happy, thus when anyone plans for a battle for tomorrow the objective or setting the goals needs to be both, on parameter of achieving the target and on perception of happiness and satisfaction.

The purpose of this chapter is to clearly understand the complex process involved in success and achievement. Knowing more about the process of success may help facilitate the process of becoming successful and reducing the stress at the same time. It will also be interesting to discuss from the perspective of mental health, which has a considerable amount of influence on the process. The mental health perspective of success and achievement plays a crucial role I believe, however not much attention is paid to this aspect. Mental health issues are common and therefore in almost all areas of life. Abnormalities, symptoms, and mental disorders adversely affect performance and learning and quality of life. Most of these abnormalities are treatable conditions. Return to normalcy is highly probable if the treatment is not delayed.

I did not give a serious thought to this aspect of life until I started working with young people. Having met so many of them I could figure out three different psychological sect which are intertwined in a manner that one does not exist without the others (1) desire to succeed (2) ability to compete and (3) conflict resolution and decision making.

As this discussion progresses we will see number of other factors which are involved in psychology of success and failure revolving around these three factors.

The context is generally discussed with psychologist and experts in organisational psychology and most often discussed in relation to work-place. 'Success' has become circumscribed to performance in work. But that's only partly true.

Mental health is the last thing people like to consider as a cause for failure or at least a significant factor involved in it. This ignorance costs dearly to the students. Sometimes the problems are not serious, but their impact on people is quite severe.

Success and failure are unpredictable. There is no rulebook to success. However, there are few common findings which suggest what may have been the cause of failure. The cause may be modifiable or non-modifiable. We will have to find out if any problem exists from childhood or if the problem has shown up later.

The most important aspect of this discussion is to be aware of 'healthy mind-healthy body.'

Your success can never be the same as my success, even when we have been competing for the same positions. Success is a personal accomplishment. Different people give different reasons, and everyone enjoys it uniquely. Experiments in psychology have shown that intelligence does not predict success; it is not guaranteed for success.

Success is excitement as well as a satisfaction

What stands between your success and failure is your mind; the hard task is to train the brain to develop a mindset for both to Achieve and Accept the outcome (whether success or failure). You may succeed but to remain successful is a challenge. Success cannot be measured in quantitative terms, i.e., it is immeasurable. A soldier fighting a war gets killed the other continues to fight and kills many; we cannot say he is more successful than the other.

Common mental health related factors are the ones, which are other mental disorder or conditions which have some or the other -specific or non-specific symptom of mental illness. e.g. presence of depression or eating disorder or subthreshold depression.

Achievement and success are described in a number of ways, and there is no consensus definition. However, one aspect of success is the accomplishment of your goals. It's a process, and the process is complex, besides several other factors, mental health issue is one of the determinants.

Overall, it appeared that stress due to an academic problem and fear of failure is a very potent factor which leads to a psychiatric disorder. Thus, there are changes in the developed brain as well as in the process of maturation, both show some amount of abnormality. Overall, these brain changes affect the psychological attributes which influence normal behaviour in human beings e.g.

- Changes in neuropsychological functioning
- Changes in memory, concentration, function, cognition, impulsivity, mood regulation, mood sensitivity to several external stimuli.
- Stress factors are some of the major spoilers of cognitive merits, precisely because the biochemical and physiological changes restrict the last minute or finish line performance. Things go wrong in anticipation-assumption and response.

You are the creator of your own destiny.

Swami Vivekanand

Believe in yourself and the world will be at your feet.

Swami Vivekanand

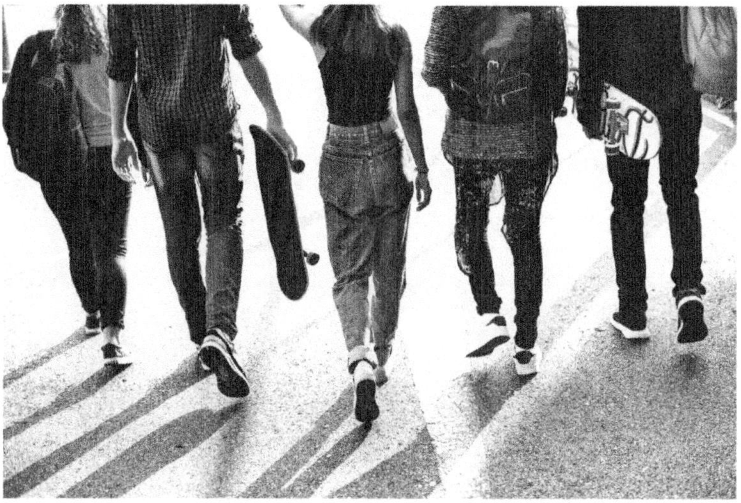

Psychiatric disorders are seen among all cultures and societies.

About 10% to 25% of students suffer from a severe level of stress the experience of psychological illness disconnects them from their own selves. Though it is a treatable condition, patients seldom receive treat- ment. One of the main barriers is the stigma which is a clinical risk factor. Mental health is not only about problems of mind but goes beyond that. When people are facing adversities, there is an increased predis- position towards mental illness and resulting chronicity. Being aware of the fact that mental health problems are treatable, one shall encourage adolescents to protect themselves by providing early treatment.

31. DESIRE TO SUCCEED

Aspiration is a fundamental psychological characteristic; every one aspires for something or the other in their life. It becomes a matter of concern or discussion when aspirations are either too high or too little. It is never a matter of great concern if it is in the middle of the scale. Human beings have the tendency to engage themselves in various activities to find out if they can survive and perform under all conditions. They usually have either an acceptance or an avoidance tendency towards a particular goal. There are a number of socio-economic and cultural determinants which shape the strong desire to see the aspirations growing. Growth of aspiration yields 'hope' and hope leads to 'survival'. Main challenge for every student is to implement the plan which is developed either by teacher/parents. In a situation of choosing or setting a career goal it is equally important to have our capacities appropriately judged by people who know and have understood us, like our parents or teachers. Developing a plan and identifying barriers is not enough, it is the implementation which is important. Life goals are what we want to achieve, and they're much more meaningful than just 'what we need to accomplish to survive'.[82] Unlike daily routines or short-term objectives, they drive our behaviours over the long run. Goal-Setting puts intentions squarely at the centre of our behaviour.[83]

- **Intelligence does not predict success; it is not guaranteed for success.**
- **Success is excitement as well as a satisfaction**
- **What stands between your success and failure is your mind; the hard task is to train it.**

32. MENTAL HEALTH AND PSYCHIATRIC DISORDERS ARE DETERMINANTS OF SUCCESS

A significant number of people suffer from either a psychiatric disorder or some problem arising due to stressful life situation. Those who have mental health problem do not perform as well as their counterparts.

Those who succeed and keep on climbing the ladder suffer from increased incidence of depression, suicide, bipolar disorder and exposure to health risks like alcoholism or smoking, obesity or hypertension.

Success and failure are like two sides of same coin of mental health, a discussion can bring requisite change to minimise the chance of failure.

Success and achievement are indeed endpoints in the backdrop of social realities. If the environment for academic growth is full of emotional neglect and stress, by the time the stress is being managed and the severity of neglect is reduced, the outcome may not be the satisfactory. The imprints of adversity remain. This negative impact may remain dormant and not present as mental health problem, but the vulnerability persists. Some people even excel in such conditions, because deprivation is a psychological drive for motivation. However, there is a tinge of negative emotion.

People have an understanding that it is the 'intelligence' which is responsible for academic success; however, intelligence alone is not the quality that makes one successful. People do not pay much attention to other mental faculties like mood, emotion and thinking. If social and emotional intelligence is high, chances of success are more. There are a number of socio-economic and cultural determinants which shape the strong desire to see the aspirations grow.

Aspirations, success and achievement are intricately related with mental health. People who are not emotionally well, do poorly in academics. It affects their life, and it consequently affects their ability to realize their dreams. Success is also not possible without a 'state of healthy mind.' The most important aspect of this discussion is to be aware of 'healthy mind-healthy body.'

Success and failure are unpredictable. There is no rulebook to success.

Your success can never be the same as my success, even when we have been competing for the same positions. Success is a personal accomplishment. Different people give different reasons, and everyone enjoys it uniquely. Experiments in psychology have shown that intelligence does not predict success; it is not guaranteed for success.

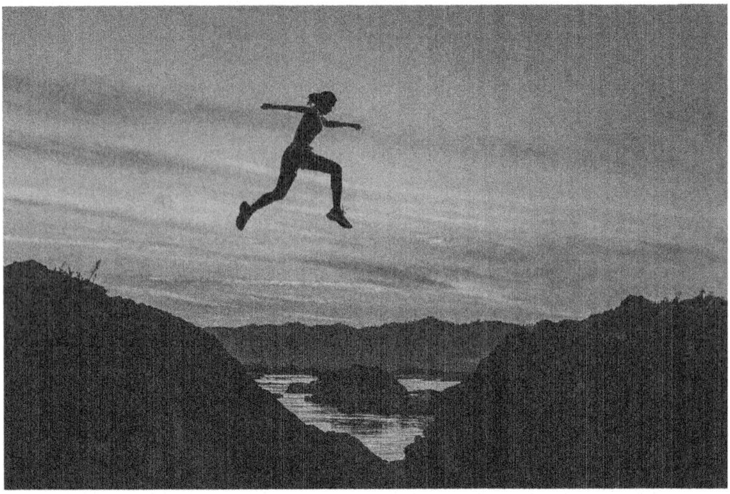

Hope is closely related to thought process. If someone is getting ex- cessive thoughts the mood will change, if someone starts feeling low, the thought process changes if the mood is normal the mathematical or intellectual characteristics are much brighter.

Emotions not only influence our thinking, intelligence and abil- ity to perceive, they also affect our internal body system.

33. EXPERIENCE OF TRAUMA AND LOSS

I recall having met number of students who came to college mental health services commonly complaining of 'failure or loss.'

On assessment I found that the student was either developing a psychiatric disorder or had an active disorder.

I find a typical pattern in the presentation problems of young students who approach a psychiatrist or a counsellor.

Interestingly majority of them had spoken about 'failure', whether in examination or in securing a job, or position in a sports team or separation in love affair. Sense of failure is a loss and 'loss' is a trauma. Thus people who do not succeed feel traumatised.

'Having failed in life' is another very strong emotion. It causes severe impact on life which can be long lasting and very difficult to deal with. Number of diseases, both physical as well as mental, which are directly or indirectly related to previous history of trauma or repeated failure.

Psychiatric symptoms of trauma keep revolving in a vicious circle. One attempt of failure leads to stress, which becomes a trigger for traumatic reaction, thus reducing resilience, coping and enhances possibility of a psychiatric disorder which again leads to failure and trauma, thus achieving success after repeated failures is very difficult to attain.

34. 'COGNITION- STRESS' DIMENSION

The role and impact of cognitive ability in relation to academic success is well documented, and a strong correlation between grades and cognitive ability was found.[84] Predictors of academic achievement often lay on a continuum with cognitive measures, intelligence and mental abilities.[85]

Cognitive system consists of certain brain areas, specific neuronal cells and chemical neurotransmission situated in frontal part of the brain and its connection with the middle part. These structures are quite stable and modifiable only with strategic and long-term treatments to some extent.

This system is a specific characteristic of every individual. It not only determines but defines that person's mental strength and acumen, ability to imagine, visualise and foresee a particular task or thought. Often people are not aware about their own power of performance. Their sense to anticipate and response can change the last minute or "finish life excellence" to make things possible. Cognitive re-structuring and remediating is a biological process for planning and execution of a task.

Stress factors are one of the major spoilers of cognitive merits, precisely because the biochemical and physiological changes restrict the last minute or finish line performance. Things go wrong in anticipation-assumption and response.

Cognition is the final common pathway for all the factors which contribute to Performance and productivity. These are features of brain which are closely associated with performance and thereby with chances of becoming successful. There is a definite centre in the middle part of the brain which is the seat of such activities, our ability to remember, reasoning and planing are maintained by cognitive functions. In fact there six type of subsets in his function like: attention, perception, memory, language, learning, and higher reasoning. The processes are interdependent and occur simultaneously. There is enough evidence to suggests that conditions in which cognitive functions are poor, perform poorer. People suffering from psychiatric disorder suffer from cognitive impairment and thus perform poorly. Cognitive features are associated to brain maturation, brain development and number of causes which lead to cognitive firmament, e.g. alcoholism.

Though it has been hard to find a drug to treat cognitive impairment, its status can be prevented if childhood development remains robust, without any neglect or deprivation. Certain treatments like cognitive behaviour therapy have shown reasonable improvement in cognitive features. Cognitive function are associated with "patterns of thought, feelings and behaviours"[86] of individuals that may continue to develop throughout their lives.[87]

These include critical thinking skills, problem solving skills, emotional health, social skills, work ethic, and community responsibility. They also matter indirectly (i.e., they correlate with other individual and societal outcomes).

Noncognitive skills are developed before and throughout children's school years. The development of these skills is dependent on family and societal characteristics.

Studies on cognitive development and on teaching and learning processes refer to a significant relationship between family involvement and academic success of children, and consequently to their school trajectory.

It is observed that the level of parental education stands out, which seems to differentiate educational strategies and how parent and child interact. Similarly mother's academic qualifications emerge as a better predictor of cognitive performance[88,89]. Impact of socio-familial variables on children's academic motivation is significant.[90,91] There is a psychological as well as a biological connection between aspiration, achievement (or success), our state of mind, ability to perform (or function) and cognitive properties. Much of information about the activity of the brain in progress or failure has become available only recently.

It is now known that the brain can be visualized by computer-generated systems. Studies have shown that several factors like the experience of trauma in childhood, or severe stress levels lead to changes in the brain. Brain maturation has undergone an evolutionary change. The evolution of humans, has bestowed the characters like foresight, or the ability to anticipate an event accurately. Numerous researchers have investigated how humans anticipate future internal contexts, specifically those related to future mental processes, such as motivational and emotional states. However, the knowledge yet remains inadequate to understand various dimensions of foresight clearly, but its close association with 'anticipation' is indicating its role in the complex decision-making process. Mental health conditions also impair cognitive ability, thereby adversely affecting the prospects of success. A significant number of people suffer from either a psychiatric ill-health of a psychiatric disorder or any problem arising due to stressful life situations. Those who have mental health problem do not perform and function well as their counterparts. Further, those who are unable to perform also have a high incidence of psychiatric disorders. Stress arising due to fear of becoming unsuccessful or staying ahead in competitive life is not specific to students and young adults. Its seen among most people. To achieve and to succeed, staying ahead of others is a strong motivation. One of the features involved in accomplishing your goals is how one takes decisions. The process of achievement, and to become successful involves synthesizing previous experience, learning, intelligence, our ability to perceive information, to be able to reproduce and perform.[92]

Intelligence and The brain function

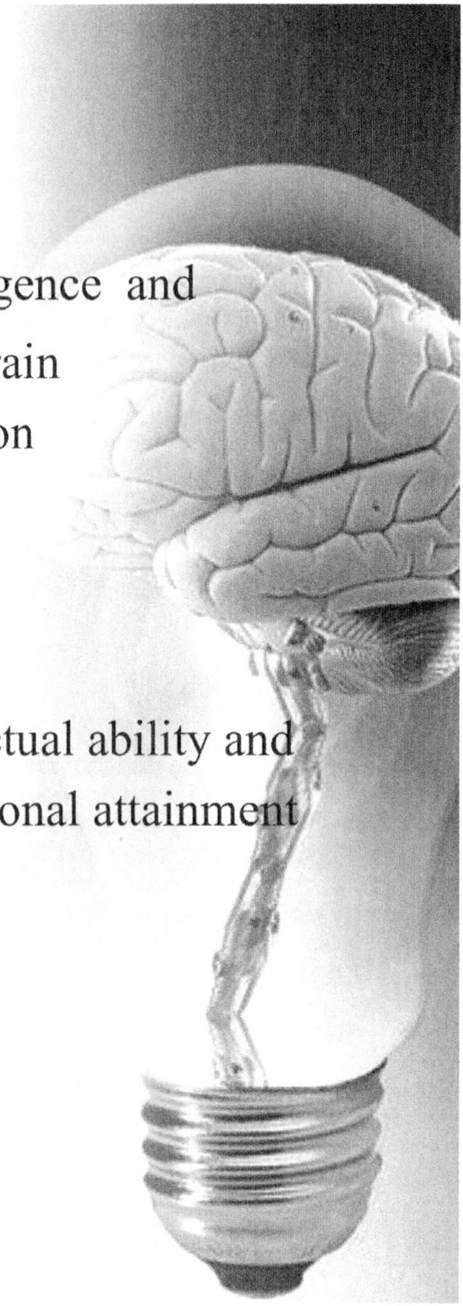

Intellectual ability and educational attainment

35. STRESS FACTOR – IS THE GAME CHANGER

IF ONE DOES NOT SUCCEED IT DOES NOT MEAN THAT ONE HAS FAILED

"TAKE RISKS IN YOUR LIFE. IF YOU WIN, YOU CAN LEAD, IF YOU LOSE, YOU CAN GUIDE."
SWAMI VIVEKANANDA

Everybody thinks about 'success' in their lives. It is a natural feeling arising from aspiration. Not that everybody succeeds, but everybody does not fail either.

Every one experiences stress, we all know that stress is related to performance. If the level of stress is severe, performance decreases. At the same time rewards of the performance also decrease, which in turn increase the stress. Thus severe stress forms a vicious circle along with poor performance, which finally leads to compromised situation to achieve success. Therefore art of managing stress is extremely important for becoming successful.

Level of stress, stress tolerance and stress management can make or break an individual's plight for becoming successful. Ability to deal with stress has huge role in performance. Almost all cognitive functions and related qualities develop along with brain maturation process; brain maturation finally remains the key factor to determine cognitive set, ability to learn, ability to use past experiences and the ability to combine several cognitive features and decide judiciously.

There are millions of examples where people have succeeded in adverse life situations and in sparse condition of physical means which are the necessities of life e.g. place to live, food to eat, electricity, transport etc. The difference lies in two factors; Motivation and Belief in oneself. The brain system is sensitive to the way one thinks. These two factors increase efforts, involvement, and experience of reward and continuity of hard work. It's also a fact that people who are socially and economically disadvantaged have hard time to receive education, employment or housing. Overall their quality of life remains relatively poorer. They may have high intelligence or ability to do hard work, but their socially disadvantaged condition affects their personality and self-esteem adversely. Schools have higher dropouts from low socio-economic groups and many are unable to achieve good marks because they have to work. While it is true that there are some gifted candidates who outshine everyone but that's a rare situation.

36. SIGNIFICANCE OF INTELLIGENCE IN ACHIEVING SUCCESS

Success is a process which involves previous experience, learning, intelligence, brain mechanism, our ability to perceive information, and to be able to reproduce and perform.

Mental health problems do not arrive only because of failure or loss. These problems are more closely associated with adjustment and coping with sudden or slow change in the environment or a potential threat to own self. These changes can be a positive event or an adverse event. Sometimes the stress is caused suddenly and in another situations it is slowing growing and thus a heightened response of the body gets no opportunity to return to a normal state.

Those preparing for a tough competition are under considerable pressure and thus at a many fold risk for developing a mental disorder. Those who do not succeed or fail have a higher number of mental disorders in comparison to those who succeed. Even those who succeed are now under stress of maintaining the position and continue climbing higher on the ladder of success, this leads to an increased incidence of depression, suicide, bipolar disorder and exposure to health risks like alcoholism or smoking, obesity or hypertension.

Therefore, a successful person who remains on edge to perform and compete all the time is exposed to several adverse reactions. Those people who are at high risk for a mental disorder easily develop one in presence of severe and continuing stressful life situation.

Positive stress also needs attention in order to minimise the risk of mental disorder.

A strong relationship exists between general intelligence and academic research about intelligence and achievement has provided a firm foundation for understanding the relationship between these two constructs.[93] Intelligence and achievement are two different but interrelated constructs. They have been studied for over a century in an attempt to explain differences in educational and life outcomes.[94] An enhanced understanding of the relationship between intelligence, both verbal and nonverbal, and achievement may contribute to improving the identification of gifted and talented children, particularly those from low socio-economic populations.[95] Since achievement is a broad and multidimensional construct and definition or understanding of the construct differs, achievement encompasses student ability and performance. It is intricately related to human growth, and cognitive, emotional, social, and physical development.[96] There is no ultimate definition of intelligence, but most researchers accept that it is an ability to solve problems (including problems of comprehension) by thinking. In other words, it is "a very general mental capability that among other things involves the ability to reason, plan, solve problems, think abstractly, comprehend complex ideas, learn quickly and learn from experience". [97] General intelligence, also known as general cognitive ability, intellectual ability, general mental ability that intelligence is not only related to the rate of learning, but the understanding of complexities.[98] The higher the level of intelligence, the easier it is to understand abstract content and comprehend the complexities of a mentally demanding career. What it does tell us is how hard one might have to work to learn specific content or, which careers will take more energy and effort if one is to pursue them with a high level of competency?[99] Academic intelligence is an ability to learn or acquire knowledge from experience. Verbal abilities have a stronger correlation with academic achievement than nonverbal abilities.[100] Furthermore, verbal abilities are related to readiness to learn, while nonverbal abilities are related to the potential to learn. If intelligence scores are used to predict future academic performance, both verbal (readiness) and nonverbal (potential) abilities should be evaluated. Students who have lower verbal scores or are not ready to learn. Firm evidence that psychometric test scores accurately predict real-world success would have considerable importance at the practical and theoretical levels. It would justify the use of such tests as educational and occupational selection tools, and as dependent variables in studies of possible genetic and neurophysiological correlates of cognitive ability differences.[101]

These students strive to demonstrate ability and avoid negative judgement of competence. Allowing students to adapt to multiple goals simultaneously falls under the heading of multitasking technology, which is beneficial.[102]

It is important to study how students are motivated, since achievement benefits are critical for school success. In many cases, achievement belief appeared to be a better predictor of school performance than the IQ or achievement test.[103]

A significant number of the population suffers from obvious or unseen mental health related abnormalities, and therefore these factors are likely to influence both cognitive and noncognitive pathways. Though it is more complex and there are differing opinions, the fact is that the cognitive properties anyway modulate all types of determinants for success. Whether it is hard work, motivation, intelligence or presence of mood changes the impact on possibility is through the cognitive pathway.

Let's consider factors like exercise and walking, or muscle-memory exercise like video games. These have demonstrated to be good to aid the possibility of success mainly in the field of business and management. And if we think how this is likely to be possible, the answer is that there is a change in brain plasticity which is associated with cognitive changes.

More research is required in the field of cognitive changes being the final common pathway for thinking, planning and doing the activity.[104]

37. ANTICIPATION

There is always a surprise, you often come across someone who was known to be a back-bencher or non-achiever, outshines everyone in performance, or player who unexpectedly becomes the game-changer due to extraordinary performance. No one knows how extraordinary performance happens. e.g when everything is all right, expected performance is no surprise, contrarily, when we know that things are not right and an extraordinary performance is displayed, it is a matter of surprise. This unexpected performance is possibly due to 'anticipation'. It cannot be explained logically, the only logic is that there are some 'processes' which, we do not yet know about. I have called such factors as x-factor for the purpose of discussion.

The process which is likely to be involved is combination of characteristics like- 'anticipation', 'assumption', and 'foresight' involved. These are 'higher functions' which are of cognitive nature and characteristic of 'wisdom', which appear unrelated to several other factors like intelligence, motivation etc. E.g you have a reknown cricket batsman going out in the field when the team is losing, he scores 6 runs on first and these second ball and crowd starts cheering up, by the time all 6 balls are bowled his score is 36 and the crowd is in frenzy (Yuvraj Singh, T20 World Cup Cricket, 2007).[105] 'Anticipatory wisdom' may give extraordinary performance.

The pathway for this process involves ability to have the foresight and anticipate. These are two characteristics which distinguish people on how they make decisions and accomplish their goals.

Though the process is complex, we can delineate a few factors which play a role at the time of performance.

How well the information stored in the memory can be retrieved?

How effectively this information or experience can be used to take make decisions?

What is the state of mental health at the time e.g. mood state or emotionality?

What is the ability of optimism and adaptability to changing a stressful situation, i.e. resilience?

How well one can handle the stress?

How well the sense of anticipation and foresight can be combined with learning from past experience?

What is the level of emotional intelligence?

Thus, the vital psychological characteristics are the level of cognitive functioning, resiliency, and managing stress.

Some of these features are from the hardware of the brain system, and others belong to a network of 'learning' to some extent both are modifiable, and that's how several techniques proposed for achieving success may be useful.

There are several reasons why this direction should also be part of our thinking process, not because of only academic exercise but to understand if anything can be changed or modified in order deal with barriers to achieving success.

38. X-FACTOR

We often wonder why some people don't succeed when they have exactly the same qualities and skills or even better than those who succeed.

The 'differences between similarities' is a great human accomplishment from the growth and development of the neuronal system. As humans, we have become privileged and superior to other primates; even our species million years back. The science of brain maturation and evolution has acquired several properties which are non-observable.

There are two specific kinds of phenomena; Those we can see and Those which exist but cannot be seen. E.g. we can see our hands working but mental activities are not visible today.

There is a third aspect of characteristics which we can only feel e.g. to have capacity to love someone or empathize, this is also a consistent feature. Still, there are characteristics like 'coming to know what might happen', 'ability to anticipate what may happen or ability to make a decision based upon the information we do not have, knowledge to retrieve data from memory and use it in conjunction with anticipation or foresight to predict certain action or behaviour.

These characteristics and some other mental features make us unique, we may have these, but we will not be sure it is there all the time.

When we are able to combine qualities like insight, judgement, skills from past experience and then decide what to do that's an x-factor which sets two people apart.

The power prediction and ability to take decision-based upon foresight and anticipation delineates how success is determined. The same person in a similar situation may not be able to use the foresight in future and then he /she will lose, this is because such higher functions of mind-&-brain is quite unpredictable.

Functions of left and right side of brain

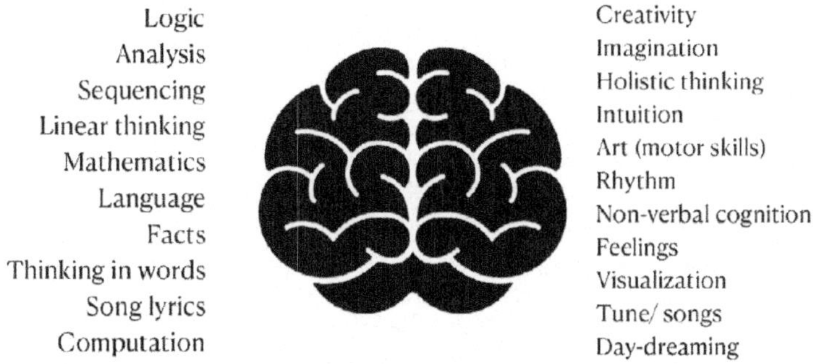

Brain regions and their functions

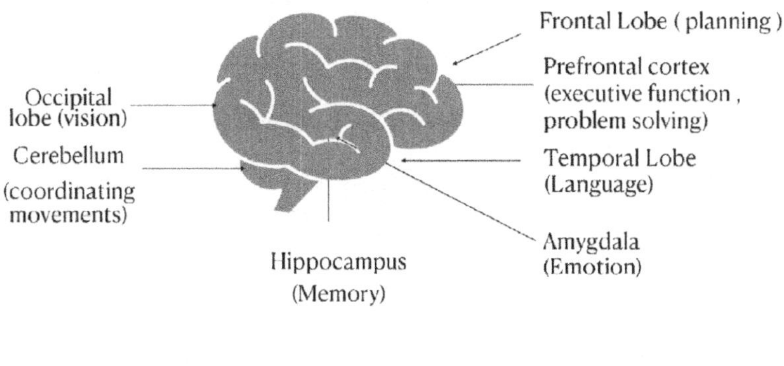

39. BRAIN MECHANISM

CHANGES IN THE BRAIN MECHANISM RELATED TO PROCESS OF SUCCESS AND ACHIEVEMENT

Mental characteristics which help achieve success are generated from the brain. It plays a vital role in determining success by facilitating strategic utilization of the mental process (qualities of mind), e.g. the ability to retrieve information from memory store at the right time.[106] It is thought that if we can 'train our brain', our chances of using the mental mechanisms will be better. Successful people possess traits like: having a vision, showing gratitude, being honest, learning from failure and having the ability to adjust well emotionally. In every single situation what makes a difference is 'decision making'.

Damage to the brain's frontal lobe is known to impair one's ability to think and make choices. Now scientists say they've pinpointed the different parts of this brain region that *preside over reasoning, self-control and decision-making.*

The part of the brain that is responsible for complex thinking is the frontal lobe—located behind the forehead. The frontal lobe controls reasoning, planning, voluntary movement, and some aspects of speech. The prefrontal cortex is the part of the frontal lobe which lies immediately behind the forehead. Various brain regions work together during the decision-making process.

'Decision-making is in the locus of your control. You have the power to break patterns of behaviour only by making better decisions. You can change your mind and your actions at any time.'[107] Anticipation is a state of expectation or excitement about an upcoming event or situation. For example, when you know an old friend is going to drop by, you probably are in a state of anticipation while waiting for them - you are excited, maybe a little nervous, and filled with expectations about the visit.

Anticipation is rooted in the portion of the brain known as the cerebellum, which controls "automatic, non-thinking" behaviour. With this anticipation always in an active state makes the human brain desire more dopamine.[108] The Amygdala is the part of the brain that stores emotional memory, and it has two parts. This is the part that is responsible for fear conditioning. The prefrontal cortex not only shows increased activity during decisions requiring self-control but during all decision-making processes.[109]

Hopefully, having a better understanding of the neuroscience behind decision-making will help everyone make decisions that lead to positive outcomes in the future and avoid self-destructive choices. Even when you're stuck in a cycle of rut-like thinking and behaviour, a change of attitude and decision-making can turn your life around.[110]

You have the power to break patterns of behaviour only by making better decisions. Various brain regions work together during the decision-making process. Other regions of the brain are responsible for serval psychological attributes which participate in process of doing right thing for becoming successful e.g. The Amygdala is the part of the brain that stores emotional memory, and it has two parts. This is the part that is responsible for fear conditioning. Anticipation is a state of expectation or excitement about an upcoming event or situation Anticipation is rooted in the portion of the brain known as the cerebellum, which controls "automatic, non-thinking" behaviour.[111]

Your genes are not the only ones that produce your mind; it's sculpted by a lifetime of experiences. Experience alters brain activity, which changes gene expression. Any behavioural changes you see reflect alterations in the brain. The maturation of the adolescent brain is also influenced by heredity factors, environmental factors, and sex hormones (oestrogen, progesterone, and testosterone), which play a crucial role in the health of neuron.

There are significant changes taking place all the time in the brain of the child in mother's womb, soon after the child is born and during the phase of development during childhood. These changes in maturation are responsible for structure and function of brain cells. Normally brain cell migrate while developing from one place to another and finally lodge themselves in the area designated for third function e.g. cells which are specific to memory function travel to collect in the middle part of the brain. Thus there can be abnormality in maturation which may reflect in nature of cell, their structure, their interconnectivity, chemical characteristics and electrical activity as well. There is a decrease in grey matter in prefrontal regions of the brain, reflecting synaptic pruning, the process through which unused connections between neurons are eliminated. Adolescence is the period during which significant improvements in basic cognitive abilities and logical reasoning are seen[112] Important changes in an activity involving the neurotransmitter dopamine occur during early adolescence.[113] There is an increase in white matter in the prefrontal cortex during adolescence, this change is especially significant for emotional regulation, facilitated by the increased connectivity between regions important in the processing of emotional information and those important in self-control.

40. HORMONE FOR HAPPINESS

Happiness is caused by pleasant sensation in the body, and these sensations are a reaction to various biochemical substances, e.g. serotonin, dopamine and oxytocin, which are present in the blood circulation, possibly producing an electrical signal in the complex brain biology. Some of these biochemical processes have been referred to as happiness hormones, like endorphin, dopamine, and serotonin.[114]

This process of happiness needs to be interpreted in the background of mental state, an important component of this mental state is mood status and cognitive abilities. Thus, in the presence of sadness of mood, hopelessness, or poor mood regulation, subjective perception of happiness is likely to be poorer. To summarise, we may set a goal for achievement, and we do everything right to achieve while having a healthy mental state, but we may still not be happy, or feel satisfied.[115]

41. MINDSET AND AMBITION

Growth of aspiration yields 'hope' and hope leads to 'survival'. Main challenge for every student is to implement the plan which is developed either by teacher/parents. In a situation of choosing or setting a career goal it is equally important to have our capacities appropriately judged by people who know and have understood us, like our parents or teachers. Developing a plan and identifying barriers is not enough, it is the implementation which is important. Life goals are what we want to achieve, and they're much more meaningful than just 'what we need to accomplish to survive'[116]. Unlike daily routines or short-term objectives, they drive our behaviours over the long run.

The psychological attributes for success and failure, e.g. being ambitious, need for achievement or aspiration for the best, do not work in isolation. These attributes form a complex which determine such outcomes.[117] If someone says that he is aspiring but could not achieve, the situation commonly leads to a sense of failure and worthlessness. The psychological factors involved in such a situation may involve factors like motivation, mood regulation, need for achievement, ability to plan, ability to sustain the efforts etc. Several studies showed that new students all over the world are usually faced with a dilemma in making a career choice decision in their lives.[118,119] The subject of aspiration and achievement has thus gained much importance.

One factor which is often referenced with great passion for success or performance of any task is known as 'mindset'. Psychologist and behavioural scientist have tried to deconstruct this aspect of human beings. However, it continues to be a complex entity. It is difficult to define it precisely. It has several connotations. One may interpret mindset to be an active route which may reflect one's confidence or aptitude, or special qualities. It is often said that one who is focused is likely to succeed, one hundred percent. When you ask why do they say so? The thought is that "He has the mindset of a winner". But we don't exactly know which mental faculty is involved.

42. PERSONALITY

Personality traits are significantly related to academic achievement. This position is based upon the observation that what an individual can do is the reflection of cognitive ability,[120] whereas, what an individual will do is a reflection of personality traits. Educators and researchers have worked on academic achievement problems for years. It is reported that besides cognitive abilities, non-cognitive factors which are known as personality traits are responsible for academic achievement too.[121] Several personality traits are related to academic achievement. There is support for the idea of evaluating personality traits as predictors of academic achievement based on several works that have been done on personality.[122]

The mental health aspect of achievement is closely related to psychological characteristics of personality. One of the interesting parts of this is the minor traits or 'typology' or 'psychological feature' in an individual's personality. This means the presence of multiple characters of mild degree but functioning as psychological traits. Personality is everyone's unique feature—the way of thinking, feeling and behaving. It includes ones behaviour and the way they solve their problems, how well they can connect with others, how they become comfortable with themselves, their ability to regulate and identify their mood. Though these traits are milder they may cause significant dysfunction. As we know everybody has a typical personality, it is a characteristic which identifies the person. More often than not, these traits become the identifying features, e.g. some people may be very obsessive, or very restless, or may suffer from frequent bouts of anger, or be very suspicious. We also know that these traits are often associated with brain related changes and level of functioning. Some of the key constructs included in the reviewed studies include: *adaptability, attitude, affect, anxiety, belief, basic skills, classroom behaviours, control strategies, cooperation, curiosity, discipline, effort, elaboration strategies, emotion, engagement, extracurricular activity, habit, help-seeking, homework, independence, etc.*[123]

Personality traits reflect people's characteristic patterns of thoughts, feelings, and behaviours. They imply consistency and stability—someone who scores high on a specific trait like Extraversion is expected to be sociable in different situations and over time. Thus, trait psychology rests on the idea that people differ from one another in terms of where they stand on a set of basic trait dimensions that persist over time and across situations. Mental health status can be assessed by symptoms reflecting functions of mind. Generally, mood state, thought, behaviour, and cognitive functions give us a fairly good idea of the presence of mental ill-health. We find 3-4 types of abnormalities, some people have frank psychiatric symptoms, which qualify for psychiatric disorders, those who have milder symptoms, will turn to become a disorder in future. There is a third group of population where they suffer from one or two behavioural traits, sometimes these are precursors of related psychiatric diagnosis. These traits may remain as such for life and accentuate during times of stress. Often people refer to them as 'personality traits'. These traits, when increased, do become part of behavioural traits responsible for compromising smooth functioning and adequate productivity of individuals

43. THOSE WHO HAVE MENTAL HEALTH PROBLEM PERFORM POORLY

- What stands between your success and failure is your mind; the hard task is to train it.
- Mental disorders are commonly associated with poor achievement.

Most psychiatric disorders present symptom patterns that cause severe impairment on the emotional, cognitive and social level. The student affected by a disease may be unable to carry out his/her academic or vocational work up to their potential.[124] Thus, adolescents who suffer from a mental disorder risk finding themselves going downhill due to psychological symptoms and negative school experiences. This results in early school leaving.[125]

The college years are a developmentally crucial period when students make the transition from late adolescence to emerging adulthood.[126] Studies suggest that 12–50 of college students are likely to have one or more common mental disorders.[127] Differences between college students and their non-college peers are generally understudied, but the available evidence shows that college students are somewhat at lower risk for developing mental disorders.[128] In any case, mental disorders in early adulthood are associated with long-term adverse outcomes in later adulthood, including persistent emotional and physical health problems,[129] relationship dysfunction.[130] These long-term adverse outcomes may be mediated by mental health problems that exist during the college years, as these years constitute a peak period for the first onset of a broad range of mental disorders.[131]

Problems regarding mental health are present in a significant number of people in the general adult population

- Psychiatric disease in about 15 to 17%
- Milder hidden psychiatric symptom – 10%
- People who are under considerable stress – 20%
- People dependent upon drugs and alcohol to lead to functional impairment- 3-5%
- Mental and physical disability – 6%
- Overall 55-56%, i.e. one out two people remain affected due to psychological health-related issue either-ill-health, stress or a mental illness.

Mental health conditions also impair cognitive ability thereby adversely affecting the prospects of success.

There are mental health factors which have been consistently ignored while deconstructing science of success. Most people have tried to explain it based on psychological factors and personal characteristics. Certainly, these factors of life, e.g. personality or motivation or commitment, conviction, hard work etc. are important, but the complexity of the science of success cannot be explained without considering mental health factor.

There are several reasons why this direction should also be part of our thinking process, not because of only academic exercise but to understand if anything can be changed or modified in order to deal with barriers to achieving success.

Mental health problems are present in significant number of people in the general adult population. It's impossible to find a situation around success or failure which does not have a close association with 'mental health' and by its natural extension, mental illness. There are some hard facts we need to think about: Almost 20% people have a psychiatric disorder. An additional 10-15% people are highly vulnerable and remain at-risk for mental ill-health. about half of the subjects who attempted suicide faced problems in their relationships.[132] Depression is the commonest psychiatric disorder among young people who die due to suicide.75% of all major disorders start developing at age 13-17 which is the prime age, and that's why students are important subjects of discussion. They are the ones who need our help.

One of the most important cause of mental disorder in students is that they face a lot of stress of parental pressure, exams, or loans depending upon the cultural situations. Studies suggest that this is pervasive. A third of the students develop suicidal ideation and/or addiction under such stress.

The presence, and sudden or new appearance of a stress source can also be considered as a triggering factor to cause a full-blown mental illness. People who are not well emotionally do not do well in academics.

On one side achieving success is a positive event however it is not free from psychological problems and those who do not succeed get agitated, fight with their own-self, blame their luck, circumstances, bosses, coaches, mentors, and everyone around themselves and rarely owning up the responsibility unless they are very insightful.

The insight sets in after a while and people start looking into what had gone wrong.

One of the main issues which students often raise is about a successful career. The desire to win and be ahead of others, defeat everyone or succeed at all costs, is not new or recent. The only thing which has changed is the social context. Today the society we live in, where people struggle to achieve and realize their dreams is far more complex. Therefore, it's not much about psychology, but about social science, economics, politics and health which determines the possibility of achievement.[133]

Achievement is a process which cannot be explained without considering all four dimensions of health - physical, social, mental and spiritual health.

Mental health components are involved in achieving success, in aspiring for success and in living with success or failure. If we try to examine, it becomes clear that:

Those preparing for a tough competition are under considerable pressure and at a many-fold risk for developing a mental disorder

Those who do not succeed have a higher number of mental disorders in comparison to those who succeed.

When I recall the young college students I have met, the most common scenario was that somebody fails in the exams or does not have the will power required to even approach it. On assessment from us, we find that the student is either developing a psychiatric disorder or has an active disorder, one whose symptoms were not given the attention that it required, hence the struggle and suffering.

I find a typical pattern in the presentation of problems by young students who approach a psychiatrist or a counsellor or mental health professional, most of the students approach because the psychiatric symptom have appeared for the first time or a psychiatric symptom may have re-appeared after a considerable period of recovery. In most of the cases the appearance of symptoms are preceded by one or more stressful factors. Sometimes such symptoms do appear without any history of stressful factors but in these cases we find that the clients are unable to remember or pin point the associated stressful factor. Thus a clear relationship emerged between the psychiatric symptoms and stressful life events interestingly majority of them had spoken about 'failure', be it in examination or in securing a job or position in a sports team or separation in love affair. Sense of failure is a loss.

'Having failed in life' is another very strong emotion, it cause severe impact on life which can be long lasting and very difficult to deal with. Number of disease, both physical as well as mental appear in the long rum which are directly or indirectly related to previous history trauma or repeated failure.

None the less, there is no rule for success and achievement and no one can predict the outcome of success with any degree of certainty. Human life is full of strength and internal resources. In some people as traumatic effect increases, their struggle for achievement increases, some such people do finally succeed.

Though it may not be success and achievement in the perspective that we are discussing here but mental mechanism is arising from 'sense of loss'. Thus 'inability to succeed' is a problem which is not restricted to success resulting from ambition or aspiration' it is also a context where 'inability to maintain status quo' is perceived as loss, the loss of what you possess and failure to achieve in what you aspire, both have common psychological and social dynamics.

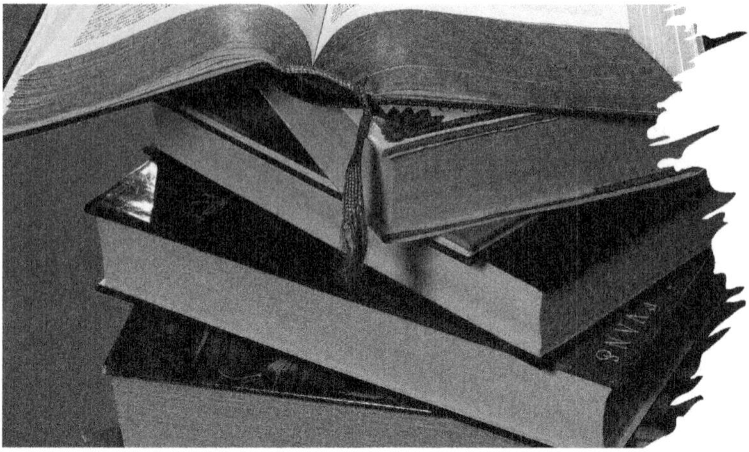

People who perform poorly in academic or other fields develop more mental health problems. The common thread between the ability to achieve, and state of mental health is the cognitive system of the brain. Those who perform poorly should watch out for their psychological helath.

44. EDUCATIONAL ACHIEVEMENT

- Education is one of the main drivers for success in life.
- Poor educational achievers develop relatively more psychological challenges

Poor attendance, particularly frequent absences for vague, non-specific physical health problems, may be related to underlying mental health needs.[134] Difficulties with academic work, social integration, adjustment to school, behaviour regulation, attention and concentration may be school-related signs of emerging or existing mental health problems in youth.[135] The impact of mental illness on school success and academic achievement is vast. High school students who screen positive for psychosocial dysfunction have three times the absentee and tardy rates of students not identified with psychosocial dysfunction—anxiety disorders—which affect 31.9 per cent of all adolescents and co-occur in approximately one-third of depressed youth.[136] They're associated with a reduced likelihood of attending college.[137] People with a lifetime occurrence of social phobia are almost twice as likely to fail a grade or not finish high school as those who have never had the condition.[138] Attention problems are the principal predictors of diminished achievement relative to expectations based on a young person's cognitive ability. Identification and treatment of mental illness improve academic success. Early detection of childhood mental health problems, timely referral, and access to appropriate services leads to improvements in both mental health and educational problems.

The global prevalence of mental health problems affecting children and adolescents is 10–20%.[139] Poor mental health was significantly associated with dropout among students in vocational and higher education.[140]

WHO study (8 country study) of full-time students; 35% screened positive for at least one of the common lifetime disorders assessed and 31% tested positive for at least one 12-month disease. Several socio-demographic and college-related factors were found associated with the prevalence of mental disorders. Some of these are, being female, having parents who were not married or deceased, having no religious affiliation, graduating in the bottom 70% of their high school class, and having primarily extrinsic reasons for going to college.[141]

These long-term adverse outcomes may be mediated by mental health problems that exist during the college years, as these years constitute a peak period when many major disorders begin to appear.[142]

One way that early-onset mental disorders may have adverse effects on adult role functioning is through educational attainment.[143] Effects of mental disorders on early termination of schooling could lead to lifelong decrements in economic and social functioning as well as in the poor health known to be associated with low socioeconomic status.[144,145,146]

Mental disorders significantly predict subsequent termination of schooling at each of the four educational milestones, e.g., primary school graduation, high school graduation, college entry and college graduation.[147] There are some common conditions which interfere with the process of academic excellence.

It is not uncommon but rather frequent that students, parents or sometimes their teachers approach a family doctor, or psychologist and discuss the poor academic progress.

Progress in educational level can inculcate a positive attitude and perception towards mental illness. Moreover, having a relative with mental illness contributes to a positive attitude concerning mental illness.[148]

People who perform poorly in academic or other fields develop more mental health problems. The common thread between the ability to achieve, and state of mental health is the cognitive system of the brain. Those who perform poorly should watch out for their psychological helath.

These have been historically known to contribute immensely in becoming successful but scientific details have emerged only very recently.

45. UNDER ACHIEVEMENT

It is not uncommon but rather frequent that students, parents or sometimes their teachers approach a family doctor, or psychologist and discuss the poor academic progress.

There are some common conditions which interfere with the process of academic excellence.

At the outset it is important to make sure that there is no illness or problem pertaining to physical health due to which the student is unable work hard or fight the stress and mood changes occurring due to the health issue. A number of conditions in physical health lead to psychological condition e.g. general weakness, loss of appetite and other symptoms which make it difficult for the student to put in the necessary effort studying. It is quite common to find someone suffering from chronic infectious disease or suffering nutritional deficiency The next step is to find out if there is any abnormality in the psychological characteristics e.g. low level of intelligence, problems with memory, and the likes. Psychological factors too may be responsible. Possibility of learning disability or problem of intelligence which may be responsible for poor academic progress.

At the same time, it is also necessary to find out if there are early signs of any psychiatric disorders e.g. excessive thinking, intrusive thoughts, panic attacks or mood changes, depression. Any such symptoms may be responsible for poor academic progress. Depression and anxiety-depression are quite common conditions, these conditions are fairly treatable with excellent recovery. Personality factors which may be interfering e.g. excessive involvement in self- or frequent mood changes. Overall, one would like to find out if any of the following conditions is responsible for the kind of difficulty the students is facing. Further, for becoming successful a lot of other qualities are also required, most of these are features of emotional intelligence and social skills. Several qualities which are involved in making people competent to achieve are in fact the attributes of mind and brain. E.g. Everyone needs to be efficient in thinking rationally, understanding the challenges and having the capacity to solve a problem. At the same time, they also need to have a particular mindset to do whatever is necessary for becoming successful.

There could be stress related factors which are interfering e.g. factors in personal life (any commitment, contrary to the objective, any relationship which may be excessively pre-occupying, or adverse family situation or poor support or financial problems.)

The stress factors can also arrive from social commitment and existential issue or activities which are non-academic e.g. sports, travel etc.

Inability to implement the plan e.g. poor attention span, or inability to focus, or inability to concentrate, forgetfulness, sleep problems or sometimes over indulgence in drug seeking behaviour. Those who succeed find it difficult to sustain because of mental health issues (high rates of mental disorder).

46. GOOD MENTAL HEALTH LEADS TO SUCCESSFUL CAREER

For centuries the topic of student mental health was swept under the rug, but as society has evolved, it's become part of the national conversation. Half a century ago, the college may have seemed impossible to students with psychiatric disabilities, but today's campuses are rapidly working to improve and expand mental health services and create environments that are welcoming to students coping with mental illness.

In western countries programs like school and college mental health highlight the significance of mental illness/health of students. Most of the universities prefer to run a clinic or program for students, these programs are fairly developed with a very high emphasis on education and information about mental health, support for academic problems, a system of referral. Most of them also run a wellness program for the overall development of the students. The programs provide excellent opportunity for screening for mental health-related programs, stress management, crisis intervention, counselling support groups but also offer facilities for consultation and follow up for students who have a mental disorder. Some students have a mental disorder before they entered the university and such facility saves their time to travel to hospitals.

Why every university needs well planned and accessible mental health care facility? To deny such facilities will be like neglecting their distress and missing an excellent opportunity for preventing forthcoming mental disorder.

Students are no different than adults as for as mental ill-health is concerned, they are more vulnerable, more responsive to treatment, better compliant to treatment programs and present a hope for mental health interventions. Mental illness is prevalent across the globe and affects multiple aspects of life. Despite advances in treatment, there is little evidence that prevalence rates of mental illness are falling.

There is accumulating evidence that mental illness is at least partially preventable, with increasing recognition that its antecedents are often found in infancy, childhood, adolescence and youth, creating multiple opportunities into young adulthood for prevention.

Adolescence is a transition from childhood to adulthood. It is characterized by rapid physiological changes and psychological maturation. It is indeed considered a vital stage of growth and development.[149] In India, 14–18 years age group constitute 11% (100.2 million) of the population. Various health policies and programmes exist in India for the holistic development of children and adolescents. However, they mainly focus on nutritional, medical and physical health including developmental aspects. Even though mental health and mental wellbeing form an important part of the health, it has not received much attention and given due importance. UNICEF and WHO agree that life skills training is essential to promote mental wellbeing and to identify and seek help during various psychosocial adversities.[150]

For many young adults, school is the best time of life. These critical years can also be undermined by depression, anxiety, and stress. Students are very likely to experience some or many stressors which may test their ability to cope: Adapting to a new environment, balancing a heavy workload, making new friends, becoming more independent, and dealing with the myriad of other issues.[158]

Stress is the most undermined syndrome in our society that is neglected since the element of mental health associated with it. Excessive stress could lead to psychological problems such as depression and anxiety. When stress is perceived negatively or becomes excessive, students experience physical and psychological impairment.[159]

The secondary school students who self-report higher levels of academic-related stress also report lower well-being on social, cognitive and physical parameters. A systematic review of 13 studies showed that in individuals undertaking higher education, self-reported levels of stress are associated with poorer quality of life and well-being.[160] Ongoing stress also precipitates the development of more serious mental health issues such as anxiety and depression.

Some students are stressed, or distressed, dealing with the developmental challenges of emerging adulthood or with life circumstances that arise while at university, like sexual assault or the death of a loved one. Student mental health is not just a postsecondary concern; it is a societal issue with ripple effects on everything from health care to the workplace and the economy.

Some are very ill or extremely distressed, sometimes with the first experience of psychosis, severe depression or obsessive-compulsive disorder. Others have milder anxiety or are suffering through their first break-up.

The problem of student mental health is much more prevalent in western countries, a survey conducted by NAMI in the United States showed that; some psychiatric disabilities are more common than others among postsecondary students. A 2012 NAMI survey titled "College Students Speak" noted that;[161]

27% of all respondents (male and female) said they lived with depression 24% said they lived with bipolar disorder.

12% said they lived with "other conditions"; these include dysthymia, eating disorders, OCD and ASD.

11% said they lived with anxiety.

5% said they lived with ADHD.

1% said they lived with substance abuse.

Overall almost one in 3 fresh college students suffer from one or the other psychiatric problem. College students in large numbers face such problems as depression, anxiety, substance abuse and eating disorders. According to the 2008 survey, 30% of students are so depressed that they find it difficult to function at school. An astonishing 49% admit to experiencing an overwhelming amount of anxiety and 6% consider suicide.

A 2013 survey of college students found that 57 per cent of women and 40 per cent of men reported experiencing episodes of "overwhelming anxiety" in the past year, and 33 per cent of women and 27 per cent of men reported a period in the last year of feeling so depressed it was difficult to function. Studies suggest that between a quarter and a third of students meet criteria for an anxiety or depressive illness during their college experience. A study by the American Psychological Association (APA) found that approximately 86 per cent of students with a psychiatric disability left school without completing their degrees. Some 80 to 90 per cent of college students who commit suicide had not received assistance from their college's counselling centre. In an APA study of 275 faculty members, 56 per cent said they didn't know how to work with students who had 'hidden' disabilities. Almost a third of all college students said they had been so depressed in the previous year that they struggled to function.

Performance and mental health issues. Many employees can and do work while experiencing mental health issues, such as depression or anxiety, with little impact on productivity. Of course, like any illness, there are situations in which the individual is not able to work due to the severity of the condition. Mental illnesses may interfere with your ability to function at work, or they may not affect at all. If your mental illness is affecting your ability to do things, such as concentrating or communicating effectively, you're probably aware of it.

DO SOME PEOPLE HAVE MORE OPPORTUNITIES AND RESOURCES THAN OTHERS?

Some people succeed who are privileged and have enjoyed all the means and luxury of life. Some people do start off with more advantages and opportunities than others. These advantages include access to high quality day care, schools, and elite colleges; being able to pay for computers, access to the Internet, tutors, college preparation courses, and dependable cars; and having family connections that can aid the process of finding a job. This doesn't mean that success is guaranteed for people who have more advantages than others, nor does it mean that none of the people who have these do not have to work harder for achieving success.

This doesn't mean that success is guaranteed for people who have more advantages than others, nor does it mean that none of the people who have these advantages work hard for their successes. Furthermore, many people who lack such advantages use their challenges as fuel to drive their ambitions."

47. COMPETITIVENESS

Competitiveness is possession of a strong desire to be more successful than others.

It is a normal and healthy psychological characteristic, it's a drive for survival, and indirectly, it means a desire to succeed.[162] The desire for success is not only amongst equals but also among unequal's. It is a mindset. It's inherent in an individual's nature, to the extent that it is important for competing to perform any task. Everything always happens quickly and more efficiently when there is competition, particularly when rewards are significant. If there is no reward, the sense of competitiveness dies. The reward may be psychological, physical, social, or economic or even health-related, like succeeding in programs to control weight. It's more widely discussed in relation to students and adolescents, primarily because it's perhaps for the first time during adolescence that they may be facing the sense of competitiveness. There is always an overdrive for succeeding, which often becomes unhealthy. Many performers may indulge in drug-seeking habit, believing they can perform better and win a competition, especially athletics. During examinations, many students start taking tablets or drugs, which keeps them awake throughout the night to study more. To satisfy their need to compete. There is a difference between 'need to succeed' and 'need to compete' one may succeed without being competitive, and one may remain in competition and face failure. This psychological drive has its health implications. Minor psychiatric problems like anxiety, and major ones like depression, self-harm, suicide, loss of sleep, alcohol and drug-seeking, are some of the unfortunate outcomes.

They were living in the hostel and used to meet every day. Both the friends had come from the same village to a city for the college education, they were neighbours in their village and very competitive. Both of them were the first from each family to go for higher education. Everyone back home were engaged in agriculture and farming. The boys came to the city carrying an extreme sense of competitiveness and both of them were under pressure from their families since it was a matter of prestige in the village. It was as though their success was going to be a testimony of which family was more powerful. Finally, after the examination the day of results were announced, both the boys scored well, but one of them had scored about 1% marks less than the other. The boy who was trailing behind could not control his anger and stormed away to his room, where he injected kerosene. He was saved by his friends.

MASTERING THE ART OF COPING: COMPETITIVENESS

Students and everybody else need to learn and master the art of competing. It is normal to be competitive, but being too hard on yourself has health consequences. When the competitiveness is emotional, there will be too much of mental preoccupation. The process of preparation suffers, attention and concentration are further reduced, and chances of failure become higher. Success in competition needs to be taken in humility because it will increase resilience and heighten the sense of satisfaction and achievement by the qualities of 'giving'. Such conditions provide a definite sense of effort, psychological mindset and motivate the person to do better. As resilience increases the power of fighting adversities also increases. To succeed in a competition the basic requirement is a strategy. One needs to assess and identify if the goal of the competition is relevant, or the competition itself is relevant or not.

Similarly, it is also essential to learn to relax instead of being overoccupied with it. Many people argue that if extra efforts are not made, there will be no chance of success, but the fact is that it is the strategic and logical planning which improves the chances of success because of enhanced cognition. Once you have a strategy, there will be clarity on how to move forward; otherwise, students go one step ahead and two steps backwards.

It is necessary to have a challenger. The challenger for the competition is always a part of the process. It is a positive aspect, and it is desirable to keep your challenger in view; if there is no challenger, there will be no competition.

Competition is healthy and rewarding as long as you do not compete with yourself.

Being competitive leads to motivational drive.

There are a few important factors related to the science of the brain and mind. There are several psychological attributes involved in the process, such as:

- Motivation
- Emotional reaction
- Cognitive factors
- Reward process and rewards centre of the brain
- Dopamine (a chemical substance in the brain, a neurotransmitter)
- Presence of a challenger
- Performance
- Well defined objective

Need to compete as well as the need to succeed is a strong motivation which is an important driver for survival; competitive behaviour is seen right from the early days of life. It motivates the organism or humans to survive. Without competition, life is complacent, which neither has any demand or requirement and therefore no success or satisfaction.

Competitiveness is not psychological alone, but it has a biological, social and cultural dimension. People behave differently in different cultures, but their core psychological demand remains the same.[163]

The process of competition begins with internal demand with a sense of purpose which may subsequently get conditioned. One may continue competitive behaviour even when there is no demand. This internal demand generates motivation; therefore, people start looking for situations of competition. Motivation increases the competing activity, which kick starts the rewarding process in the brain; if an act of competitiveness is rewarding the sense of competitiveness persists, it does not cease.

Brain regions and their functions

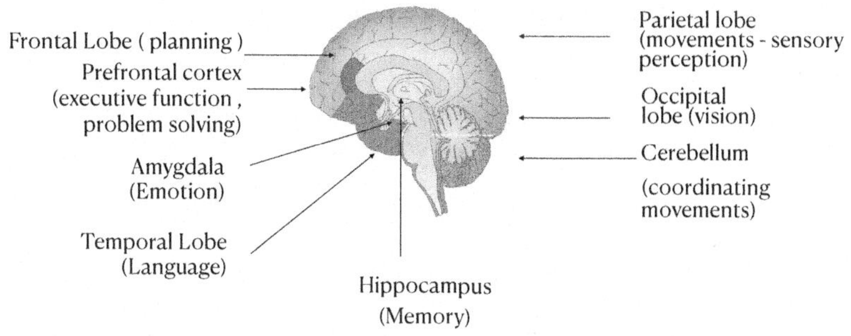

Neuroplasticity

Brain plasticity, also known as neuroplasticity, is a term that refers to the brain's ability to change and adapt as a result of experience. Neuro refers to neurons, the nerve cells that are the building blocks of the brain and nervous system, and plasticity refers to the brain's malleability.

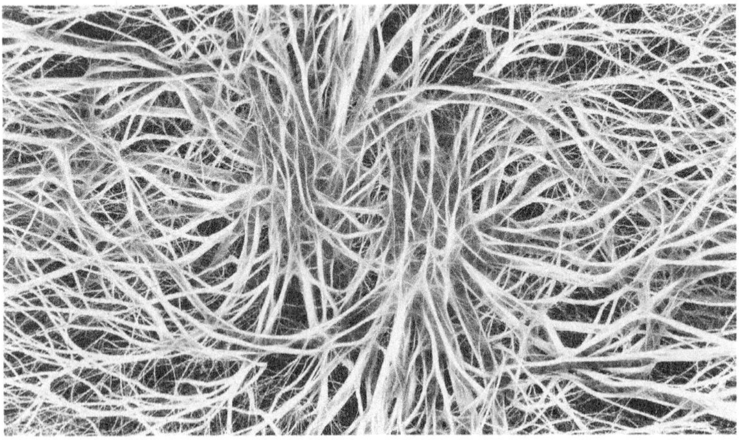

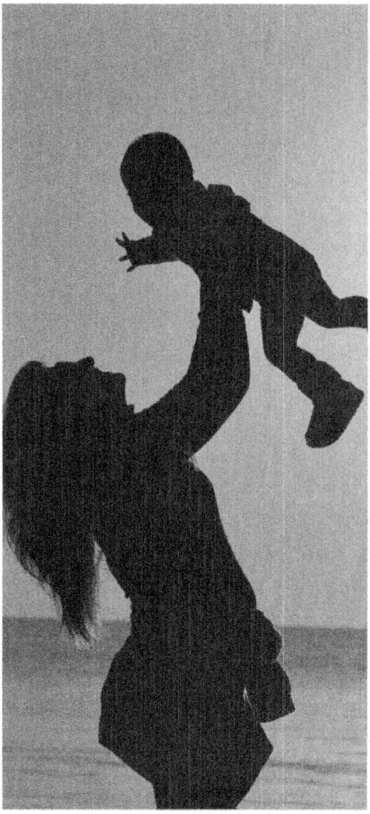
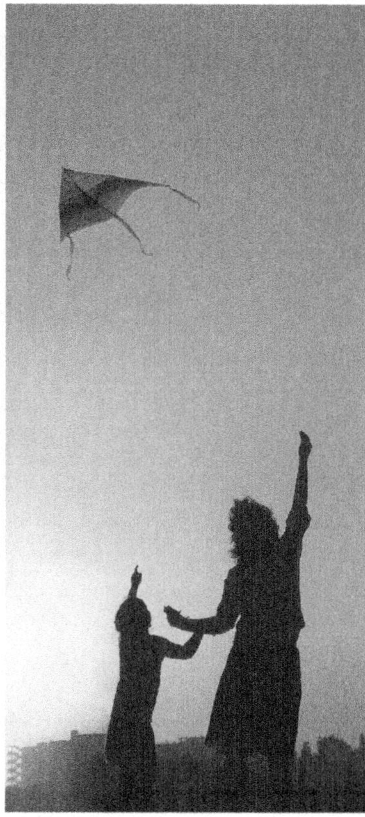

Mother child bond and Childhood development

Social conditions
genetics
poverty
social support
resources

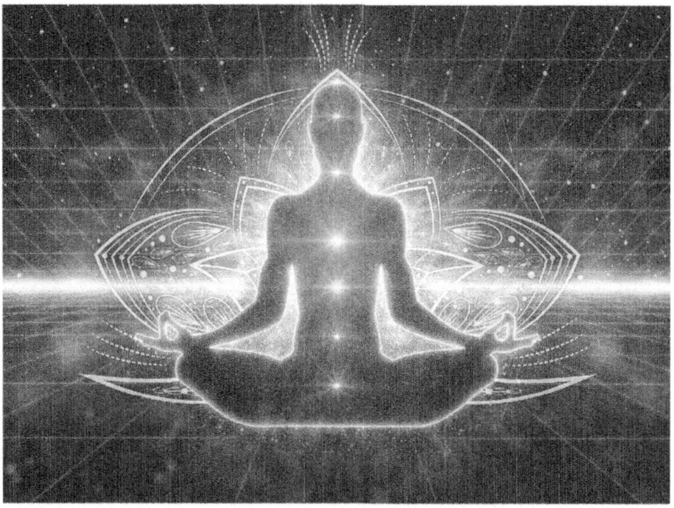

Spiritual insight

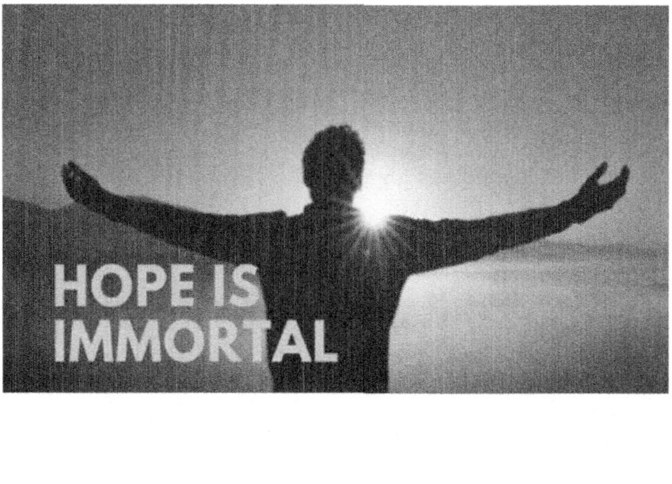

CHAPTER 5
BRAIN MECHANISMS

48. BRAIN STRUCTURE

The Brain has Three main parts: the cerebrum, cerebellum and brainstem. Cerebrum: is the largest part of the brain and is composed of right and left hemispheres. It performs higher functions like interpreting touch, vision and hearing, as well as speech, reasoning, emotions, learning, and fine control of movement.

The brain has two halves or hemispheres: right and left. The right hemisphere controls the left side of the body, and the left hemisphere controls the right side. In most people, the left hemisphere regulates language and speech, and the right hemisphere controls non-verbal, spatial skills. If the right side of the brain is damaged, movement of the left arm and leg, vision on the left, and/or hearing in the left ear may be affected.[164] Injury to the left side of the brain affects speech and movement on the right side of the body. Each half of the brain is divided into main functional sections, called lobes. There are four lobes in each half of the brain: the Frontal Lobe, Temporal Lobe, Parietal Lobe, and Occipital Lobe. Other important sections of the brain are the Cerebellum and the Brain Stem. Although not usually divided into lobes, the cerebellum and brain stem both have different parts. Each of the brain hemispheres and lobes, cerebellum, and brain stem has specific functions, and they all work together:

As advancement in brain sciences, improved causes for mental disorders were more clearly understood. It was recognised that different parts of the brain are involved in mental disorder and that the region of frontal area and middle part of the brain regulate memory, thinking, emotion and intellect.

The frontal lobe is located at the front of the brain and is associated with reasoning, motor skills, higher-level cognition, and expressive language.[165, 166] The cerebral cortex is the part of the brain that functions to make human beings unique.

The parietal lobe is located in the middle section of the brain and is associated with processing tactile sensory information such as pressure, touch, and pain. The temporal lobe is located on the bottom section of the brain. The limbic system is part of the brain involved in regulating behaviour and emotions. The structures and interacting areas of the limbic system are involved in motivation, emotion, learning, and memory. The limbic system is where the subcortical structures meet the cerebral cortex. The limbic system operates by influencing the endocrine system and the autonomic nervous system. These structures form connections between the limbic system and the hypothalamus, thalamus and cerebral cortex. The hippocampus is important in memory and learning, while the limbic system itself is central in the control of emotional responses.[167]

The thalamus, hypothalamus (production of important hormones and regulation of thirst, hunger, mood etc)[168] and basal ganglia (reward processing, habit formation, movement and learning) are also involved in the actions of the limbic system, but two of the major structures are the hippo campus and the amygdala.[169] The occipital lobe is located at the back portion of the brain and is associated with interpreting visual stimuli and information. The midbrain is often considered the smallest region of the brain. Connections made in the hippocampus also help us associate memories with various senses. The basal ganglia are a group of large nuclei that partially surround the thalamus. These nuclei are important in the control of movement. The red nucleus and substantia nigral of the midbrain have connections with the basal ganglia. The human brain is remarkably complex, and researchers are still working toward understanding many of the mysteries of how the mind works. By better understanding how different parts of the brain function, you can also better appreciate how disease or injury may impact certain functions.[170]

The hippocampus is one site in the brain where new neurons are made from adult stem cells. This process is called neurogenesis and is the basis of one type of brain plasticity. So it's not surprising this is a key brain structure for learning new things.

The amygdala is located right next to the hippocampus, the left and right amygdalae play a central role in our emotional responses, including feelings like pleasure, fear, anxiety and anger. The amygdala also attaches emotional content to our memories, and so plays an important role in determining how robustly those memories are stored. Memories that have strong emotional meaning tend to stick.

The frontal lobe is located near the forehead and plays a vital role in motivation and memory. The frontal lobe is part of the brain's cerebral cortex. Individually, the paired lobes are known as the left and right frontal cortex. The frontal lobe is the part of the brain that controls important cognitive skills in humans, such as emotional expression, problem solving, memory, language, judgment, and sexual behaviours. It is, in essence, the 'control panel' of our personality and our ability to communicate.

The limbic system is a set of structures in the brain that deal with emotions and memory. It regulates autonomic or endocrine function in response to emotional stimuli. The limbic system are involved in motivation, emotion, learning, and memory. The limbic system is where the subcortical structures meet the cerebral cortex. The limbic system is the part of the brain involved in our behavioural and emotional responses, especially when it comes to behaviours we need for survival: feeding, reproduction and caring for our young, and fight or flight responses.

You can find the structures of the limbic system buried deep within the brain, underneath the cerebral cortex and above the brainstem. The thalamus, hypothalamus (production of important hormones and regulation of thirst, hunger, mood etc.) and basal ganglia (reward processing, habit formation, movement and learning) are also involved in the actions of the limbic system, but two of the major structures are the hippocampus and the amygdala.

The neuron is the basic working unit of the brain, a specialised cell designed to transmit information to other nerve cells, muscle, or gland cells. Neurons are cells within the nervous system that transmit information to other nerve cells, muscle, or gland cells. Most neurons have a cell body, an axon, and dendrites.[171]

As the brain develops, neurons become more and more intricately connected, and these increasingly complex interconnections lead to increase in complexity in the behaviour. Different regions of the brain and several functional activities are involved in this process, e.g. the part of the brain located in the front (Grey matter of the pre frontal cortex), amygdala, hippocampus, cingulate gyrus, reticular activating system, visual cortex etc.[172, 173]

49. WHAT IS THE FUNCTION OF BRAIN?

The functional activity involves chemical and electrical activities of the brain cell and its communication with other cells. It matters how different parts of the brain are connected, what is their sensitivity to various chemical or hormonal substances, and how effective is the passing of information from one region of the brain to another.

Emotional intelligence is critical to life success. The part of the brain that regulates emotion, the amygdala, is shaped early on by experience and forms the brain's emotional wiring. Early nurturing is important to learning empathy, happiness, hopefulness and resiliency.

Social development, which involves both self-awareness and a child's ability to interact with others, also occurs in stages.[174]

Role of the brain in the mental disorder has been recognised since Hippocrates in the fourth century (B.C). It was called the great interpreter of consciousness; it was thought that mental disorder arose from an unhealthy brain.[175]

As advancement in brain sciences, improved causes for mental disorders were more clearly understood. It was recognised that different parts of the brain are involved in mental disorder and that the region of frontal area and middle part of the brain regulate memory, thinking, emotion and intellect.[176] Most recently, neuroscience has begun to uncover some of the intricate and less apparent relations between the mind and the brain, as investigative approaches from biochemistry, psychology, and genetics converge on an understanding of the physiology of mental illness.[177]

Most of the abnormalities take place during the process of brain maturation. The process of brain maturation is highly influenced by 'experiences' gained during growth and development. These experiences can be emotional or social conditions, the ability to think, reason and imagine all originate in the cerebral cortex.[178]

Neurotransmitters are endogenous chemicals that enable neurotransmission. It is a type of chemical messenger which transmits signals across a chemical synapse, such as a neuromuscular junction, from one neuron (nerve cell) to another 'target' neuron, muscle cell, or gland cell.[179]

Information transmission within the brain, such as takes place during the processes of memory encoding and retrieval, is achieved using a combination of chemicals and electricity. It is a very complex process involving a variety of interrelated steps, but a quick overview can be given here.[180]

A neurotransmitter is defined as a chemical messenger that carries, boosts, and balances signals between neurons, or nerve cells, and other cells in the body. These chemical messengers can affect a wide variety of both physical and psychological functions including heart rate, sleep, appetite, mood, and fear. Billions of neurotransmitter molecules work constantly to keep our brains functioning, managing everything from our breathing to our heartbeat to our learning and concentration levels.

Neurotransmitters are often referred to as the body's chemical messengers. They are the molecules used by the nervous system to transmit messages between neurons, or from neurons to muscles.

Communication between two neurons happens in the synaptic cleft (the small gap between the synapses of neurons). Here, electrical signals that have travelled along the axon are briefly converted into chemical ones through the release of neurotransmitters, causing a specific response in the receiving neuron.

50. BRAIN CHANGES IN MENTAL DISORDER

The brain as a site for abnormality in mental disorders is known since historical times. When a person has a mental disorder, certain changes occur in the brain. Brain and mind are not separate from each other.

Brain changes are seen in mental disorders, but not all changes in these functions signify a mental disorder. Billions of neurons make up a structure weighing just three pounds in the average adult. Brain structure, as well as brain function, continues to evolve throughout its maturation.

Mind and brain have been conceptualised as two individual systems working together which explain human behaviour, consciousness, intellect and wisdom.[181] It is only during the past fifty years when sophisticated instruments became available for taking a closer look inside the brain that the complexity of this relationship has started unfolding. People's behaviour, emotions, thoughts, hopes, and dreams are produced by a variety of neurons throughout the nervous system working in consonance.[182] These changes are, to some extent, responsible for symptoms of mental disorder.

Abnormalities in the mental state, e.g. cognition or memory function, behaviour, mood, or thinking have been correlated with certain abnormalities in the brain. Similarly, symptoms suggestive of mental disorder and corresponding changes in the brain have been examined, e.g. estimating the changes in chemical substances like neurotransmitters, imaging or scanning, etc.

Brain change has also been studied for the effects of social changes, resulting from several conditions like housing, employment, trauma, work culture or migration, etc.

Mental disorders are associated with disturbances in six primary domains of brain function: Thinking, Perception, Emotion, Signalling, Physical, and Behaviour.[183] Each of these brain functions is the result of millions of cells (neurons) communicating with each other through various circuits, using various chemical messengers called neurotransmitters (e.g. serotonin, dopamine, etc.)

Brain structure, as well as brain function, continues to evolve throughout its maturation. The health of brain cells refers to the maturation of each cell, its structure, its relationship with another neuron, the architecture of the neuronal network, the arrangement of several neurons in their physical locations, and function of chemical substances, called neurotransmitters.[184]

Each neuron is protected by a sheath made up of protein structure. Brain maturation also depends upon the health of mothers during pregnancy and nutrition of the baby. Many functions, like mathematical calculations, music, or learning, involve complex functions of the brain. It is a matter of great inquisitiveness how we get the power of imagination or learning many languages or communicating with people.

Due to advances in technology, we can now examine the brain with the help of x-rays and recording of electrical activities of the brain cells. It becomes clearer that our thought, actions, and feelings arise from a complex change in functions of the brain, which plays an important role in its regulation. Findings from research about the brain offer new insight for determining if a lost function can be restored. The brain has an enormous capacity to learn. Distinct brain patterns visible on neuroimaging reveal patterns of response that correlate with the ability to cope with psychological stress. It is revealed in the studies that certain parts of the brain involved in functions like the prefrontal cortex is the site responsible for decision making.

Brain functions are primarily responsible for the symptoms of mental disorder. It is now known that risk factors for many common mental disorders include social inequalities. Bigger the inequality, higher is the risks of developing mental illness.[185] The idea that certain risk factors make it more likely that children will experience poor mental health show how frequently, and under what conditions.

HOW ADDICTION OVERPOWERS THE BRAIN

We may think that addiction has nothing to do with our brain. But this is not true. The fact remains that when drugs enter the body, it changes the way the brain works.

Addictive substances can cause harmful changes in how the brain functions.[186] These changes can last long after the immediate effects of the drug even when the intoxication wears away. Intoxication is the intense pleasure, calm, increased senses or a high caused by the drug. Intoxication symptoms are different for each substance. Over time people with addiction build up a tolerance, meaning they need larger amounts to feel the effects of the drug.

Our brains rely on a delicate balance of chemicals and processes. Alcohol is a depressant, which means it can disrupt that balance, affecting our thoughts, feelings and actions – and sometimes our long-term mental health. This is partly due to 'neurotransmitters', chemicals that help to transmit signals from one nerve (or neuron) in the brain to another.[187]

The relaxed feeling you can get when you have that first drink is due to the chemical changes alcohol has caused in your brain. For many of us, a drink can help us feel more confident and less anxious. That's because it's starting to depress the part of the brain we associate with inhibition.

But, as you drink more, more of the brain starts getting affected. It doesn't matter what mood you're in to start with, when high levels of alcohol are involved, instead of pleasurable effects increasing, it's possible that a negative emotional response will take over.

Alcohol can actually increase anxiety and stress rather than reduce it. Unfortunately reaching for a drink won't always have the effect you're after.

Over time, the brain adapts in a way that actually makes the sought-after substance or activity less pleasurable. There is a system of rewards in the brain which gives us pleasure.[188] Unfortunately, as addiction increases more and more, the brain craves for more rewards. Dopamine is an organic chemical in our body which gives pleasure and acts as a reward for motivation.

51. REWIRING OF BRAIN: NEUROPLASTICITY

Earlier it was believed that brain cells do not regenerate once dead during adulthood and that the brain was a 'non-renewable organ', it slowly dies as we age. Back in 1990, research showed that in contrast to the prevailing belief, that the brain could indeed change after a person had reached adulthood. Neuroplasticity is a term that is used to describe the brain changes that occur in response to experience.

Brain plasticity, also known as neuroplasticity, is a term that refers to the brain's ability to change and adapt as a result of experience. Neuro refers to neurons, the nerve cells that are the building blocks of the brain and nervous system, and plasticity refers to the brain's malleability.[190]

Generally, brain cells are tightly held together in a specific design. Neuroplasticity is a process which reorganises the brain cells and enhances their activities.[191] This mechanism explains how the brain can participate in increasing its power which can increase the effects of several properties necessary to achieve success. There are methods which improve neuroplasticity which in turn will also create better conditions for intellectual and cognitive functions. Brain plasticity refers to the lifelong changes in the structure of the brain that accompany the experience. This term suggests that the brain is pliable, like plastic, and can be moulded into different forms, at least at the microscopic level. Brains exposed to different environmental experiences are moulded in different ways.[192]

Earlier it was believed that brain cells do not regenerate once dead during adulthood and that the brain was a 'non-renewable organ', it slowly dies as we age. Many human qualities could not be explained based upon this theory, particularly the individual's ability to learn and become wiser as age advanced.[193]

Back in 1990, research showed that in contrast to the current belief at that time, the brain could indeed change after a person had reached adulthood. Neuroplasticity is a term that is used to describe the brain changes that occur in response to experience.[194] There are many different mechanisms of neuroplasticity, ranging from the growth of new connections to the creation of new neurons.

The brain can form new connections, new pathways, and change how its circuits are wired; neurogenesis is the even more amazing ability of the brain to grow new neurons. It also refers to the brain's ability to adapt and develop beyond the usual developmental period of childhood—neuroplasticity changes with age. Brain cells are protected by a protein material which is called neuro protectives heath, an abnormality in this exposes the cells to the possibility of damage Neuroplasticity is involved in the process of learning and continues to create new neurons by performing mental activities. This can restore lost connections between neurons and retrieve functions that have not been used in some time. It can enhance memory and enhance overall cognitive skills.

There are ongoing attempts to search for medications which can improve neuroplasticity. Scientists have also reported that those who walked at least about 5 miles weekly had significantly greater grey-matter volume. The study found that people who walked roughly six to nine miles in a week had greater grey matter volume nine years later than people who did not walk as much.[195] Meditation is a simple way to increases grey matter volume in the brain.[196] Mindfulness meditation is paying precise, non-judgmental attention to the details of our moment to moment experience. Mindfulness in meditation is often practised sitting with eyes closed, cross-legged on a cushion, or a chair, with the back straight.

Playing Action Video Games increases Grey Matter Volume: Researchers observed playing certain types of action video games (AVGs) has its effect on grey matter volume. They found that playing action video games for two months for at least 30 min per day can significantly increase grey matter volume.[197] Exploring virtual environments help people to learn, remember, and even explore real-world environments. Video games could be therapeutically useful for patients with mental disorders in which brain regions are altered or reduced in size. However, the impact of playing violent video games need further study. In internet game addiction, individuals showed a significant reduction of grey matter.[198] Hence, the impact of playing a video game can be either positive or negative, depending on the content of the games and the nature of addiction.

Psychology has identified 'willpower' as a product of the interaction-between genes and environment and early childhood training. These are essential elements for success in school and beyond. While overall levels of will power vary from person to person, acquiring a new skill, or mastering a current one usually takes many hours. But people vastly underestimate the positive impact 'a practice', even 15 minutes per day can have. It's far better to allocate a small amount of time each day to practising something, rather than spending hours on your craft one day per week. The repetitive daily habit ends up having a higher and deeper impact on your brain than long but infrequent practice.[199]

With age, grey matter in the brain decreases. Scientists have demonstrated that with age brain structure can be altered upon prolonged exposure to novel experiences. The neural pathways and synapses can be changed by yoga, meditation, exercises, training, and diets. This positive change can happen at the cellular level or the level of collection of cells in a more substantial part of the cortex. There are several different methods known to increase the process of neuroplasticity, e.g. physical activity and good physical fitness.

Most exciting observation has been the finding of increased grey matter due to the practice of yoga and meditation. Meditation, yoga, omega-3, and many other therapies can increase the grey matter in the brain.[200,201]

- *Until fairly recently, the adult brain was considered largely fixed and stable*[202]
- *Current perspectives suggest a dynamic brain which changes physically by both internal and external factors*[203]
- *Significant structural differences between patients and healthy individuals.*[204]
- *There is much that is still unclear about the relationship between neuroplasticity and mental health.*
- *Although there is not yet consensus, contribution of multiple factors, rather than a single explanation is likely to be the case.*[205]

BRAIN CHANGES DURING STRESS

The brain of people who are constantly exposed to stress and stressful factors, either due to a sudden event or due to long-standing stress, develops several abnormalities. There is clear research evidence that stressful factors interfere with biochemical factors, release several hormones, and lead to abnormal functioning of brain cells

It will not be a surprise if we run into someone who is in a hurry to meet a deadline, someone who is worried about a big presentation and any dear friend who is dreading his final exam day. Anyone who has had those days knows what stress is.[206]

The brain of people who are constantly exposed to stress and stressful factors, either due to a sudden event or due to long-standing stress, develops several abnormalities. There is clear research evidence that stressful factors interfere with biochemical factors, release several hormones, and lead to abnormal functioning of brain cells. Several scientists also feel that changes in the brain function or a neuronal connection, make them vulnerable, and these changes can be the cause of a psychiatric illness are seen in response to stress. Important changes seen are given below.[207]

Stress affects various areas of brain and disorders, their chemical and physiological character.

It affects various brain structures as well as functions; the most important change takes place in the central part of the brain, neurochemical substances, and certain hormones. This occurs in response to the threat perceived by the brain, stress activates a brain network involving the hypothalamus, the pituitary gland, and the adrenal cortex directly to release stress hormones.

Such hormones include several cortisone-like compounds called glucocorticoids, and the most prominent one in humans is cortisol.[208]

If there are physiological effects of stress on the brain, in response to any incident, amygdala (the emotional centre of the brain) sends the signal to the hypothalamus. This results in the release of hormones, which help our body to FIGHT or FLIGHT. This explains why our heart starts beating faster, the adrenaline rush we feel and our increased sensitivity to the environment. Afterwards, cortisol is released, which makes up for the energy that we have spent. This hormone level will come down once the stress is over.

Glucocorticoids have a profound effect on both the body and brain. The brain accomplishes regulation of glucocorticoids, and learning experiences have a profound effect on this control system.

It is not stress but persistently raised cortisol levels that adversely affect the brain in the long-term. In a normal amount, cortisol maintains healthy body functions, but in higher concentrations, cortisol can harm the brain's normal functioning. It can disrupt the synaptic regulation resulting in decreased reactivity to the environment, damage neurons, and can also cause brain atrophy. This brain atrophy is primarily seen in the prefrontal cortex, which is responsible for judgment, planning, problem-solving, and memorising skills. These areas will be negatively affected.

Chronic stress creates free radicals that are very harmful to neurons. Excessive cortisol releases a neurotransmitter called Glutamate, which is essential and healthy in a normal amount. When glutamate is produced in excess, it turns into neurotoxin and releases oxygen free radicals which are highly reactive. Just like free oxygen which is highly reactive causes metals to rust, the presence of free radicals in the brain damage the neurons.

A decline in brain function is very distressing in itself as our memory is affected and our emotional reactions (due to the amygdala in operation constantly) can result in frequent crying and feeling of being on the edge and irritable.

Since Amygdala is the most active centre when our brain is dealing with stress, it constantly fires signals. Now the exciting thing about amygdala is that every time it fires signals, it stores it in memory; therefore, it will immediately identify the stimulus in future that generated anxiety/fear previously. It will act faster to the same stimulus in the future, hence creating a vicious fear anxiety cycle in which the person is trapped.

By (contributed by Sidhhansh Shrivastava MD)

Raised levels of cortisol, decrease or completely stops the production of Brain-Derived Neurotrophic Factor (BDNF), which is a protein that helps keep the brain cells healthy and also helps in the production of new brain cells. Therefore, stress not only kills brain cells, but it also halts the production of new ones.[209]

Stress depletes the essential chemicals in the brain known as neurotransmitters, e.g. Serotonin and Dopamine. This results in the decreased levels of Serotonin which is required for maintaining normal happiness. Now you know chronic stress results in Depression. Dopamine, which is responsible for the mind's natural 'high' and motivation, also decreases when a person is in stress resulting in lack of motivation to pursue anything.[210]

The brain and mind are often used synonymously. However, this is not true. The brain-like the heart and lungs is a physical organ of the body, but our mind is not. It is the mind which rules our thoughts and emotions.

One of the main functions of the mind is to save human life from any psychological stress, threat, or trauma, which generally happens in everyday life. It has always been a question about how we protect our self, how do we continue to function in a normal way no matter what our external condition is. That's where the concept of mind comes into being.

Our mind stands between the brain and body and the external environment; we continue to feel, behave, and remember because of our mind. It was proposed that the significant part of the structure of mind belongs to the unconscious portion regarding which we are not aware, but it continues to work and protect ourselves. The unconscious mind comprises of mental processes that are inaccessible to consciousness, but these influence judgments, feelings, or behaviour. The unconscious mind is the primary source of human behaviour. Our emotions, motives, and decisions are powerfully influenced by our past experiences and stored in the unconscious mind. The unconscious mind contains our biologically based instincts for the urges for sex and aggression. Those features that the conscious mind wants to keep hidden from making us aware are repressed into the unconscious mind. These are mostly unpleased-ant, like repressed feelings and memories which we would like to forget.

The human mind has been a subject of research from different perspectives in various fields of science and art. What is the need is to combine these perspectives by improving our understanding of the human mind. The nervous system is necessary for mental development and functions, but equally important is the social interaction between people and the impact of their surroundings and culture. Man's mind is responsible for keeping the traumatic memories away from the position that it could interfere with life, and whenever it does, that is in the state of abnormality. It also is a safe deposit of our wishes, dreams, and aspirations which remain unfulfilled but the mind makes such arrangements that these items do not appear in our awareness and thus do not trouble us. Mind also remains responsible for all neurological as well as mental mechanisms which involve various crucial functions like memory, emotion, intellect, intelligence, awareness, and insight. An abnormality in any one or more of these parameters suggests the beginning of abnormality of mind, which may originate from the mind itself. Or it may reflect the abnormality of the brain because the function of the brain is under the mind's control. There are several biological changes in the brain which are important. These biological substances create an effective connection between brain and mind.

52. COGNITION

Cognition can be defined as the processes of knowing, remembering and reasoning. Cognition is about content of these processes, such as concepts and memories. But what exactly are thinking and knowing? And how do they relate to attention, memory, and reasoning?[211]

Cognition is an important area of research in wide range of psychiatric disorders, e.g. schizophrenia, mood disorders and neurocognitive disorders.[212] It has started unlocking various secrets of psychotic disorders such as revealing the biological underpinnings, explaining the causes, the course, the outcome and strategy of treatments. Cognition in broad sense means information processing. It means a relatively high level of processing of specific information including thinking, memory, perception, motivation, skilled movements and language. The site of its origin lies in middle part of brain, where neuronal circuitry activities take place. E.g. hippocampus. It refers to functions like perception and intellectual aspects. There are some specific functions which are assessed to determine cognitive status. E.g. ability to learn necessary skills, solve problems, reason and make judgement, ability to retain and recall events, ability of doing mathematical task, or language competency, orientation, etc. are its important functions.[213]

Cognition is the characteristic of mind, and this field of science is also referred to as cognitive psychology or cognitive sciences. In simple terms it is an attribute of mental function which regulates individual's memory, intelligence, planning and execution, to think and foresee or anticipate. Though this branch is known in Vedic sciences in India since thousands of years, in the field of western school of psychology it became popular subject for study of mental disorder in early nineteenth century. Ancient Indian scriptures contain very rich psychological theories that are intertwined with religious and philosophical content.

Working memory plays a crucial role in cognitive tasks such as reasoning, learning and understanding.[214] The executive function refers to ability to use abstract concept, to form an appropriate problem solving test, to achieve future goals, to plan one's action, to work out a strategy and to execute these tasks.[215] Attention and information processing refers to ability to identify relevant stimuli. Important domains of illnesses represent abnormality in cognitive function.

It is based upon observations of growth and development children. Modern method of investigating brain cells, its structure and functions using neuropsychological tests and brain scans or imaging studies have provided pathbreaking information in neuroscience. Processes involved in cognition are interdependent and occur simultaneously. Contemporary science explains 3 types of cognitive theories, based on, *Cognitive developmental* theory, socio-cultural theory, information processing theory.[216]

53. CONCENTRATION AND MEMORY

Memory is an information processing system that is made of a sensory processor, short-term (or working) memory, and long-term memory. This can be related to the neuron. The sensory processor allows information from the outside world to be sensed in the form of chemical and physical stimuli.[217]

form of chemical and physical stimuli.[218]

Memory can be defined as a function of mind and brain. It is a highly advanced system of brain cells and the connection between cells. Memory is involved in processing vast amounts of information. This information takes many different forms, e.g. images, sounds or meaning. This function is known as brain activity for receiving information, processing and distributing it to a different part of the brain and storing it, and retrieving it as and when required.

One of the most common complaints of students is their inability to concentrate. It's a prominent symptom which indicates a feature of the first entry point to the memory system. Though poor concentration is common and it is not an illness, people who complain about poor concentration have a higher chance of developing psychiatric problems. There is a nagging worry at the back of the mind if poor concentration will eventually affect their memory.[219] From a mental health perspective, poor concentration occurs because the information is not registered in the memory system and therefore, not stored as required for its retrieval. Several psychiatric problems are associated with it, e.g. abnormal response to a stressful events, any mental shock or trauma, mood difficulties or depression. It hardly appears in isolation. There are almost always other symptoms present which may indicate the most likely reason for poor concentration, e.g. trouble sitting still, difficulty thinking clearly, frequently losing things or difficulty remembering where things are, inability to make decisions, failure to perform complicated tasks, lack of focus, lacking physical or mental energy to concentrate, making careless mistakes. Poor concentration is also one of the features commonly seen in brain disorders, e.g. Alzheimer's disease, dementia, alcoholism, head trauma etc. These disorders generally appear in older people. In the case of young students, stress and depression are more common conditions. There are some hormone-related conditions like low functioning of the thyroid gland, which creates symptoms like poor concentration and difficulty in rec-collection. If the poor concentration is due to stress or any psychiatric condition, it improves, after adequate treatment.

The memory system is a delicate functioning of the brain. Several structures in the middle part of the brain constitute a compact unit which is responsible for memory functions. The brain cells in this system are designed to possess qualities for information receiving, processing, interpreting and storing. Memory can be impaired if this part of the brain is injured. It is common to come across someone who had developed blood clots in the brain, or brain changes due to age or alcoholism, complaining of poor memory.[220] Memory can be defined as a function of mind and brain. It is a highly advanced system of brain cells and the connection between cells. Memory is involved in processing vast amounts of information. This information takes many different forms, e.g. images, sounds or meaning. This function is known as brain activity for receiving information, processing and distributing it to a different part of the brain and storing it, and retrieving it as and when required.

The system of memory in the brain is fascinating. It receives the information through our senses like hearing (auditory), visual, touch, smell, and taste, which is then collected in the nerve cells and processed further (by a filtering system). This system determines the nature of information which needs to be retained for a long or short-term.

Memory is an information processing system with explicit and implicit functioning that is made of a sensory processor, short-term (or working) memory, and long-term memory.[221] This can be related to the neuron. The sensory processor allows information from the outside world to be sensed in the form of chemical and physical stimuli.

The memory system also decides which information is to be utilised depending upon the purpose. The memory system can combine various information and produce composite output, for example, problem-solving activity.

The memory system is actively involved in the learning process; everything we learn is stored in the brain. The network of nerves are two types:

One, which brings the information from various organs to the brain and second, which takes the information/instructions from the brain to the organs. When information comes into our memory system (from sensory input), it needs to be changed into a form that the system can cope with so that it can be stored.[222]

There are three main pathways in which information can be processed and stored

1. Visual (picture)
2. Acoustic (sound) and
3. Words or Semantic (meaning).

The way we store information affects the way we retrieve it. Information can only be stored for a brief duration in short-term memory (STM) (0-30 seconds).

Some memories are capable of enduring much longer, last days, weeks, months, or even decades. Most of these long-term memories lie outside our immediate awareness, but we can draw them into consciousness when they are needed. The long-term memory (LTM) can last a lifetime. In order to form new memories, information must be changed into a usable format, which occurs through the process known as encoding.[223] Once the information is successfully encoded, it must be stored in the memory for later use. Much of this stored memory lies outside the realm of our awareness most of the time, except when we need to use it. The retrieval process allows us to bring stored memories into conscious awareness. Some memories are very brief, just lasting seconds, and allow us to take in sensory information about the world around us.[224] Often a question is asked if one has a strong memory. There is no such thing as a weak or strong memory. When we can focus or pay attention, i.e. we can concentrate, the information is appro-privately taken inside the brain to be retrieved later. It means, if we cannot reproduce information which was given only a few minutes back, there was likely a problem of concentration. There can be an abnormality in receiving information or in filtering and processing it to send to the memory storage, or the anomaly can be at the place where the information is stored. There can also be some abnormality in the system which brings it out. Therefore, if we do not remember, there can be a problem in this loop.

Memory thus involves:

- Reception of information;
- Processing or filtering of this information;
- Storage of the information for long periods; and
- System by which it is retrieved or made available.

The ability to access and retrieve information from long-term memory allows us to use these to make decisions, interact with others, and solve problems. But how is information organised in our memory? The specific manner in which information is held in long-term memory is not well understood, but research studies have shown that these memories are arranged in groups. For example: if a student is told to perform an experiment and follow specific steps, and he reproduces it in the same sequence, as required, this means he can arrange and rearrange the information.

Memory activity takes place in the middle or central part of the brain in which specific brain areas take part. Brain cells or neurons are responsible for this activity, and the entire sequence is a biochemical activity in which the chemical substance connecting the neurons play a crucial part.

Working memory serves as an encoding and retrieval processor. The function of long-term memory is to store data through various categorical models or systems.

The problems of memory can affect all ages. In children, it is related to the development of the memory system; in adults, it is associated with several physical disorders, e.g. disease of the thyroid gland. In the elderly, memory problem commonly arises either due to depression or brain related problem arising due to old age or high blood pressure.

Studies demonstrate that students with working memory difficulties have an extremely high risk of making poor academic progress.

They represent approximately 10% of their age group in mainstream schooling.[225] Without early intervention, working memory deficits cannot be made up over time and will continue to compromise the likelihood of academic success.

There are several test batteries which can be used to assess working memory, as the Working Memory Index in the WISC. However, most assessment instruments that are currently available require considerable experience in the administration, scoring and interpretation of these tests.[226]

In young age, the problems of memory are more likely to be of psychological origin; however, it could also have a physical background; e.g. head trauma, congenital neurological problem, or epilepsy.

It is imperative to find out if there is any abnormality in the brain due to injury or accident. Hormonal problems are not uncommon; therefore, one should make sure that physically, everything is all right.

If there is a problem of alcohol abuse or drug dependence, it needs to be treated.

It is one of the worst situations when no one, neither the student nor the doctor or the parents realise or investigate the problem and seek timely help.

Excessive sleeping pills have the worst effect on brain function and create memory problems. It needs to be treated similarly to the treatment of alcoholism. Hopefully, controlled sale of these medications will make a difference.

If one is suffering from the problems of mood or going through a phase of depression or having a memory problem; it is advisable to see a doctor and not to wait for it to change or go away on its own.

If there are any other symptoms, a discussion with your doctor is necessary. All physicians can carry out screening for memory. It is more common among people after the age of 45 or 50 years. However, more than approximately 20% of people suffering from depression in adulthood present with problems like inability to focus, concentrate or remember.

Make a self-assessment if you are passing through a stressful condition, acknowledge if anything adverse is happening in your life or your family, or if there is any tension in your personal life.

Students who have memory problems can go for specialised memory tests which are available in hospitals as well as with clinical psychologists. These are sophisticated tests which can be of immense utility to the students. Psychiatric consultation is useful for assessment of conditions like low intelligence, learning disability or problems with attention and restlessness, e.g. (ADHD) or depression. These problems can interrupt the ability to think, hamper attention, memory and decision-making abilities. Intelligence is also strongly influenced by the environment. Factors related to a child's home environment and parenting, education and availability of learning resources, and nutrition, among others, all contribute to intelligence.

INTELLIGENCE AND LEARNING

- *Anyone who is intelligent may not be intelligent in all type of tasks or abilities*
- *Intelligence is a representation of multiple capacities that people have; however, the test that measures intelligence, the IQ test, does not measure all types of capabilities.*

Intelligence is the ability to think, to learn from experience, to solve problems, and to adapt to new situations. Intelligence is critical because it has an impact on many human behaviours.[227, 228]

The central theme in the definition of intelligence includes the ability to learn from experiences and adapt to changing environments. It consists of the ability to reason, plan, solve problems, abstract thinking, and understanding complex ideas.

Intelligence is defined in many ways: the capacity for logic, understanding, self-awareness, learning, knowledge, reasoning, planning, creativity, critical thinking, and problem-solving. More generally, it can be described as the ability to perceive or infer information and to retain it as knowledge to be applied towards adaptive behaviours within an environment or context.

Intelligence quotients or IQ is a test for assessing or measuring the level of intellectual development. Some people are more intelligent, and some others possess a lesser degree of it. Most people have a middle range of intelligence. Complex research has led to a standard measurement which can reflect an accurate state of intelligence in relation to age. It becomes further complex when we consider several other factors which affect the level of intelligence, e.g. environment or family history. However, with extensive research work, it is now possible to measure the level of intelligence on a numerical scale as well as on several qualitative dimensions. Thus intelligence is represented as (1) total or global intelligence – measured in numeric terms (2) qualitative subgroups, e.g. ability to perform in mathematics, language or writing skills.

Intelligence is a representation of multiple capacities that people have; however, the test that measures intelligence, the IQ test, does not measure all types of capabilities. It also depends on the type of test used. There have been extensive studies to settle this question about what intelligence is and how to measure it.

Many tests are developed which can measure intelligence in children, adolescents, adults and older adults. These tests are mostly free from cultural influences which brings uniformity. An intelligent person is similarly smart everywhere. However, to some extent, culture plays a role in how people express various aspects of intelligence, e.g. an illiterate person will find it challenging to convey intelligence in numerical terms, that does not mean he is not intelligent. Mostly, once developed it remains unchanged. It has been a temporary understanding that IQ is unchangeable; however, recent research has challenged this position. Further, these tests don't measure all kinds of intelligence, e.g. such tests can't identify differences in social intelligence. Social intelligence is the capacity to know oneself and to know others or the expertise people bring to their interactions with others. Everyone who is intelligent may not be intelligent in all type of tasks or abilities, besides a global level of intelligence people have higher level of intelligence for a specific task and they may also have limitation in a particular task. e.g. musicians have high cognitive/intelligence this is a special ability, while, there are others who have selective dysfunction for writing, reading or other related activities. This is because of the brain structure and function.

- Brain volume, speed of neural transmission, and working memory capacity are related to IQ.
- The human brain is wired to develop and make use of social categories and schemas. Schemas help us remember new information but may also lead us to falsely remember things that never happened to us and to distort or misremember things that did.
- A variety of cognitive biases influence the accuracy of our judgments.
- The brain plays an important role like: different parts of brain regions, their connecting wiring, nature of brain cell, level and nature of regional functioning play a roll many have investigated whether it is a fixed characteristic assigned at birth or if it can change over time.[229,230]
- There is also evidence for specific intelligence(s), measures of specific skills in narrow domains, including creativity and practical intelligence. Emotional intelligence refers to the ability.

EMOTIONAL INTELLIGENCE

Reasoning, Planning, creativity, critical thinking and problem-solving.

Everyone has features to their mental capacity which gives them the ability to think, feel, calculate or solve problems. These features do not arise individually they are interlinked e.g.; the ability to feel is also related to the ability to think. or the ability to solve a problem also depends upon how quickly we are able to identify the problem.

Intelligence is a global representation of many different characteristics. Some people have exceptional qualities, e.g. someone can be a mathematician par-excellence and other may be an outstanding musician. Similarly, emotional intelligence (EI) is a special quality.

As individuals the success of our profession today depends on our ability to read other people's signals and react appropriately. Emotion is a wide range of observable behaviors, expressed feelings, and changes in the state of mind and body. It is the ability to deal with other people successfully. Feelings, emotions, our likes, and dislikes, give our individual lives meaning and make us happy or unhappy, satisfied or dissatisfied, while Numerical Intelligence i.e. IQ, is the ability to acquire and apply knowledge and skills. Emotional Intelligence is the ability to deal with other people successfully. It is measured and expressed as emotional quotient 'EQ'.

This make us more effective. Psychologist have defined it only since last one hundred years but the concept of emotional intelligence as specific feature of a robust and righteous human being and is known since thousands of years.

Recently, EI is valued across the workplace as an essential component in determining the leadership effectiveness, mainly, when leaders are dealing with teams at the workplace. They can inspire team members to work efficiently in order to achieve organisational goal. EI helps build stronger relationships, succeed at school and work, and achieve desired career and personal goals. It can also help connect with one's own feelings, turn intention into action, and make informed decisions about issues that matter most.

- Self-Awareness
- Self-Regulation
- Motivation
- Empathy
- Social Skills Other features include:
- Communication.
- Leadership.
- Initiating or managing change.
- Conflict management.
- Building bonds.
- Collaboration and cooperation.
- Team capabilities.

EQ is enormously important. **it helps recognise, understand and manage** our own emotions, and it also helps recognise, understand and influence the emotions of others.

It is 'intelligent regulation of mood' as well as 'application of intelligence with appropriate emotional overtones'.

Several characteristics have been described for a person who has high emotional intelligence, e.g. Awareness, social skills, optimism, satisfaction, empathy, passionate, motivated, high self-regulation, belief system, high moral and ethical values etc.

Over all the features of EI represent

- Coping ability
- Resilience
- Well-adjusted personality
- Ability for mood regulation
- Self-awareness
- Inter-personal relationship

EI affects our lives in many ways e.g. people with high EI have greater mental health, job performance, and leadership skills although no causal relationships have been shown and such findings are likely to be attributable to general intelligence and specific personality traits rather than emotional intelligence as a construct.

There are several ways to enhance EI, some of it can be done undertaken by self and others can learn by training. E.g. Knowing your values, holding yourself accountable, practicing being calm, remaining self-motivated. Such leaders work consistently toward their goals, and they have extremely high standards for the quality of their work. Thought regulation and regulate mood variation, ability to sustain criticism, and being authentic.

The EI is a quality which makes people more robust and effective due to a number of social and inter-personal skills. People with high EI have qualities which help them connect with others. These qualities are socially highly respected and appreciated and majority of people therefore look forward to enhancing it while others comfortably live with their role devoid of high EI.

'I have no special talents. I am only passionately curious.' — Albert Einstein,

SOCIAL INTELLIGENCE

Social Intelligence develops from experience with people and learning from success and failures in social settings.

Human evolution has differentiated us in a number of ways from what people were in the past.

What exactly changed overtimes is not only the anatomy, intellect and intelligence but behaviour emotion and understanding as well.

One interesting change has been the size of the brain in human beings in relation to their body between humans and non-humans species, it is said that we possess a developed brain not only in size but in number of characteristics like adaptability to social conditions or adaptability to appreciate a social change, ability to perceive the social spurs. It is exactly the quality to understand 'what goes on in someone else's mind' and how to respond to that situation.

The concept of 'social intelligence' that is used here goes beyond the standard psychological definition

Main features of social intelligence are:

- Conversational Skills.
- Knowledge of Social Roles, Rules, and Scripts
- Effective Listening Skills.
- Understanding What Makes Other People different
- Role Playing and Social Self-Efficacy.

Depending upon these characteristics social intelligence can be enhanced to some extent, though most of the skills are also genetically determined. There are definite changes in the brain which appear during the period of growth in adolescence.

The ability to make sense out of the actions of others is critical to people's daily functioning. Strong relationships improve our immune system and help combat disease. Loneliness and weak relationships are one of the major sources of stress, health problems and depression. Our relationships affect every area of our lives–from colleagues to spouses to friends to kids. Social cognition is the key property to reflect social intelligence, thus social intelligence indicates, mental capacity in social terms the original definition is 'the ability to understand and manage men and women and boys and girls, to act wisely in human relations'.[231]

To become someone with more effective Social intelligence generally have the followings:

- Communicator
- Listener
- Conversationalist
- Better participant
- Better perception of surroundings
- Learning to interpret human emotions
- Networking organisations or speaking groups,

26 qualities of Righteous people

The divine qualities	Tranquility
Fearlessness	Staying away from fault finding
Purity	Compassion
Wisdom	Absence of greed
Charity and self	Humility
Devotion to God	Modesty
Self study	Firmness
Penance	Radiance
Simplicity	Forgiveness
Truthfulness	Fortitude
Renunciation	Cleaniness
Unenvious	Lack of false ego

Qualities of righteous people[232] A lesson and Vedic learning Quoted from http://speakingtree.in

In chapter 16 of Bhagwat Gita Sri Krishna has described Twenty-Six Divine qualities in order to impress that 'jivas' or embodied beings who exclusively engage in divine activities and fully renounce demonic activities are awarded 'Moksha' or liberation from material existence.

'Abhayam' meaning fearlessness, for in knowing one is eternal there is nothing to ever be afraid of. It means getting over the anxiety arising about losing someone or something or getting over the apprehension of damage to the physical body or emotional disruption caused by some undesired event.

'Sattva-samsuddhi' denotes purity of heart consisting of pure goodness undefiled by passion and hatred. Freedom from both aversion and craving lead to such purification.

'Jnana-yoga-vyavasthitih' means situated in the knowledge resulting from discriminating the soul from physical matter. This means realising the ultimate truth about the oneness of the individual consciousness and the cosmic consciousness the Brahman

'Danam' is the charity done for the people who are worthy of it, from one's legitimate means. If you give away anything that is not yours, the same does not qualify as Danam. 'Damah' is self-restraint, controlling the mind to be uninfluenced by sense objects. It aims at achieving control over all the cravings of the senses and acting out of needs and not wants.

'Yagna' is Vedically authorised ritualistic ceremony for propitiation and devotion to the Supreme Lord, without any self-interests. Aimed at remembering the almighty and spreading the knowledge to all others without any vested interest. In modern times, it can be cultivated by developing regular worship of the almighty individually as well as with the community.

'Svadhyayah' means devoted study of spiritual text. The religious scriptures are the repositories of knowledge and guide for moral and spiritual conduct. They are not only to be read but also contemplated upon during introspection. It may pertain to study of any spiritual text of any religion that connects you to a higher realm.

'Tapa' is austerity and penance. The Righteous people develop their qualities through austerity and fasting. This helps attain self-regulation and focus.

'Arjavam' is simplicity, straight forwardness to others in thoughts, words and deeds. Clarity in thought, straight forwardness in words and simplicity in action are the hallmark of this quality.

'Ahimsa' is non-violence to all living entities by thought, word and deed. People underestimate the violence caused by thoughts and words. Non-violence should be followed in totality. One should refrain from thinking, saying or doing anything that may have a negative impact on other.

'Satyam' is truthfulness meaning speaking what is true and beneficial to all beings. It is not a passive quality and has to be followed along with non-violence. Words that may be truthful but because violence are not to be said.

'Akrodah' is freedom from anger. A righteous person does not harbour short-term or long-term resentment towards others and does not get angry. Anger is harmful even if not expressed.

'Tyagah' is renunciation of whatever is opposed to soul realisation. Anything that is sensual, material, needs to be renunciate. At a worldly level, it means detachment from the material things by not craving for them.

'Shantih' is tranquillity, which means keeping the senses peaceful and impervious to agitation. The agitated mind is prone to violence, aversion and desire. The mind should be pervaded with peace and tranquility.

'Apaisunam' is aversion to fault finding and slandering. The approach of a righteous person should be positive. He should not indulge in unhealthy criticism of others and learn to reform only through positive feedback.

'Daya' is compassion and empathy for the distress and misery of others. A righteous person understands the misery of others and tries to help them in overcoming the same.

'Aloluptvam' is absence of greed for sense gratification. A righteous person does not seek repetitive and undue satiation. He is content with what he can get rightfully through right conduct.

Mardavam is gentleness and humility that comes with attainment. False pride or arrogance of any sort is unwarranted as it blinds the person and feeds the ego.

Hrih is modesty, the feeling of shame at the thought of anything inappropriate. A righteous person would not do anything that brings shame, lawlessness or disorder. He is a proponent of harmony.

Acapalam is determination to remain firm against temptations presented to one. Assertion of one's beliefs and sticking to right conduct despite threats is difficult but unavoidable for a righteous person.

Tejas is radiance, lustre. A righteous person glows with wisdom and radiates his innate qualities. One can identify him even in crowd.

ksama is forgiveness. The absence of vengeful feelings against those who have harmed you leads to inner peace. This also includes forgiveness to oneself.

'Dhritih' is fortitude. A righteous person is able to withstand all adversity with unsurpassed strength. He does not complain or give up but continues to move on the divine path.

'Shaucham' is cleanliness both internally and externally to be spiritually worthy. The righteous person bathes regularly and meditates regularly to achieve the purity of both body and mind by scrubbing out the negativity.

'Adrohah' is absence of envy. A righteous person believes in the collective growth. He is not moved by the progress of others who may move ahead of him in any feat. However, he supports them and learns from them.

'Natimanita' meaning absence of false ego. A righteous person is driven by innate qualities of the true self. He does not indulge in promoting or satiating the demands of his ego, the outer self that has a habit of dictating things on the basis of habit, experience or learned behaviour. It does not practice self-preservation and aggrandisement.

THE MELLINNIALS MORE GREY MATTER: NEXT GENERATION

The brain of Millennials is uniquely wired. Younger brains are craving multi-sensory approaches to life, and technology can give them just that. Additionally, because of this 'sensory overload', they are better at filtering information and processing it in ways that make us ever more productive.

The new generation is always discussed by the previous generation and the common findings in their mind is that the boys and girls of today are smarter and have more brain power.

What does it mean? It's not just an impression but an observation and observatory findings are also scientifically significant. Cognitive ability has shown important changes. We find them doing mental activity faster. They are also used to play with number of gadgets at the same time.

It is interesting to find how the environment leads to changes in the brain; the present generation who are in their teens are tech-savvy. They have excellent ability for receiving information and problem solving and at the same time, they can handle more than one stimulus or task at the same time, i.e. multitasking however there is a flip side of it. These young students experience more problem with mental health and higher levels of anxiety, depression, and thoughts of suicide.[234] Young people today are more likely to be depressed and to self-harm, than they were ten years ago, however,[235] there is a significant increase in the mental health problem now than a decade ago. This generation carries much higher levels of perfectionism, and that these elevated expectations may be to blame.[236, 237] Research has found that it is necessary that their problems are seen in perspective and they receive help which they deserve. They have several psychological challenges, e.g. reduced coping and inability to manage stress. Their symptoms are very distressing; they suffer from difficulty in memorising and concentration; Frustration; Inability to regulate their emotion; Difficulty in forming an inter-personal relationship; Difficulty in handling romantic relationship; Self-esteem and self-confidence. These problems affect academic progress. The symptoms are distressing for family members as well.[238] Students are stressed while making adjustments often in a new place. Some students become homesick, missing their family, and friends. A lot of energy goes into trying to make sense of the new environment. Students may feel confused and bewildered from time to time. Students are entering into new surroundings which will affect them. Understanding student and parental expectations about the kind of contact that will be maintained is essential. All these problems affect growth, development and quality of life. Some of the issues remain for an extended period, which may lead to a psychological and social burden. Students need to learn how to prevent mental health problem.

Self-help and seeking help are the two components necessary for managing mental health. Sometimes simple skills to deal with difficulties in a student's life can be a turning point.[239] Across generations, younger people report experiencing the most stress and the least relief—they report higher stress levels than older generations[240, 241]

BRAIN OF MILLENNIALS IS DIFFERENTLY WIRED.[242]

Younger brains are craving multi-sensory approaches to life, and technology can give them just that. They believe that because of this 'sensory overload', we're better at filtering information and processing it in ways that make them ever more productive. Social sharing makes them feel good – so we've learned to harness that power across all aspects of life. But how have they managed to get their approach to technology to actually change our brains? A study carried out in Canada found that the average human attention span is now shorter than that of a goldfish, sadly all down to smartphones, apparently. In the year 2000, we could concentrate for 12 seconds. Now, that's down to just eight – as opposed to a goldfish's nine. Microsoft actually reckons that millennials have much more capacity to multitask. While they can't concentrate for long periods, the more digital a person's lifestyle – often synonymous in itself with being a millennial – the more they can direct their attention to multiple sources at once and give their attention to lots of places in intermittent bursts.[243] Research in brain development among millennials is fairly new. The brains of people in this generation are physically developing differently because of their almost constant interaction with technology. These changes in the organ could affect millennials' communication skills. They are much faster in their engagement with technology, information processing, easier time management with multifaceted communication.

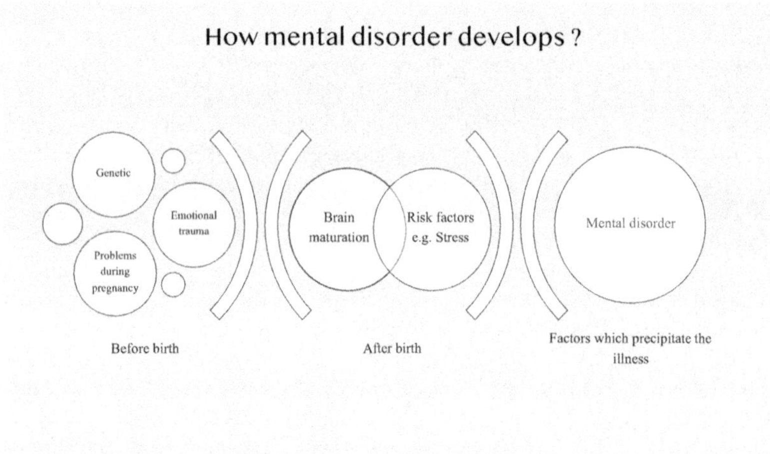
How mental disorder develops ?
Genetic
Emotional trauma
Problems during pregnancy
Brain maturation
Risk factors e.g. Stress
Mental disorder
Before birth
After birth
Factors which precipitate the illness

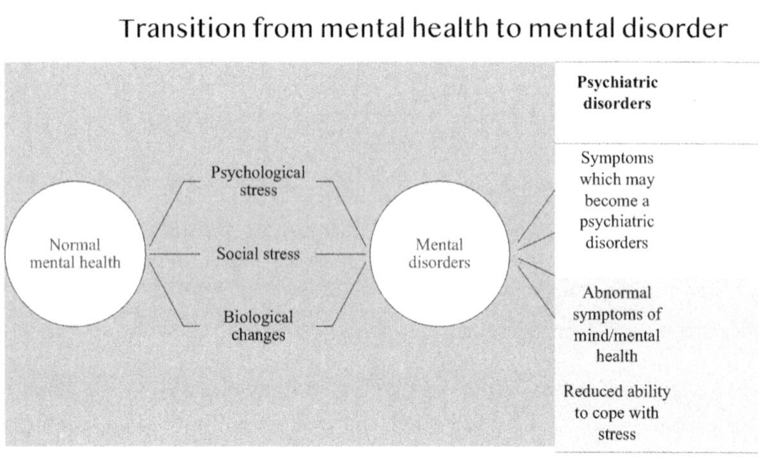
Transition from mental health to mental disorder
Normal mental health
Psychological stress
Social stress
Biological changes
Mental disorders
Psychiatric disorders
Symptoms which may become a psychiatric disorders
Abnormal symptoms of mind/mental health
Reduced ability to cope with stress

SECTION 2

Magic of Mental Health

CHAPTER 6

BREAKING THE BARRIERS: SUCCESS AFTER MENTAL ILLNESS

54. SUVARNA (PEOPLE WITH MENTAL ILLNESS ALSO SUCCEED)

Suvarna was 20 years old and had just enrolled for a business management course in Bangalore. His father was a government employee with a modest income and prominent social status. His family was in Lucknow where his parents lived with his older brother. Swarna was a bright student and the parents had very high expectations of him.

They were taken by shock and surprise when he returned home unannounced from the university, to declare that he had decided to drop out of the course, and go on a journey exploring life. He had decided to not take any monetary help from them and would find work to fend for himself. He had his journey chalked out and had also reached out to an ashram [hermitage] in Rishikesh. Since he wanted to convey this personally to his family, he had made the visit home, and his mind was set on the decision.

Of course, this was a rude shock for the family. His mother was furious and the father was short of words and in a state of shock. Indian parents consider it their solemn duty to pay for and look after their kid's education. Not doing so was considered a social slur. It was not just a matter of money, their hopes were tied to it.

This cultural system is taxing for the children too. They many times have left home for the first time, to attend to the best university. So migration to a new city can be a challenge too. This is not without the emotional and financial burden. This cultural and psychological dynamics is flowing through generations which has its roots in poverty and deprivation. The assumption that they are expected to return home with pride and prosperity, can be a burden too.

Suvarna was in a distraught state of mind and so were his parents. All seemed lost and unable to understand Swarna's condition. Tears flowed and emotions ran high. This brought Mr Brinda, in the scene. He was the family's close friend who ran a small cloth merchandise business. He held a two hour long conversation with Swarna and tried his best to remind him how this decision could have multiple consequences, which would favour none. The money borrowed to pay for his education would be in vain. Incomplete qualifications, would hamper his career growth. All explanations during the discussion were not fruitful, since Suvarna's mind was set on his decision. 'God has chosen this path for me, I am meant to take it, so let me go', was his argument. Nobody knew that his emotions had changed, he was neither feeling happy, nor sad, neither concerned, not attached nor detached, nothing at all, he was fixed on his goals, studies were out of the question at present. He needed to go and experience the truth of life.

Suvarna only agreed to one thing. He would meet up with the family physician. Family doctors were good as their names, they were almost a part of the family, knowing about most things going on in the patient's family. After understanding Suvarna's state of mind, his firm suggestion was that they should let him choose his own path. He explained that the situation would be worse if they lose track of Swarna's whereabouts if they try to be stern with him, since he was firm on his plans. The doctor had a good sense of Suvarna's state of mind.

What if Suvarna left the house without disclosing the location he was moving to? This would increase the family's stress tenfold. The doctor further explained that in the long run of life, one year's gap was not going to matter. The situation should be compared to the possibility of a wasted year if someone failed an examination. Good sense prevailed, and his parents changed their attitude and kept their fingers crossed. They let him go. A lot of religious rituals followed, astrologers, priests, visits to temple whatever was possible and whatever they believed in. Swarna was going around the country, for an entire year, spending time in solitude and experiencing several things which he never revealed.

Often, we do not realise that the mind is not constant. It takes over several other functions that change the way we think and feel. This is not a mental disorder, let's make no mistake. These were slow-growing mood changes in a normal human being, who had started thinking differently. Could he have developed a mental disorder if his wishes were thwarted, no one can say. Social and emotional intervention, family support and open communication helped him overcome his difficulties. Should all such situations be treated similarly, then the answer is 'NO'. Whenever any such problem arises, it is essential to understand and provide space.

This outcome seems very good but there is a lot which happened between the time that Swarna left home and completed his education. He went around several places and stayed in Ashrams with some people. We do not have any information about his whereabout during that one year period. It was well kept promise though, he returned and joined his college but the sad part of his life was when he got into the habit of drugs and started using heavy doses of cannabis.

He managed his health and mood for one year with a lot of difficulties. He went through frequent mood changes, was irritable, felt frustrated and angry over trivial matters. He completed the course but in the final years, the pressure was too much and he crashed. He was losing himself in his thoughts and went around the city purposelessly, alone. He remained aloof and stopped talking to anyone. Self-care was grossly neglected and he had even stopped bathing. He lost appetite and would go hungry for days together, lying in the hostel room, he was depressed and sleepless, his mental state was deteriorating every passing day. Even during this state of mind he had found himself a girlfriend, but after spending some time with her he soon lost interest. She was surprised but had no choice, since he stopped seeing her. One day he again invited her for a coffee, when he revealed to her that he was trying to find some sure and easy method of committing suicide. That was when she promptly took charge and managed to take him to the hospital where he was admitted. He spent about 10 days and treated with antidepressant. After being discharged from the hospital, he was in a good mood but his suicidal thoughts did not go away and after 3 months he was admitted once again. He was found behaving bizarre and pacing up and down in the hostel. This time he spent two months in the hospital. He was not able to stop the cannabis and he still enjoys it.

It took four years to get out of depression and addiction to several drugs except cannabis. He completed the degree with honours.

He progressed quite fast after completing his education.

He was a bright student so he made up and covered the lost ground. He is taking a maintenance dose of an antidepressant, using cannabis as well and settled in his life.

He was lucky – everything became alright, he managed the illness, education as well as career. There are very few in such good conditions, the strength of Swvarna personality is that he recognised that he was getting stressed, He got the idea that something was going wrong, he was not aware and did not approach for treatment. In a state of hopelessness he decided to go out on exploration. No one knew he was already having a cannabis -related problem. He went around for one year, but could not be saved from getting an episode, This is a delayed intervention – a condition of treatment delay. Regrettably the parents, doctor or the relative no one could identify the symptoms that he was quite argumentative, losing his capacity to understand things and also suffered from hopelessness. This caused a treatment delay. He became sick and he was treated successfully. The excellent life is an outcome of 'early intervention'. He had such a good response despite a delayed treatment. The kind of symptoms he displayed when he came home are the 'prodromal state' or symptoms of ultra-high risk state or we may call him simply a person who was displaying early stage of illness.

Early treatment can transform your life and restore the lost ground of the illness but delayed treatment almost always takes always its share from the pie of the outcome.

TREATMENT OUTCOME

The day he was first hospitalised it was quite an ordeal for his parents. They were emotionally shaken, and unable to understand what had gone wrong. Their lack of knowledge about mental illness was one of the reasons they could not gauge the seriousness of the situation. They had travelled a thousand kilometres, to understand and take care of their son. When they met the doctor his explanation seemed like medical jargon for them. The explanation of chemicals and serotonin as cause of depression was truly tough to understand or make sense. The only mental illness they had known was when someone was hospitalised after becoming violent. They only knew that if someone is mentally ill, he is taken to a mental hospital. That was the image of mental illness. Of late, examination related stress has been under discussion so they knew about it but they never expected that their son could be in such a condition because he has been performing well in his college. They found it difficult to live there after Suvarna was discharged and wanted to bring him back home, to Lucknow. Though they insisted he outright refused and did not ever consider it.

It was a painful time. He refused to listen and insisted for his parents to return. Parents were left with little choice.

The parents asked the doctor during their meeting,

'Why is my son depressed?'

'We do not know exactly' said the young doctor who maybe around thirty in age. The mother was not surprised, she understood that the doctor needed more experience to give a definite opinion. She was sure that a senior doctor will certainly know.

After 2 days, they were asked to come in the afternoon, because a family meeting was organised with the consultant. It's a part of clinical practice in mental health, because family is important in providing information and taking responsibility for management after discharge. Relatives of a patient always have several questions and they are never satisfied if such a meeting does not take place. Working with family is a necessary part of the treatment. Treatments like psychoeducation, family therapy, family counselling etc are well-researched fields of psychiatry.

Let me explain:

1. Suicide is a preventable cause of death, despite which its incidence is increasing worldwide. A study conducted in India concluded

that the majority of subjects on recovery from the suicide attempt perceived that their suicide attempt could have been prevented by family members, or people close to them. The analysis revealed that 80% of suicide attempters felt that their suicide attempt could have been prevented. Sixty-four per cent of the study subjects perceived that family members and near and dear ones could have helped in preventing their attempt while 16% of the study subjects perceived that society could have helped.[244]

2. The World Health organisation dedicated its report in 2001 with a prestigious document, setting the agenda for health care for coming days, to mental health. This report, 'New Understanding, New Hope' was edited by an Indian, Professor R. Srinivasa Murthy. This report highlights the role of the family in the treatment of schizophrenia. It cites the studies and concludes the following: 'In developing countries, response to treatment is more positive, medicine dosages are lower, and the duration of treatment is shorter. In the total care of the patients, the support of the families is important. Some studies have shown that a combination of regular medication, family education and support can reduce relapses from 50% to less than 10%.'[245-248]

   In one study, three groups of patients were studied. One did not receive any active treatment and remained on placebo, the second group of the patients were given a drug called chlorpromazine and the third group was given chlorpromazine plus 'family intervention'. Family intervention means care in which family is actively involved and family members support the patients emotionally. After one year of treatment, the number of patients who relapsed (they again develop symptoms almost same as they had when they developed the illness) was calculated. Only 2%–23% patients relapsed in the group, which was given family therapy in addition to medication, as against 20%–25% in the group which received the only medication and 55% in the group which did not receive any active treatment(placebo).

   It is important to talk about the mental health and the role of family and culture benefiting both conditions; development of mental disorder as well as its prevention and treatment.

3. The two disciplines, family therapy and substance abuse treatment, bring different perspectives to treatment implementation.[249] Addiction impacts negatively to almost all family members living with the subject and at the same time problems in the family like, scene or experience of violence, emotional deprivation, mental illness in parents is closely related to development of addiction problem.

4. Many of the risk factors for major depression are not amenable to change. Aspects of emotional support are significantly associated with depression outcome.[250] A broad array of parent and family factors is associated with youth risk for depression, ranging from parental pathology to parental cognitive style to family emotional climate. Families have mostly not been incorporated into clinical treatment research with depressed adolescents, with only 32% of treatments including parents in treatment in any capacity.[251]
5. It is no secret that alcohol and family problems frequently go hand in hand. Alcoholism impacts every aspect of a family, including physical, emotional, financial, and legal. Research has shown that adolescents from single-parent households are more prone to delinquent behaviours, including drug and alcohol use.[252]

While treating the young adults and adolescents with depression it is important to consider the involvement of family. Families provide valuable information which helps in diagnosis and treatment.

It is necessary for clinicians to think:

1. Whether the family is working in the best interest of the depressed young man. By raising this question, I am not trying to be disrespectful to our culture and traditions, in which entire energy of parent's life is invested in their children. However, in several situations we even meet families which are detrimental to the patient's welfare. There are social situations in which we find negative emotions, conduct and callousness or indifference on part of parents. As doctors we need to be sure that discharging a patient in a family environment which is not healthy for the patient is inappropriate and a mistake. We need to work with family, either to deal with the negative factor or to find an alternative placement where the patient can live without the emotional burden and fear. It is hard to think in this direction because, the life of adolescents and students in early adulthood is highly dependent on parents. They have no financial independence or autonomy and they cannot look after themselves. In some cases, it is other way round, where several university students are under pressure to look after their parents.

55. WHY STUDENTS DEVELOP MENTAL HEALTH PROBLEMS?

Students go through several conflicts e.g. in the growth and development of body and mind during adolescence and teenage, they are passing through a severe psychological turmoil which compromises their capacity to deal with changes, adversities, and stressors. They are in this age 'transitioning' from one stage to another in anatomy or their shape and size, sexuality when they are trying to understand sexual characters and sexual functions, sexual organs and romanticism. They also undergo changes in hormones, brain chemistry, and emotion regulation. It is important for teachers and parents to be aware of how these problems appear in order to identify them at the earliest.

The experience of psychological illness disconnects them from their own selves. Though it is a treatable condition, patients seldom receive treatment. One of the main barriers is the stigma attached to it which is a clinical risk factor. We are unable to deal with stigma because people do not speak up and do not talk about their experiences.

Mental health is not only about problems of mind but goes beyond that. When people are facing adversities, there is an increased predisposition towards mental illness and resulting chronicity. Being aware of the fact that mental health problems are treatable, one shall encourage adolescents to protect themselves by providing early treatment. I believe that it is not an impossible task to incorporate mental health into their curriculum of academia. Knowledge will empower them to fight ignorance.

- Social inequality is slowly decreasing. The country has maintained an average enrolment ratio of 95% for students in the age range of 6 to 14 years from 2007 to 2014.
- Changing social and economic challenges, migration from villages to cities, lack of educational support is some of the causes which have made student's life very stressful.
- The social stress is unmasking the biological risk and vulnerability, which finally leads to a psychiatric disorder. A WHO study conducted in 8 countries showed that 35% students had at least one psychiatric disorder in previous 12 months as tested by screening.
- A national mental health survey of India estimates the current prevalence of mental disorders in the age group of 18–29 years at 7.39% (excluding tobacco use disorder) and lifetime prevalence at 9.54%.

- The prevalence of mental disorders (excluding substance use disorder) in the age group of 13–17 years is reported to be 7.3%.
- The burden associated with common mental disorders (depressive and anxiety disorders) rises abruptly in childhood (1–10 years). And peaks in adolescence and early to middle age (10–29 years).
- Suicide death rates in India are among the highest in the world (WHO)
- Thity-seven per cent college students in India are suffering from depression or some form of mental illness.

MENTAL DISORDERS ARE COMMON AMONG STUDENTS

- The global prevalence of mental health problems affecting children and adolescents varies between 10 per cent and 20 per cent.[253]
- Poor mental health was significantly associated with dropout among students in vocational and higher education.[254]
- Several socio-demographic and college-related factors were found associated with the prevalence of mental disorders. Some of these are, being female, having parents who were not married or deceased, having no religious affiliation, graduating in the bottom 70% of their high school class.[255]
- The college years are a developmentally crucial period when students make the transition from late adolescence to emerging adulthood.[256]
- Studies suggest that 12%–50% of college students are likely to have one or more common mental disorders.[257]
- Differences between college students and their non-college peers are generally understudied, but the available evidence shows that college students are somewhat at lower risk of mental disorders.[258]
- In any case, mental disorders in early adulthood are associated with long-term adverse outcomes in later adulthood, including persistent emotional and physical health problems.
- These long-term adverse outcomes may be mediated by mental health problems that exist during the college years, as these years constitute a peak period for the first onset of a broad range of mental disorders.
- One way that early-onset mental disorders may have adverse effects on adult role functioning is through educational attainment.

- Effects of mental disorders on early termination of schooling could lead to lifelong decrements in economic and social functioning as well as in the poor health known to be associated with low socioeconomic status.
- There are four dimensions of health, physical, mental, social and spiritual. Though widely accepted, spiritual health does not figure in the official definition of health by WHO. The revision was proposed as 'Health is a dynamic state of complete physical, mental, spiritual and social wellbeing and not merely the absence of disease or infirmity.' Similar elaboration of spiritual health has been included in the medical textbooks of India. Spiritual component of health has been recognised by National Health Portal, Government of India, a gateway for authentic information.

Multiple social, psychological, and biological factors determine the level of mental health of a person at any point of time. For example, violence and persistent socio-economic pressures are recognised risks to mental health. The clearest evidence is associated with sexual violence.

56. FROM MENTAL HEALTH TO MENTAL ILLNESS

Today, on one hand problems related to stress are increasing among all sections of the society. People suffering from stressful situations do not just develop a psychiatric problem but a large number of people develop several types of physical problems too. Heart disease, diabetes, arthritis, obesity, and many more. This fact remains undiscussed most of the time, consequently, people's awareness remains poor.

Psychological stress is also an important cause of loss of productivity and ability to function. Thus, mental health challenges are the conditions which require the earliest possible intervention. When you review the history of psychiatric disorder, you will find that almost all patients have suffered from psychological stress or mental ill-health or psychologically challenging situation. However, everyone who has a psychological problem does not develop a mental disorder. It is obvious that the presence of stress of psychologically minor problems offers a great opportunity for the prevention of mental illness. Identification of such individuals at an early stage is extremely important. If we miss this opportunity and a transition of health to disease sets in mental health starts deteriorating, and later an intervention or treatment does not provide sufficient restoration of a healthy state.

57. PSYCHOLOGICAL ATTRIBUTES

We have seen that psychological attributes play an important role in all aspects of life, whether employment or personal life. They lead to unhappiness and dissatisfaction. These traits also determine the status of our physical and mental health.[259] It is important to note that these adverse factors are not self-limiting conditions.

Textbooks and scriptures are full of such descriptions with a hope to educate people, caution them to control their unhealthy desires and drives. Those authors believed that education teaches to self-regulate and helps people minimise the consequences of harmful psychological traits.

Traditionally growing children are taught how to develop good personality, moral and social conduct by the families and/or schools.

Many are born with psychological traits which may be unpleasant and negative. These traits may remain:

Silent or dormant and not interfere with life and people may function well.

Such traits may accentuate in time of stress and interfere with life, may become harmful for self and others.

May start becoming abnormal from very early in life and people live with such experiences.

These traits may progress to develop a mental disorder which mostly remains untreated.

They present with risk for social conditions and physical health.

May lead to severe social and spiritual abnormality.

These traits have to be identified and treated.

There are effective methods to deal with these symptoms.

There are several strategies used for correction which are known as positive psychological intervention (PPI). However the challenge is to implement these interventions, design them in a culture-specific and socially acceptable manner which people can adopt and comply with.

Focus on psychological traits have significantly increased due to incorporation of 'well-being' as a criteria for health. The current definition of health has evolved.

It now:

1. incorporates 'state of well-being'. It states that health is not just 'absence of illness.' Being illness-free or not having a disease is not health.

This shift in concept has changed the approach for treatment as well as prevention of illness, be it physical or mental. Its understanding now includes the level of functioning or inability to function. At the same time, it introduces happiness as a part of health and well-being.

2. The new definition has incorporated spiritual health which is the fourth dimension of health.

The psychological traits have also been identified as markers of behaviour to determine the future course of education and employment. Characteristics like belief and truth, righteousness and compassion have been guiding principles for life. Most research has been on positive attributes possessed by individuals labelled as either psychological strengths, character strength, or psychological assets.[260]

In modern science, this field is referred to as Positive Psychology.[261] Positive psychology focusses on assessing well-being and not ill-health. It is now being applied in the health care context for individuals suffering from several physical disorders like heart diseases or cancer.[262] Considering overall context, one can easily say that most problems due to inadequate psychological characteristics affect personal health, family relationship, academic life, employment and social functioning.

Whether it is a religious discussion, spiritual discourse or educational curriculum, all have defined good human characteristics as necessary component for a virtuous man who displays good moral and social conduct. Disciplined people have followed it and non-compliant have been defiant. These traits or conducts are so important that on several occasions it has not only become matters of life and death due to physical illness, or provoke fights, aggression and social disruption but also cause historical damage.

Over the last few decades, many psychological treatments were developed for common mental problems.

There are several types of psychological interventions indicated for different nature of problems which provide good outcome.

These intervention categories include humour, gratitude, building character strength, optimism, mindfulness, kindness, and active constructive response.

Accordingly, positive psychological interventions have shown to be effective and beneficial for various clinical conditions also. Of particular importance is the cognitive behaviour therapy, problem-solving therapy and interpersonal therapy.[263,264]

Cognitive therapy is a treatment which enables patients to correct false self-beliefs that can lead to negative mood and behaviours.[265]

Researchers have identified more than 20 character strengths, grouped in six components of virtues: namely *wisdom, courage, humanity, justice, temperance and transcendence.*

Overall, it means that psychological characteristics affect: *physical, mental and spiritual health along with the level of functioning which includes social and occupational health.* People are born with psychological characteristics which can affect our stress response. Further, several people may have poor ability to deal with problems in real life.

To have proper functioning in life we need to address:

1. How the emergence of adverse consequences can be minimised? E.g. if someone is suspicious, what needs to be done so that he does not develop paranoia or jealousy, or delusional thoughts.
2. How people can strengthen the characteristics of psychological nature which allows them to deal with negative events or stressful factors in their surroundings?

There is no doubt that these cannot be left untreated. While some can live with these problems without having serious consequences several others will see consistent deterioration in their health, behaviour, and conduct.

These psychological characteristics may also indicate the kind of diseases one may develop? This aspect has been discussed in the chapter of 'type A' personality.

Some of the methods helpful in dealing with psychological characteristics, besides approaching cognitive, behavioural or interpersonal therapy by mental health professionals are:

1. Psychological measures – for managing the state of mood
2. Cognitive restructuring for solving problems.
3. Social-skills for enhancing engagements with people.
4. Physical health by lifestyle intervention, exercise and nutrition.
5. Behavioural methods for optimising sexuality and risk behaviour, impulsivity, e.g. addictive potential.
6. Spiritual interventions to develop foresight, contentment and optimism.

These factors form principles of management, but the main question still needs to be addressed; 'What exactly should a person do?'

Management

People are suffering from a mental disorder and many individuals are a victim of an undiagnosed illness or having only a few symptoms, while a significant number of people suffer from problems due to psychological attributes.

It is important to know that change in behaviour and personal conduct has to be made for bringing improvement to deal with psychological problems. These changes have to be done by the person himself as well as the contacts in the surroundings.

What needs to be done?

The first step is to know that problem exists.

Knowing that the challenges due to risk factors, risk behaviour and risk situations widely affect the health, well-being, finance and families, there is no doubt that people must identify psychological challenges and deal with it in consideration of 1. personal gains and also 2. social gains.

Second is, to create awareness and deal with ignorance. Awareness about this aspect of life is extremely important. Awareness will increase with education. Acquiring new knowledge will further increase the ability to identify the presence of such abnormalities and therefore the first step is awareness, education and identification. Most people go to schools, colleges, work on social media, electronic media etc. The world has changed in terms of knowledge translation or communication; There are a variety of options to reach out to people.

After the problems are identified, they need to be dealt with at a personal level but the 'personal strength' is dependent upon several collaterals in the surrounding e.g. the employer, teacher, parents, in-laws, friends. Adopting methods to develop skills mentioned above will allow an individual to effectively deal with such problems. Many times a person is equipped and empowered with the idea to deal with stressors but on several occasions, they can change only when others can change, therefore the strategy to improve will have to be developed at all these levels not just by the person himself e.g. if someone is facing job stress due to breakdown of the team with which he is working, precious little can be done if the administration/organisation does not get involved; that means the organisation has to change its human resource and professional development policies, similarly if there is a relationship problem, both the partners have to share the responsibility.

To be compliant: the fourth step required is to have a logistical arrangement to start making changes. Making change is extremely difficult. Unfortunately, the evidence that positive change can be made with education and awareness is very poor e.g. one will be disappointed if we try to think; how many have stopped smoking, abusing, become regular or disciplines in food, lunch, dinner or breakfast habits, stress management, improvement in communication and may more? It can be done, but it needs a specific strategy to bring the positive change in on oneself.

Depending upon the severity professional help may be accessed. Overall solving of the psychological problems needs building capacity for multiple types of coping skills, remain disciplined and comply to resolve the conflicts without delay and develop the mindset for compassion, truth and faith.

It is well recognised that the thought process precedes our mood state and therefore learning to solve problems shall regulate the mood state associated with it. The following activities will be helpful while achieving the objectives stated above:

Discipline,
Prayer or meditation,
Exercise,
Discourse or debate,
Volunteerism and
Nutrition.

Is it possible? Do we have options from developing individual strength?

Untreated, undetected symptoms/problems have huge adverse consequences. It has an impact on social life, health and finance. The society has become complex because social pressures have increased, society is more complex and people feel the pressure all the time. e.g. the social problems of the society like unemployment, poverty, discrimination, inequality, delayed justice, abuse, institutional arrangement, work culture etc. all these social situations always increased personal unhappiness, health risk and family stress.

Given these constrains the only modifiable factors remains **change yourself,** becoming more proactive and struggling for doing everything necessary to improve your functioning which may be otherwise compromised due to adverse psychological characteristics.

58. MENTAL DISORDERS

Mental disorders are different from psychological distress or a mental health problem. It arises from a complex interplay between a person's genetic makeup and the environment in which they live or have been exposed to at different times in their lives.

Abnormality of mental health can be seen in any of the mental or social functions or more than one of these functions. E.g. a person can feel depressed, or feel anxious, may lose weight, be sleepless, may start forgetting or may remain lost in his thoughts or may indulge in excessive thinking.

Most symptoms of mental disorders reflect in changes in sleep pattern, emotion, mood, concentration, energy level, feeling of pleasure, anxiety, aggression, violence, problems related to memory, sometime loss of control on self, abnormal thoughts and problems related to perception and interpretation of changes in vision, hearing, etc. Mental illness takes many forms, including eating disorders, which influence eating behaviour and are accompanied by negative thoughts about body shape and weight. Although suicide is not itself considered a mental illness, it is often the result of some underlying mental illness.

A vast majority of individuals with mental illness continue to function in their daily lives and can lead a good quality life.

But some people may become so sick that they may need hospitalisation to ensure their safety.

Living with mental illness is hard, and for some, it's unbearable. E.g. about 40% to 80% suicides are directly attributable to untreated mental illnesses[266]. Successful treatment of mental disorder effectively minimises the adverse consequences, but untreated illness complicates life, increases the risk of violence, suicide and deteriorating physical health.

Most mental disorders are treatable. If treated early, the patients recover to lead a normal life. Unfortunately, here we come across a wall. Treatment facilities are severely lacking all over the world, in addition to the lack of awareness and the stigma associated with mental disorders. If people are aware, it can be identified early. If not treated in time, it is likely to have a negative impact on social and personal life. It also leads to a severe loss of productivity.

Treatment of mental disorder is best done by a combination of methods—which involves counselling, resolving conflict, providing proper education about psychological health, talking to families, therapy, talk therapy, medications. Sometimes people have to be hospitalised to ensure their safety. Mental illness is treatable. The vast majority of individuals with mental illness continue to function in their daily lives and can lead a quality life.

In case of major mental disorders like psychosis, schizophrenia, major depression, bipolar disorder or alcoholism and addiction majority of the patient recover well when treated early. Most mental disorders recover and achieve good outcome. Good outcome is defined as a state of recovery in which the person does not have any symptoms or side effects, is able to function in his job and fulfil social, family and personal responsibilities. This level of recovery can be sustained forever only if it is achieved when the patients are treated early and adequately. However it is also true that not everyone recovers to this stage, only about 40%–45% achieve good outcome in early treatment. Out of which about 10%–15% do carry forward some or the other symptom and loose a significant level of functioning.[267]

Children of people with mental disorders are also affected. They sometimes remain emotionally disconnected and do not get opportunities for education and progress, mental illness is more commonly seen among children of people with mental disorder, possibly due to genetic vulnerability and social-emotional consequences.

The spouse bears a huge burden not only social and economic one but also in personal, marital or sexual life.

59. DEVELOPMENT OF SYMPTOMS SUGGESTING ABNORMALITIES

All psychiatric symptoms are neither a mental disorder nor do they necessarily develop into a mental disorder. Large number of people in society remain at risk for mental disorder however only a few of them develop and illness. Mental disorders present with both mental as well as physical symptoms. The symptom suggesting any psychological problem may have several correlates. Most of these symptoms appear as changes in behaviour, mood, thought, inability to understand things surrounding them or changes in memory. These attributes are part of our psyche and represent normal traits of personality. The symptoms of mental disorders are often developing gradually and sometimes difficult to differentiate or recognise.

These symptoms may be present in low intensity and many people continue to live with it. These symptoms also do not interfere with daily life activity.

The initiative to identify people at-risk for developing a mental disorder is one of the important developments in psychiatry. Current initiative is to identify people much before they develop any signs or symptoms. Several risk factors make people vulnerable to develop a mental disorder and therefore identification of specific risk factors is necessary. However, it is difficult to find out specific risk factors because mental disorders are caused by a number of factors from social, psychological and cultural fields. Vulnerability for mental disorder has characteristic features e.g.

1. Majority of such individuals have non-specific symptoms and some of them may develop increased severity of symptoms within a few months.
2. It is now known that the changes in the brain of at-risk individuals have possibly begun in early stages of life.
3. Majority of such individuals suffer from significant decline in their social functioning, ability to carry out intellectual work and social interaction.
4. Generally in a period of approximately two years, about 20%–30% of these individuals go on to develop frank and full-blown mental disorder.
5. When treated early a better response to treatment and lesser adverse effects are observed in such cases.
6. These individuals are better rehabilitated back in mainstream of life.

7. Vulnerability can be reversible to some extent i.e. the symptoms can diminish almost completely and social functioning can be improved, if treated early.
8. So far there is no specific medication which is effective in treatment to control symptoms as well as to restoring social and vocational functioning.

We don't know any predictors and it is almost impossible to distinguish those who may develop a mental disorder from those who may not. Furthermore, it must be realised that a person who is at-risk remains under stress and functions poorly, they need help, and most importantly the suffering needs to be alleviated.[268]

Concept of mind continues to remain philosophical. Defining mental health is challenging. Everyone has the ability to automatically manage all physical and mental functions appropriately, however, sometimes due to a number of reasons certain changes may occur. The functions like sleep, appetite, mood regulation or ability to adjust to a situation may either increase or decrease. Such changes are called abnormalities and these abnormalities may become health problems if the changes persist for a few days or months.

Main factors which can lead to such abnormalities arise from:

1. A state of any mental tension, or stress,
2. Presence of adverse social or psychological conditions
3. If anyone in the family has been suffering from problems of mental health e.g. problems of mood or problem of memory or ability to remember.

Everyone finds it difficult to distinguish an abnormal mental state from a normal mental state. This difficulty leads to a delay in the identification of mental health-related problems and consequently, the abnormality becomes long-standing and more severe. It is then very difficult to treat it and therefore it is very important to identify the problem at the earliest.

A number of factors stand as a potential risk for causing a mental disorder. Several situations too may lead to an abnormal state (i.e. at-risk individual, risk factors and risk situations). A mental state can become abnormal and manifest in any one or more areas of its functioning as described above. Mental health problems obviously arise in those areas which are governed by mental health and the functional inadequacy can reflect in physical health, emotion, thought, perception, memory, judgment, behaviour, understanding concepts and ability to reason, plan and execute any task. It can also be seen in the field of social interaction, ability to work or earn, ability to function. Many a times social situations around an individual indicate a possibility of problems relating to mental health e.g. domestic violence, divorce, separation, failure, resignation from work. Abnormal behaviour is also perceived as behaviour due to which people experience distress and it prevents them from functioning in their daily lives. Many times behaviour of an individual often remains ambiguous even to trained professionals. Furthermore, to a large extent, cultural expectations for 'normal' behaviour in a particular society influences the understanding of 'abnormal behaviour'.[269]

Most of the risk-taking behaviours and psychological problems among children and adolescents emerge during the adolescent period which can be prevented with the help of universal preventive and promotive school mental health programme. Crime, violence, sexual promiscuity, drug abuse, academic competition, bullying, and school dropout are on the rise among the youth.

When abnormality starts in mental health certain symptoms start appearing. These symptoms are suggestive of the kind of psychiatric problem one may develop. If people are aware about these symptoms it will be easy to catch these problems at an early stage. It's crucial because early recognition will lead to early treatment which will eventually lead to better response to treatment and outcome.

A clinical condition where mild symptoms are present which sometimes progress to a full-fledged illness is called prodromal state. Prodrome is a medical term for early signs or symptoms of an illness or health problem that appear before the major signs or symptoms start.

These early symptoms are seen in all types of mental disorder. These symptoms present an opportunity for prevention.[270] Early symptoms are not very specific for future mental illness e.g. if a person is presenting with depressive symptoms, the possibility of developing depression or any other mental disorder is however generally the constellation of symptoms and other clinical features can provide a clue for the nature of disorder which is likely to develop.[271]

Signs appearing in a prodrome include trouble with memory or problems paying attention and staying focused, mood swings, stress, confusion and problems in thinking are common. Other symptoms in the prodrome include: Low mood or mood swings, Increased anxiety, Sleep disturbances, Unusual fatigue, Difficulties concentrating or focusing, Feeling suspicious, Disorganised thoughts or confusion, Sensitivity to noise, lights, and other sensations, Withdrawal from others.

Typically, people begin with symptoms of withdrawing themselves from surrounding or friends or family members, remain reclusive, become excessively irritable or anxious, or sometimes develop episodes of rage or anger. The anger may be provoked or unprovoked which is disproportionate.

Many people start forgetting normal events or if the problem has been existing since long they may decline in their performance doing house-hold work or performing in their job. Newer habits like excessive smoking or alcohol consumption or binging is not uncommon. The symptoms do point out the direction of developing a specific psychiatric disorder but it may change during the course e.g. a prodromal symptom of depression or mood is most likely to develop into an illness like major mood disorder but some of such cases may develop into schizophrenia.

Looking at the trajectory of mental disorder it's clear that risk factors as well as protective factors play an important role. Childhood adversity, trauma and inability to deal with stress, coping ability of individuals, positive or negative environment, emotional health, and family dynamics tilt the balance in favour or otherwise, for mental disorder. Most important factor remains the person himself and his ability to deal with environmental factors. High resilience is protective for mental health. Thus, any modality which can either minimise impact of environmental stress or enhance individual's capacity to deal, will be suitable for prevention of mental disorder much before the development of any symptoms.

Abnormality can be seen in any function related to psychological or physiological (bodily or internal systems) or brain functions e.g. sleep, appetite, sexuality, hunger, motivation, disturbance of perception, thought, etc. and reduced memory.

It is easy to recognise presence of a psychiatric disorder.

The concept of mental health is so omnipresent that we do not give a conscious thought to it in our day to day life. But all our abilities and actions are connected to it. Our mental health bestows us the capacity to trust, show compassion and carry out our duties. It is our mental health which determines how passionately we shall pursue a desire, how diligently we handle our projects and our contribution towards larger goals of the society we live in. An abrasion in mental health or undue pressure due to stress disturbs the equilibrium between the brain and mind. Mental health is all composite, we cannot own a sound mental health without good physical health.

60. SOME HARD FACTS ABOUT MENTAL DISORDERS/ILLNESSES

1. Mental illness like physical illness can disrupt your life. Their effect range from mild to severe on a person's thoughts and behaviour making even handling simple things in life difficult.
2. Mental illness is the reduced ability for a person to function effectively over a prolonged period of time because of: significant levels of distress, changes in thinking, mood or behaviour feelings of isolation, loneliness, and sadness the feeling of being disconnected from people and activities.
3. Mental illness is known to occur in all age groups, among both genders' males and females and among those living in rural, urban areas or in every country or culture.
4. It occurs among people of all age groups, children, adolescents, adulthood or older people. It can strike at any time. People of all cultures, from all educational levels, from all income levels can be affected.
5. There are people who are more at risk to develop a mental disorder than others e.g. those who have mental disorders in the family, those who face social or economic inequalities or have a physical illness.
6. Women' students, people from downtrodden communities, people in extreme poverty or facing discrimination are vulnerable to mental disorders.
7. By and large, most of the mental disorders are treatable conditions, with scientific advances occurring at a fast pace more effective treatments are becoming available.
8. Mental disorders are not contagious, but it affects everyone around the person who too suffer.
9. It causes significant social and functional disability, economic loss, poor quality of life, absence from work.
10. Sometimes mental disorders can be serious when suicide or violence can take place.
11. These are caused by multiple factors within our body, and social environment, our ability to cope with stress and sometimes from hereditary factors.
12. Mental illness usually begins during adolescence and young adulthood. This is a stage when extreme care and vigilance should be maintained. However, mental illness can be experienced by older people too.

13. Mental illness is not the same as feeling distressed because of normal reactions to difficult situations, such as:
14. The death of a loved one, job loss, a romantic breakup,
15. A sudden change of circumstance, like moving to a new area, attending a new school, going through a divorce.

61. MENTAL ILLNESS IS TRULY A 'SOCIAL ILLNESS' TOO

We need to explore if there is anything which has affected the growth and development of the depressed person or is there any factor which is interfering with the progress while under care. A host of family factors are known to be associated with psychological disorders, mainly depression. E.g. parent's mental illness, family violence, addiction in a family member, physical, emotional and sexual abuse etc. An attempt is made to correct what is possible to deal with. Of course, there are families who do not want to believe in the advice and suggestions. They feel they are the best judges of the psychiatric condition or do not want to accept the illness itself. They do not know what harm they are doing by taking the adolescents back to the pathological situation of the family and try to discipline them by using the power invested in them by the social traditions. It's never helpful and often the consequences are severe.

E.g. A 16 years old girl drank 'Baygon' (an household insecticide). She informed her mother about it and said that she was feeling nauseas. She started vomiting after sometime. Her mother rushed to her family physician who had her admitted in a local hospital. She was kept under observation awaiting a psychiatric opinion. After two hours in the evening her father came and plunged in a fight with the hospital staff and the family doctor. He of course did not spare his wife. He said he knew his daughter well enough and that she cannot do such a thing. She may be worked up about something. Finally, he had her discharged from the hospital against medical advice. After a week she slashed her left hand with a kitchen knife in front of her father. His reaction was that he slapped her and went out of the house. She became severely depressed and received no treatment. After one month she jumped from her third-floor apartment and died.

Its only lose-lose game. Regrettably, the medical team is helpless legally, socially and economically to help people where the relatives are not considering best interest of the patient.

We can seek involvement of the family in the treatment. One method as an example could be to teach them more about depression and include them as responsible members of the treatment team. These are simple steps and most parents are excited to know that it is a possibility. In this manner they also get a chance to be with their loved ones while the treatment is going on.

Coming back to the parents of Swarna, they were sitting outside the ward, awaiting their turn to speak to the doctors. Many other relatives were present there too. The number of people was a consoling factor that our son is not the only one suffering. This seems to be a good treatment centre and many affected people seek help here. They would have loved to talk with some parent in a hope of understanding more about their experience and problems if any, with the therapy. But by the time they could find someone willing to talk, they were called in.

They were seated with three others from the treatment team, a junior doctor, a nurse and social worker.

The doctor briefly explained what was going on in the course of treatment of the patient. They were asked if they had any questions. The confusion and worry was the same why their son had developed depression?

Was he short of money or food, was anyone bothering him? Was he in any relationship or connection with any girl, what was the reason?

They tried to ask questions like this and tried to explore but the answer was negative. This was too much, the father felt he can help his son only if he knew what to do.

But here is a situation that he was not having any idea what should be done.

The meeting was rather frustrating.

They returned without any answer except what was told to them when they had met the junior doctor, that depression was because of a 'chemical imbalance in the brain'.

Since Swarna had refused to come home with the parents, they returned on the day of discharge and lived a stressful and anxious life.

They wanted to know what was going on Swarna's life and he did not want to share. There were frequent anger, anxiety and frustrating dialogues during an occasional phone call, the son wanted his independence and the father wanted to be a part of his everyday life. Their relations strained and gradually declined. Swarna developed another episode of depression and got hospitalised again. He informed his parents almost after a week and convinced them not to come since he was fine.

He later on did well and settled.

About 15% to 20% students are suffering from depression and more than 15% have suicidal thoughts at any time.

It is a matter of concern but it's also an opportunity, the first break symptoms or when depression appears for the first time, its recognition is a gamechanger in life.

62. PSYCHIATRIC DIAGNOSIS

There are about 200 types of psychiatric diagnosis. International agencies have developed well-structures criteria for identification and diagnosis. Most of the people in the world follow the ones developed by either the World Health Organisation or the American psychiatric Association.

Besides the psychiatric diagnosis, psychiatric symptoms are also important. Each of these symptoms should be considered seriously. Its severity may not amount to a diagnosable degree but the symptoms alone can cause significant deterioration in quality of life and performance

In order to accomplish this one needs to have a clear idea about:

1. Normal mental health
2. Mental health related problems – not amounting to mental disorder and
3. Mental disorders.

A number of factors stand as a potential risk for causing a mental disorder. Several situations too may lead to an abnormal state (i.e. at-risk individual, risk factors and risk situations). A mental state can become abnormal and manifest in any one or more areas of its functioning as described above. Mental health problems obviously arise in those areas which are governed by mental health and the functional inadequacy can reflect in physical health, emotion, thought, perception, memory, judgment, behaviour, understanding concepts and ability to reason, plan and execute any task. It can also be seen in the field of social interaction, ability to work or earn, ability to function. Many a times social situations around an individual indicate a possibility of problems relating to mental health e.g. domestic violence, divorce, separation, failure, resignation from work. Abnormal behaviour is also perceived as behaviour due to which people experience distress and it prevents them from functioning in their daily lives. Many times behaviour of an individual often remains ambiguous even to trained professionals. Furthermore, to a large extent, cultural expectations for 'normal' behaviour in a particular society influences the understanding of 'abnormal behaviour'.[272]

Most of the risk-taking behaviours and psychological problems among children and adolescents emerge during the adolescent period which can be prevented with the help of universal preventive and promotive school mental health programme. Crime, violence, sexual permissiveness, drug abuse, academic competition, bullying, and school dropout are on the rise among the youth.

When abnormality starts in mental health certain symptoms start appearing. These symptoms are suggestive of the kind of psychiatric problem one may develop. If people are aware about these symptoms it will be easy to catch these problems at an early stage. It's crucial because early recognition will lead to early treatment which will eventually lead to better response to treatment and outcome.

Symptoms

Though the symptoms are specific to disease there are some symptoms which are common and represent a group of mental disorders. Mainly these symptoms arise in the function of behaviour, mood, thinking, memory, understanding, suicidal ideation etc.

Some of the symptoms which one should watch out for are listed below:

Sleep or appetite changes — Dramatic sleep and appetite changes or decline in personal care.

Mood changes — Rapid or dramatic shifts in emotions or depressed feelings.

Withdrawn behaviour — recent social withdrawal and loss of interest in activities previously enjoyed.

Drop in functioning — An unusual drop in functioning, at school, work or social activities, such as quitting sports, failing in school or difficulty performing familiar tasks.

Problems thinking — Problems with concentration, memory or logical thought and speech that is hard to explain.

Increased sensitivity — Heightened sensitivity to sights, sounds, smells or touch; avoidance of over-stimulating situations.

Apathy — Loss of initiative or desire to participate in any activity. Feeling disconnected — A vague feeling of being disconnected from oneself or one's surroundings; a sense of unreality.

Illogical thinking — Unusual or exaggerated beliefs about personal powers to understand meanings or influence events; Nervousness — Fear or suspiciousness of others or a strong nervous feeling.

Unusual behaviour – Odd, uncharacteristic, peculiar behaviour, there are online tools available to screen the possibility of abnormal mental states.

Abnormal mental state is caused by 'complex interaction' of several factors which represent changes in body system and brain function, presence of any physical illness, abnormal psychological state, stressful life events, adverse childhood experience, adverse social conditions, and the experience of trauma. Anything can trigger a mental health problem.

LIST OF PSYCHIATRIC DISORDERS

Psychiatric diagnosis as per Diagnostic and Statistical Manual fifth edition (DSM-5) from the American Psychiatric Association

Anxiety disorders	Occasional anxiety is an expected part of life. You might feel anxious when faced with a problem at work, before taking a test, or before making an important decision. But anxiety disorders involve more than temporary worry or fear. For a person with an anxiety disorder, the anxiety does not go away and can get worse over time. The symptoms can interfere with daily activities such as job performance, school work, and relationships. There are several types of anxiety disorders, including generalised anxiety disorder, panic disorder, and various phobia-related disorders.
Attention-deficit/ hyperactivity disorder	**Attention-deficit/hyperactivity disorder** (ADHD) is a disorder marked by an ongoing pattern of inattention and/or hyperactivity-impulsivity that interferes with functioning or development. **Inattention** means a person wanders off task, lacks persistence, has difficulty sustaining focus, and is disorganised; and these problems are not due to defiance or lack of comprehension. **Hyperactivity** means a person seems to move about constantly, including in situations in which it is not appropriate; or excessively fidgets, taps, or talks. In adults, it may be extreme restlessness or wearing others out with constant activity. **Impulsivity** means a person makes hasty actions that occur in the moment without first thinking about them and that may have a high potential for harm, or a desire for immediate rewards or inability to delay gratification. An impulsive person may be socially intrusive and excessively interrupt others or make important decisions without considering the long-term consequences.
Autism spectrum disorder	**Autism spectrum disorder** (ASD) is a developmental disorder that affects communication and behaviour. Although autism can be diagnosed at any age, it is said to be a 'developmental disorder' because symptoms generally appear in the first two years of life. Difficulty with communication and interaction with other people Restricted interests and repetitive behaviours Symptoms that hurt the person's ability to function properly in school, work, and other areas of life Autism is known as a 'spectrum' disorder because there is wide variation in the type and severity of symptoms people experience. ASD occurs in all ethnic, racial, and economic groups. Although ASD can be a lifelong disorder, treatments and services can improve a person's symptoms and ability to function.

Bipolar disorder

Bipolar disorder (formerly called manic-depressive illness or manic depression) is a mental disorder that causes unusual shifts in mood, energy, activity levels, concentration, and the ability to carry out day-to-day tasks.

There are three types of bipolar disorder. All three types involve clear changes in mood, energy, and activity levels. These moods range from periods of extremely 'up', elated, irritable, or energised behaviour (known as manic episodes) to very 'down', sad, indifferent, or hopeless periods (known as depressive episodes). Less severe manic periods are known as hypomanic episodes.

Bipolar I Disorder— defined by manic episodes that last at least 7 days, or by manic symptoms that are so severe that the person needs immediate hospital care. Usually, depressive episodes occur as well, typically lasting at least 2 weeks. Episodes of depression with mixed features (having depressive symptoms and manic symptoms at the same time) are also possible.

Bipolar II Disorder— defined by a pattern of depressive episodes and hypomanic episodes, but not the full-blown manic episodes that are typical of Bipolar I Disorder.

Cyclothymic Disorder (also called Cyclothymia)— defined by periods of hypomanic symptoms as well as periods of depressive symptoms lasting for at least 2 years (1 year in children and adolescents). However, the symptoms do not meet the diagnostic requirements for a hypomanic episode and a depressive episode.

Borderline personality disorder

Borderline personality disorder is an illness marked by an ongoing pattern of varying moods, self-image, and behaviour. These symptoms often result in impulsive actions and problems in relationships. People with borderline personality disorder may experience intense episodes of anger, depression, and anxiety that can last from a few hours to days.

Depression

Depression (major depressive disorder or clinical depression) is a common but serious mood disorder. It causes severe symptoms that affect how you feel, think, and handle daily activities, such as sleeping, eating, or working. To be diagnosed with depression, the symptoms must be present for at least two weeks.

Some forms of depression are slightly different, or they may develop under unique circumstances, such as:

Persistent depressive disorder

(also called **dysthymia**) is a depressed mood that lasts for at least two years. A person diagnosed with persistent depressive disorder may have episodes of major depression along with periods of less severe symptoms, but symptoms must last for two years to be considered persistent depressive disorder.

Postpartum depression	is much more serious than the 'baby blues' (relatively mild depressive and anxiety symptoms that typically clear within two weeks after delivery) that many women experience after giving birth. Women with postpartum depression experience full-blown major depression during pregnancy or after delivery (postpartum depression). The feelings of extreme sadness, anxiety, and exhaustion that accompany postpartum depression may make it difficult for these new mothers to complete daily care activities for themselves and/or for their babies.
Psychotic depression	occurs when a person has severe depression plus some form of psychosis, such as having disturbing false fixed beliefs (delusions) or hearing or seeing upsetting things that others cannot hear or see (hallucinations). The psychotic symptoms typically have a depressive 'theme', such as delusions of guilt, poverty, or illness.
Seasonal affective disorder	is characterised by the onset of depression during the winter months, when there is less natural sunlight. This depression generally lifts during spring and summer. Winter depression, typically accompanied by social withdrawal, increased sleep, and weight gain, predictably returns every year in seasonal affective disorder.
Bipolar disorder	is different from depression, but it is included in this list is because someone with bipolar disorder experiences episodes of extremely low moods that meet the criteria for major depression (called 'bipolar depression'). But a person with bipolar disorder also experiences extreme high – euphoric or irritable – moods called 'mania' or a less severe form called 'hypomania'.
Disruptive mood dysregulation disorder	**Disruptive mood dysregulation disorder** (DMDD) is a childhood condition of extreme irritability, anger, and frequent, intense temper outbursts. DMDD symptoms go beyond a being a 'moody' child—children with DMDD experience severe impairment that requires clinical attention.
Eating disorders	There is a commonly held misconception that eating disorders are a lifestyle choice. Eating disorders are actually serious and often fatal illnesses that are associated with severe disturbances in people's eating behaviours and related thoughts and emotions. Preoccupation with food, body weight, and shape may also signal an eating disorder. Common eating disorders include anorexia nervosa, bulimia nervosa, and binge-eating disorder.
HIV/aids and mental health	HIV, or human immunodeficiency virus, is the virus that causes AIDS: HIV attacks the immune system by destroying CD4 positive (CD4+) T cells, a type of white blood cell that is vital to fighting off infection. The destruction of these cells leaves people infected with HIV vulnerable to other infections, diseases and other complications. A person infected with HIV is diagnosed with AIDS when he or she has one or more opportunistic infections (which occur when your immune system is damaged by HIV), such as pneumonia or tuberculosis, and has a dangerously low number of CD4+ T cells (less than 200 cells per cubic millimetre of blood).

Obsessive-compulsive disorder

Obsessive-Compulsive Disorder (OCD) is a common, chronic, and long-lasting disorder in which a person has uncontrollable, reoccurring thoughts (obsessions) and/or behaviours (compulsions) that he or she feels the urge to repeat over and over

Post-traumatic stress disorder

Post-Traumatic Stress Disorder (PTSD) is a disorder that develops in some people who have experienced a shocking, scary, or dangerous event.

It is natural to feel afraid during and after a traumatic situation. Fear triggers many split-second changes in the body to help defend against danger or to avoid it. This 'fight-or-flight' response is a typical reaction meant to protect a person from harm. Nearly everyone will experience a range of reactions after trauma, yet most people recover from initial symptoms naturally. Those who continue to experience problems may be diagnosed with PTSD. People who have PTSD may feel stressed or frightened, even when they are not in danger.

Substance use and mental health

Did you know that addiction to drugs or alcohol is a mental illness? Substance use disorder changes normal desires and priorities. It changes normal behaviours and interferes with the ability to work, go to school, and to have good relationships with friends and family. In 2014, 20.2 million adults in the U.S. had a substance use disorder and 7.9 million had both a substance use disorder and another mental illness. More than half of the people with both a substance use disorder and another mental illness were men (4.1 million). Having two illnesses at the same time is known as 'comorbidity' and it can make treating each disorder more difficult.

Coping with traumatic events

A traumatic event is a shocking, scary, or dangerous experience that can affect someone emotionally and physically. Experiences like natural disasters (such as hurricanes, earthquakes, and floods), acts of violence (such as assault, abuse, terrorist attacks, and mass shootings), as well as car crashes and other accidents can all be traumatic. Researchers are investigating the factors that help people cope or that increase their risk for other physical or mental health problems following a traumatic event

(Summarised from National Institute of Mental health, USA)[273]

CHAPTER 7
CLINICAL CONDITIONS

63. INTERNET USAGE

Internet usage in modern times has gone far beyond the limits and boundaries. It is the concern of many parents; particularly parents of adolescents, in the recent past. Assessment of the problematic internet use or Internet Addiction (IA) is necessary because it is associated with several psychiatric disorders which leads to impaired functioning of a user.[274]

Several personality traits like shyness, socially anxious personality and low self-esteem are associated with an abnormal pattern of internet usage.

The internet-related behavioural problem has been described under many names, whatever name we want to use. The fact is that it creates stress, leads to irresistible behaviour, mental preoccupation and inculcates a sense of unusual urgency. The time duration of getting pleasure starts decreasing significantly. Controlling the impulse becomes a problem; the ability to regulate our emotions is diminished. This process mainly happens to some people who are having an inherent risk of running into such tendencies which is to some extent because of a unique structure in which their brain is wired or programmed. Addiction or dependence is also a biological affair. The content of the web is surfed at high speed, keeping one engrossed, but the pleasure is short-lived. This gradually grows into an addiction which veers out of control. There is a constant struggle between your desire to control and your inability to control. Significant brain changes are involved in the genesis of this addictive behaviour.[275]

There are several names used for internet-related psychiatric or behavioural disorder proposed in the scientific community like Internet addiction disorder, pathological internet use (PIU), problematic Internet use, excessive Internet use, Internet dependence, compulsive computer use and virtual addiction and so on. The consequences are almost similar and its extremely difficult to wean-off this behaviour.[276, 277]

Several premorbid traits like shyness, social anxiety, low self-esteem are associated with problematic internet usage. Depression and its association with internet use have been proved in recent studies. Few Indian studies have also substantiated this association.

64. ANXIETY STATE AND ANXIETY DISORDER

Anxiety is a part of our life. Students may feel anxiety before sitting for an examination, adults may worry about issues in job, their relationships and other domestic problems. Anxiety disorders take place when anxiety intensifies and refuses to go away making even routine life difficult.

This century is referred to as a century of anxiety, its common among all ages, be it a child or an elderly living anywhere in this world. Anxiety is a normal reaction to stress and can be beneficial in some situations. It can alert us to dangers and help us prepare and pay attention. It is perfectly normal when it happens in response to day to day stressful situations. Such conditions return to normalcy without causing much distress or leaving behind any seeds for long-term implications. Whereas anxiety as a mental disorder can become a matter of concern sometimes, it may reach a state when you are unable to control it. There are several symptoms which appear and make life difficult to live, these symptoms interfere in everything or most of the things that we do in our daily life.

Anxiety disorders differ from normal feelings of nervousness or anxiousness and involve excessive fear or anxiety. Women are more likely than men to experience anxiety disorders. In the episodes of anxiety people develop fear in anticipation.

Anxiety refers to the anticipation of a future concern and is more associated with muscle tension and avoidance behaviour. It involves excessive worry that persists and interferes with daily activities. Often it is related to many other symptoms such as restlessness, feeling on edge or easily fatigued, difficulty concentrating, muscle tension or problems sleeping. It may also interfere with job responsibilities or minor events of day to day living. Anxiety can be very incapacitating at times.

A lot of help can be given by talking to people in the family and friends, seek professional counselling or visiting the family doctor. Medications are also helpful. Untreated problems make people's life difficult, their ability to function and socialise reduces, their participation in a number of activities declines. People are not able to utilise their full potential and therefore it must be treated without delay.

Anxiety is considered to be excessive when it swells out of proportion to the challenge or stress or when it results in significant distress and impairment. It is viewed as a normal part of childhood. Children experience fear, nervousness, shyness, and avoidance of places and activities that persist at times despite the helpful efforts of parents, caretakers, and teachers. It can alert us to dangers and help us prepare and pay more attention.

Separation anxiety is often thought of as something that only children deal with; however, adults can also be diagnosed with a separation anxiety disorder. People who have separation anxiety disorder have fears about being parted from people to whom they are attached. They often worry that some sort of harm or something untoward will happen while they are separated. This fear leads them to avoid being separated from them and avoid being alone.

Strange as it may seem even children can suffer from anxiety disorder. Difficulty in coping with studies, concern about weight, having fewer friends, lack of intimacy with parents, and being treated differently from siblings can be the associated factors of anxiety disorders. Childhood anxiety disorders are temporary but in some, they can be chronic and persistent. Depression is more than eight times as likely in youths with anxiety disorders than in those without anxiety disorders. Worrying is normal. However, when we worry too much and go overboard it can be a generalised anxiety disorder. Anxiety disorder is treatable, and a number of effective treatments are available. Treatment helps and most people lead normal productive lives.

There are several types of anxiety disorders, including generalised anxiety disorder, panic disorder, and various phobia related disorders.

Generalised anxiety disorder involves persistent and excessive worry that interferes with daily activities. Often the worries focus on everyday things such as job responsibilities, family health or minor matters such as chores, car repairs, or appointments. This worry and tension may have physical symptoms, such as restlessness, feeling on edge or easily fatigued, difficulty concentrating, muscle tension or problems sleeping.

People with generalised anxiety disorder (GAD) display excessive anxiety or worry, most days for at least six months, about a number of things such as personal health, work, social interactions, and everyday routine life circumstances. The fear and anxiety can cause significant problems in areas of their life, such as social interactions, school, and work. Some of the symptoms the patient may experience are:

Feeling restless, wound-up, or on-edge Being easily fatigued Having difficulty concentrating; mind going blank Being irritable Having muscle tension Difficulty controlling feelings of worry

Having sleep problems, such as difficulty falling or staying asleep, restlessness, or unsatisfying sleep.

Anxiety disorders can run in families, suggesting that a combination of genes and environmental stresses can produce the disorders. The causes of anxiety disorders aren't fully understood. Life experiences such as traumatic events appear to trigger anxiety disorders in people who are already prone to anxiety. Inherited traits also can be a factor.

For some people, anxiety may be linked to an underlying health issue. In some cases, anxiety signs and symptoms are the first indicators of a medical illness.

Examples of medical problems that can be linked to anxiety include:

Heart disease Diabetes Thyroid problems, such as hyperthyroidism Respiratory disorders, Drug misuse or withdrawal from alcohol, anti-anxiety medications or other medications Chronic pain or irritable bowel syndrome Rare tumours that produce certain fight-or-flight hormones. Sometimes anxiety can be a side effect of certain medications. It's possible that your anxiety may be due to an underlying medical condition. Researchers are finding that both genetic and environmental factors contribute to the risk of developing an anxiety disorder. Although the risk factors for each type of anxiety disorder can vary, some general risk factors for all types of anxiety disorders include:

Temperamental traits of shyness or behavioural inhibition in childhood. It can also develop in a repressed childhood.

Exposure to stressful and negative life or environmental events in early childhood or adulthood. A history of anxiety or other mental illnesses in biological relatives.

Some physical health conditions, such as thyroid problems or heart arrhythmias, or caffeine or other substances/medications, can produce or aggravate anxiety symptoms; a physical health examination is helpful in the evaluation of a possible anxiety disorder.

Factors given below may increase your risk of developing an anxiety disorder:

- Trauma.
- Stress due to an illness.
- Having blood relatives with an anxiety disorder.
- Adolescents in crisis of transition to teen age.
- Other mental health disorders.

65. PANIC DISORDER

Another type of anxiety disorder is panic disorder. This may cause panic attacks where the patient experiences intense uncontrollable fear for a short time which brings his life to a standstill. Panic disorder can be dangerous, needing repeated hospitalisations.

A panic attack is a type of anxiety which appears in 'attacks' or 'episodes'. Panic disorder can be serious condition needing repeated hospitalisations. It presents like an emergency medical condition because of difficulty is respiration and increased heart rate. Panic disorder is an anxiety disorder characterised by reoccurring unexpected panic attacks. Panic attacks are sudden periods of intense fear that may include palpitations, sweating, shaking, shortness of breath, numbness.

Many people suffer from anxiety in the form of panic attacks. It is a situation which starts suddenly associated with perspiration and breathing difficulty, many times, it is difficult to differentiate it from any heart or lung problem. During an attack several of these symptoms occur in combination: palpitations, pounding heart or rapid heart rate, sweating, trembling or shaking, feeling of shortness of breath or smothering sensations, chest pain, light-headed or faint, feeling of choking, numbness or tingling etc.

Some people feel like they're having a heart attack or suffocating or fear that they are dying. However, a panic attack goes away on its own. It can be a normal reaction to a stressful situation or a part of another mental illness. They may avoid places, sensations, or activities that remind them of a panic attack.

Attacks can occur unexpectedly or can be brought on by a trigger, such as a feared object or situation.

During a panic attack, people may experience:

Heart palpitations, a pounding heartbeat, or an accelerated heart rate, sweating, Trembling or shaking, Sensations of shortness of breath, smothering or choking, Feelings of impending doom, Feelings of being out of control, Palpitations, pounding heart or rapid heart rate, Sweating, Trembling or shaking, Chest pain, Feeling dizzy, light-headed or faint, Feeling of choking, Numbness or tingling, Chills or hot flashes, Nausea or abdominal pains, Feeling detached, Fear of losing control, Fear of dying. As symptoms are severe, many people who experience a panic attack believe they are having a heart attack or any other life-threatening illness. They rush to the hospital emergency room.

Panic attack and panic disorder are not the same. Panic is one of the symptoms which appears in several other conditions, both medical as well as psychiatric. It is diagnosed based upon history and clinical finding,

Typically people remain preoccupied with the possibility of another attack any time. It generally begins in adulthood, after 20, Sometimes children also suffer from it. It is a chronic condition. Most people do not know that they are suffering from a real disorder. The illness is more common among females; it can interfere in daily life activities primarily due to fear of another attack and uncertainty that help may not be available.

Panic is associated with several other symptoms, most commonly anxiety of going in an open space or fear of going in a closed space. Some people have a fear of being in crowds, standing in line, or going into shopping malls. They are afraid of having another panic attack or of not being able to escape.

Mostly the people develop other symptoms of anxiety between two episodes, there are no biological teats for this condition and doctor diagnose it with certainty based upon clinical details.

It can also be seen in:

A health problem such as an overactive thyroid (hyperthyroidism), or heart or breathing problems. depression or another mood disorder. Heavy alcohol use. Using too much nicotine or too much caffeine. Taking certain medicines, such as those used to treat asthma and heart problems. Misusing drugs.

Living with high levels of stress for a long time.

The condition responds very well to treatment. There are medication which have shown excellent results. Besides medication, cognitive behaviour therapy, a type of behavioural intervention or psychotherapy is also effective. A family physician can give these medicines.

Panic disorder involves repeated and unexpected panic attacks. A panic attack is a feeling of intense fear or terror that lasts for a short period of time and reach their peak within minutes. Some people feel like they're having a heart attack or suffocating or fear that they are dying. However, a panic attack goes away on its own. Panic attacks can be a normal reaction to a stressful situation or a part of another mental illness. With panic disorder, panic attacks seem to happen for no reason. People who experience panic disorder fear more panic attacks and may worry that something terrible will happen as a result of the panic attack. They may avoid places, sensations, or activities that remind them of a panic attack.

Attacks can occur unexpectedly or can be brought on by a trigger, such as a feared object or situation.

During a panic attack, people may experience:

Heart palpitations, a pounding heartbeat, or an accelerated heart rate

As symptoms are so severe, many people who experience a Sweating Trembling or shaking Sensations of shortness of breath, smothering or choking Feelings of impending doom Feelings of being out of control Palpitations, pounding heart or rapid heart rate Sweating Trembling or shaking Feeling of shortness of breath or smothering sensations Chest pain Feeling dizzy, light-headed or faint Feeling of choking Numbness or tingling Chills or hot flashes Nausea or abdominal pains Feeling detached Fear of losing control Fear of dying panic attack may believe they are having a heart attack or other life-threatening illness and may go to a hospital ER. Panic attacks may be expected, as a response to a feared object, or unexpected, apparently occurring for no reason

66. DEPRESSION

Depression is an illness characterised by persistent sadness and a loss of interest in activities that you usually enjoy, accompanied by inability to carry out daily activities. Depression can happen at any age but often begins in adulthood. Depression is now known to occur in children and adolescents, although it sometimes presents with more prominent irritability than a case of low mood.[278]

There are effective treatments for depression, but nearly 50% of people with depression do not get any treatment. Depression is a significant public health problem globally as well as in India. A considerable number of people suffer from depression in our country. They develop a severe and longstanding illness. Often people misunderstand that it is a disease of rich people of the society; contrarily, it is more common among the marginalised and impoverished population, in both rural as well as urban regions. It is not an illness found only amongst adults, but it also affects children, adolescents and the elderly. It causes severe economic loss in the family. The WHO office of the south-east Asian region has written an account of depression in India which elaborates on the scientific research carried out in India.[279] Its worst outcome sometimes is suicide when people decide to kill themselves. While it is easy to diagnose depression among adults, it may be more challenging to diagnose the same among adolescents. This is mainly because many symptoms overlap with some of the regular changes which take place during adolescence.[280] Fortunately, it is treatable. The proper and right treatment can yield amazing results.[281,282]

HOW COMMON IS DEPRESSION?

In India, the National Mental Health Survey 2015-2016 reveals that nearly 15% Indian adults need active intervention for one or more mental health issues and one in 20 Indians suffers from depression. It is estimated that in 2012, India had over 258,000 suicides, with the age-group of 15–49 years being most affected.

Depression is more common in women than men. The report on Global Burden of Disease estimates the point prevalence of unipolar depressive episodes to be 1.9% for men and 3.2% for women, and the one-year prevalence has been estimated to be 5.8% for men and 9.5% for women.

Depression is a widespread illness affecting people of all ages, genders, different socioeconomic groups and religions in India and all over the world. Globally, one estimated 300 million people were affected by depression.[283]

SYMPTOMS OF DEPRESSION AND ITS IDENTIFICATION

Recognising depression in young people can be more complicated than recognising depression in adults. It includes changes in feelings, physical health, thinking and behaviour. It is more common in the age group of 15 to 30 years.

Many people with depression also suffer from anxiety symptoms, disturbed sleep and loss of appetite and may have feelings of guilt or low self-worth, poor concentration and even medically unexplained symptoms. Depending on the number and severity of symptoms, a depressive episode can be categorised as mild, moderate, or severe. An individual with a mild depressive episode will have some difficulty in continuing with everyday work and social activities. Their overall functioning is compromised. During a severe depressive episode, it is doubtful that the sufferer will be able to continue with social activities and employment, or domestic activities.

A severe form of depression is predominantly of biological origin. Sometimes it is not associated with any stress factor. This condition is called major depression or endogenous depression.

Depression occurs in response to seasonal changes because of its relationship with the biological clock (circadian rhythm). It is particularly common in colder countries.

Depression is characterised by a cluster of specific symptoms, with no significant differences between adult or adolescent depression except for irritability, which is more common among children and adolescents. Symptoms of depression can vary from mild to severe.

WHAT IS THE CAUSE OF DEPRESSION?

No one exactly knows why it happens, but many factors are at play pushing a person into depression. Depression results from a complex interaction of social, psychological and biological factors. People who have gone through adverse life events (unemployment, bereavement, psychological trauma) are more likely to develop depression. Current research suggests that depression is caused by a combination of genetic, biological, environmental, and psychological factors.[284] Neurotransmitters are chemical messengers that help the brain cells. To communicate with each other. These chemical substances i.e. neurotransmitters, which are found related to depression are involved in chemical communication between the two cells. These chemicals help regulate many physiological functions. Depression can, lead to more stress and dysfunction and worsen the affected person's life situation. Low levels of neurotransmitters is observed in depression and sometimes people are more susceptible to depression. Neurotransmitters: serotonin, norepinephrine, dopamine. Changes also take place in cognitive functions like concentration and memory.

Resilience seems to play a significant preventive role in adolescent depression; many high-risk children (combining familial predisposition and exposure to adversity) do not develop the disorder. Individual factors reported to serve as a protective role against the development of depression in high-risk adolescents include inherited factors and high intelligence, as well as potentially modifiable factors like emotion-regulation skills, grief coping mechanisms, and positive thinking styles.[285] Depression can be challenging to diagnose in teens because adults may expect teens to experience mood swings. They may consider it a natural part of growing up. Also, adolescents do not always understand or express their feelings very well. They may not be aware of the symptoms of depression and may not seek treatment

HOW IS DEPRESSION TREATED?

Depression is treated with various types antidepressant medications. However, drugs have limited effects if the treatment is not combined with psychotherapy or behavioural therapy. The procedure consists of medications, measures to enhance the patient's coping ability and dealing with conflicts and actions to reduce social and environmental stress. Missing out on any one of these three would lead to incomplete recovery of health. A positive outcome of such treatment shall not be possible; further, if the treatment remains inadequate consequently patients remain at a risk of 1. Relapse or 2. Continuity of symptoms. Social treatment would consist of measures to develop a rapport with employers to help build a clear strategy.

Depression is common in older people but often overlooked and untreated. Depression among older people is often associated with physical conditions, such as heart disease, high blood pressure, diabetes or chronic pain; difficult life events, such as losing a partner; and a reduced ability to do things that were possible when younger. Older people are at a high risk of suicide. Depression is treatable, with talking therapies or antidepressant medication or a combination of these.one can do several things to manage depression: Talk to someone you trust about your feelings. If you think you are depressed, seek professional help. Keep up with activities that you have always enjoyed, or find alternatives if previous activities are no longer possible. Stay connected with people. Keep in contact with family and friends.

Eat at regular intervals and get enough sleep. Exercise regularly if you can, even if it's just a short walk. Avoid or restrict alcohol intake and only take medicine as prescribed by your health-care provider.

If you sometimes feel that life seems so hard that it is no longer worth living, take this matter seriously. The pain seems overwhelming and unbearable. You may feel hopeless, point in living. remain consumed by negative and disturbing thoughts. You cannot imagine any solution to your problems other than suicide. Or You imagine death as a relief. Or may start thinking everyone would be better off without you, considering yourself as worthless, feel lonely even in company of friends you need to remember that you are not alone.

Many other people have gone through what you are going through and are alive today. It is okay to talk about suicide. It can help you feel better. You are not to blame and it can happen to anyone. You can get better.

There are people who can help you. You can do several things[286] Talk to a trusted family member, friend, or colleague about how you feel. If you think you are in immediate danger of harming yourself contact the emergency services or a crisis line, or go there directly. Talk to a professional, such as a doctor, mental health professional, counsellor or social worker.

67. UNDERSTAND PEOPLE WITH SUICIDAL IDEAS

The world can be a better place if communication between people is better. Understanding the people, being compassionate and caring are key qualities which can improve life and even save the life of a person one loves. It could be your child or student.

It is important that parents and teachers start making an effort to understand the calibre and the abilities of their children. To simply pressurise them and blame them for their poor performance in academics is only going to add on to their problems. This will make them suffer in silence and make them feel lonely. Loneliness and stress combined together can slowly lead them to depression. There are counsellors, psychologists and even close friends who are more than willing to help them cope with whatever they are facing. Feelings of grief, anger, guilt, betrayal, and relief are normal reactions. High school can be a rewarding time for young people. But for some students, it can also be emotionally difficult, especially in 9th grade during the transition to high school and again in 12th grade during the transition out of high school. The stresses of high school and the mental and emotional stage of adolescence can combine with risk factors and enhance the possibility, for suicide, such as depression, and increase the risk of suicide for some teens. Parents and school staff can help identify students at risk of suicide and help them get treatment before a tragedy occurs. Many high school students reported that they had seriously considered suicide in the past year.

An overwhelming surge of emotions that never seem to end – that's what some who have attempted suicide try to describe to those who want to understand why they feel the way they do. Those who are contemplating suicide might feel as though there is no way out of their situation. They are bombarded with feelings of hopelessness, fear, isolation, hatred toward themselves, and so much more. The pain they feel is often immeasurable, to a point where they see no other option than to end their lives.[287] But many people who have attempted suicide will say that they wanted to live. They really didn't want to die; the desire to remain with loved ones remained very strong. They simply didn't see any other option.

Some of the initial feelings may include shock or numbness, strong feelings of, anger or confusion, emotional withdrawal from others, feelings of depression and loneliness, difficulties with everyday routines, such as eating and sleeping, guilt. With time, the intense feelings start reducing.[288]

WHO CAN BE AT RISK FOR A SUICIDE ATTEMPT?

People with a specific feature are at a higher risk for a suicide attempt.

Risk assessment is complex. It must be clearly understood that many factors collectively work together in possibilities of an attempt increases.

Several factors present at the same time in a person may not lead to suicide; however, a single factor alone may be a precipitating factor or a leading factor for a suicide attempt. But it is also true that risk will be higher if a more significant number of risk factors are present. It is further interesting to understand that it is not possible to predict suicide only based on several risk factors. Presence of risk factor serves as a caution for the prevention of suicide. If one is feeling suicidal and is known to be at risk, care and treatment should not be delayed.

- Family history of suicide
- Family history of child maltreatment
- Previous suicide attempt(s)
- History of mental disorders, particularly clinical depression
- History of alcohol and substance abuse
- Feelings of hopelessness
- Impulsive or aggressive tendencies
- Cultural and religious beliefs (e.g. belief that suicide is a noble resolution of a personal dilemma) and Cultural and sociodemographic factors
- Isolation, a feeling of being cut off from other people
- Barriers to accessing mental health treatment
- Easy access to lethal methods
- Unwillingness to seek help because of the stigma attached to mental health and substance abuse disorders or suicidal thoughts.

WHAT ARE THE PROTECTIVE FACTORS WHICH CAN HELP

There are several factors which can help protect a victim from attempting to end their life. Sometimes discussing or sharing one's feelings with another person who is close or someone you trust, can help. Suicide is preventable if one can open communication or get treatment for a probable victim.

Protective factors buffer individuals against suicidal thoughts and behaviour. To date, protective factors have not been studied as extensively or rigorously as risk factors. Identifying and understanding protective factors are, however, equally as important as researching risk factors.

Effective clinical care for mental, physical, and substance abuse disorders can be life-saving. If a person is feeling suicidal because of drug or alcohol abuse, the best support one can provide a de-addiction centre or mental health clinic. There should be easy access to a variety of clinical interventions and support for seeking help.

Family and community support (connectedness): Adolescents and children, can be close to their family members. They have strong emotional ties. If a family member suspects that one of their loved ones might be suicidal, it is best to talk to that person and see that the person is never left alone.

Skills in problem-solving, conflict resolution, and non-violent ways of handling disputes: At times, violence and conflict

Family and friends may come across people who have negative reactions towards them. For example, some may see suicide as a mark of failure. Others may not know how to respond because suicide is seen as a socially unacceptable cause of death. Some people simply avoid the issue out of embarrassment.[289]

68. ADOLESCENTS

ADOLESCENTS MENTAL HEALTH CONTINUANCE IN TEEN AGE
Adolescence is considered as a period of transition from childhood to adulthood. It is characterised by rapid physical growth and significant physical, emotional, psychological and spiritual changes. According to WHO adolescents are young people between the ages of 10 and 19 years. It is the stage of life during which individuals reach sexual maturity. It is the period of transition from puberty to maturity, period of rapid physical growth, sexual and psychological changes. Adolescents constitute about 20% population in India

Teenagers can experience crises. Adolescence is a traumatic time. Parents may feel confused and frustrated in their interactions with the teenager. The parents may disagree and argue about what should be done, thus losing them credibility. However, sometimes parents may feel the need to seek help from mental health professionals. Schools may try to help, but may blame the student, who will eventually drop out if they feel school is boring, unsupervised or humiliating for them. Some children may only go to school to be with friends who have access to drugs, cars, cigarettes and so on. The possibility of drug or alcohol use may be overlooked by doctors, counsellors or parents, as they are afraid or reluctant to give their child a drugs screen. They may take the child's word that they are not using alcohol or drugs. Also, a teenager may admit to drinking, but not to taking drugs. Drugs and a negative peer or social group can seriously affect a teenager's life and put them on a negative pathway. Many adolescent girls are sexually active but lack information and skill for self-protection.

Adolescents have crucial reproductive health needs: menstrual hygiene, contraception (including emergency contraception) safety from sexually transmitted diseases and HIV and communication gap exists with parents and other adults especially on these issues. The 70% of the deaths in adulthood is linked to habits picked up during adolescence (risk-taking behaviour, substance abuse, eating habit and conflict resolution). Habits and behaviour picked up during adolescence have lifelong impact. Adolescence is the last chance to correct the growth lag and malnutrition. Adolescent girls definitely constitute socially disadvantageous group in our society, especially in rural areas. Lack of 'connectedness' with parents and other adults prevents transmission of health messages and crucial skills leading to adoption of risky behaviour, substance abuse, early sexual debut and sexually transmitted diseases. Adolescent mothers are at a higher risk of miscarriages, maternal mortality and give birth to stillborn and under weight babies. Adolescent nutritional problems are common throughout the country.

They have to encounter a series of serious nutritional challenges not only affecting their growth and development but also their livelihood as adults.

Sometimes, the way adolescents present their problem appears similar to what is seen in early phase of psychosis (many call it as nervous problem or break down). They behave in a manner which is disorganised, develop thoughts which does not make sense, sometimes start hearing voices when no one is speaking, may become irritable and give you a sense that they are unpredictable for doing anything irrational. Studies conducted among adolescents have found that the prevalence of 'psychotic experiences' in this age group is between 17% and 18%. These are frequently associated with states of emotional disturbances (mood or anxiety disorders) and it has been stated that in 90% of these cases, no declared psychotic disorder is developed. Psychotic experiences reported by young people are rarely interpreted as isolated and declared psychoses: in actual fact, they may throw light on the existence of neurotic psychopathology.

Adolescence is a crucial period for developing and maintaining social and emotional habits important for mental well-being. These include adopting healthy sleep patterns; taking regular exercise; developing coping, problem-solving, and interpersonal skills; and learning to manage emotions. Supportive environments in the family, at school, and in the wider community are also important. Multiple factors determine the mental health of an adolescent. Factors which can contribute to stress during adolescence include a desire for greater autonomy, pressure to conform to peers, exploration of sexual identity, and increased access to and use of technology. Other important determinants for the mental health of adolescents are the quality of their home life and their relationships with their peers. Violence (including harsh parenting and bullying) and socio-economic problems are recognised risks to mental health. Children and adolescents are especially vulnerable to sexual violence, which has a clear association with detrimental mental health. Some adolescents are at greater risk of mental health conditions due to their living conditions, stigma, discrimination or exclusion, or lack of access to quality support and services.

There is no magic pill for the treatment of behaviour problem but it is heartening to know that about half of the adolescents grow out of such problems fully, and the other half persist with a minor or major psychiatric problem which can be treated with some success. Professional help is necessary. It is helpful if parents can observe the behaviour at an early age and do a proper intervention, it's difficult to define the term proper' but it means a respectful treatment in relating to them. Adolescents need to be heard. On many occasions their fears are genuine but they are denied the opportunity to express. Traditions, excessive control, the presence of stress, unpleasant family environment, etc contribute to the occurrence of such episodes. When the critics erupt it is important to ensure safety for everybody, there is the high incident of consuming pills or trying to run away from the house or attempt suicide. It is also important to remember that the difficulty arises more because of consequences and complications of adolescent crisis rather than from the crisis itself. If the crisis is not attended to the behaviour continues, they are conveying a clear signal to be understood and the attempt should be made. At the same time treatment of anxiety is also important. In our society where treatment for behavioural problems is not easily available and it is also not the mindset of people to approach mental health professionals for what they call it as 'day-to-day' difficulties. The best answer is to remain vigilant, identify early and intervene on a priority basis by talking and educating, we must provide an answer to emotional problems. Finally, for severe cases no doubt a psychiatric intervention would be necessary.

69. EATING BEHAVIOUR

Eating disorder is also a severe condition. Most people suffer from mild form of the illness and never realise the problem. The symptoms which are low intensity also lead to extreme behavioural symptoms, and psychological distress. People with problems of eating disorder remain mentally preoccupied and their mindset revolves around eating or binging.

Many more people suffer from problems of eating behaviour which do not qualify for 'diagnosis' and remain as low intensity symptoms. Often people consider it as 'typical feature' of a person. However it is important to understand that these symptoms increase or become severe when people face severe psychological stress or adverse social conditions. It is important to recognise the presence of eating disorder but at the same time it is also important to recognise people who are 'vulnerable' to it. Eating disorders are not merely disorders of eating behaviour but these disorders represent certain biological changes in the body which lead to abnormal behaviour patterns. Very few pay attention to eating disorders thinking that it could be a lifestyle choice. If you notice abnormal eating behaviour in your loved one which is causing trouble in his or her life it could signal a psychological problem where treatment is necessary. At times eating disorders can be dangerous even causing death. The late Princess Diana was reportedly suffering from one.

Eating disorder (ED) is a serious psychiatric disorder which is progressively increasing in the younger generation, which alters cognitive function, judgment, emotional stability, and restrict the life activities of an individual.

There are three types of eating disorders, anorexia nervosa, bulimia nervosa, and binge-eating disorder. Anorexia nervosa is a slow-growing disorder of behaviour with serious biological changes. It is an intense desire of keeping the body weight at the minimum even if they are already very thin. People suffering from this problem refuses to maintain normal weight by restricting the food intake, this behaviour, as well as the distress associated with it, become so severe that they start forcefully taking out food by purging or vomiting the food they had eaten. They remain mentally preoccupied with thoughts of reducing weight. Along with the symptoms of eating behaviour depression, anxiety, rumination, obsession, fearfulness are other very common features. This illness becomes so severe that more than 20% to 30% years of life is often spent in hospitals. This ailment is more common among females, about 10% people die due to medical complication arising due to lack of food intake. Such patients make several attempts of self-harm due to sadness and frustration arising out of distress due to the illness. Anorexia nervosa can cause heart and kidney problems, low blood iron, bone loss, digestive problems, low heart rate, low blood pressure, and fertility problems in women.

Bulimia nervosa involves periods of uncontrollable binge-eating (stuffing themselves with food) followed by purging (eliminating food, such as by vomiting or using laxatives). Such people always feel their body weight is higher no matter what the actual weight is. They feel worthless and sad. Health problems caused by bulimia nervosa may include kidney problems, dehydration, and digestive problems. Forced vomiting can damage a person's teeth, mouth, and throat. People who experience binge-eating disorder may feel they can't control how much they eat and feel distressed, depressed, or guilty after binging. They keep the binging pattern secret. People who experience lower self-esteem or poor body image, perfectionism, dealing with stress may be more likely to experience an eating disorder. Many people who experience an eating disorder are scared to go through treatment because they may believe that they will have to gain weight. Many also feel a lot of shame or guilt around their illness, so the thought of talking about very personal experiences can seem overwhelming.

BINGE EATING

Eating disorder is also a severe condition. Most people suffer from mild form of the illness and never realise the problem. The symptoms which are low intensity also lead to extreme behavioural symptoms, and psychological distress. People with problems of eating disorder remain mentally preoccupied and their mindset revolves around eating or binging. These people plan, collect means, find a situation which is favourable and finally succeed in carrying out excessive eating despite their desire not to do so. This pattern of behaviour persists. Most of the management is behavioural, e.g. change in situation, selecting food habits, engaging with people to discuss the distress, watching out for mood symptoms and suicidal thoughts which should be treated as described earlier.

70 ATTENTION DEFICIT DISORDER.

Many children develop problems of concentration and at the same time some of them also develop difficulty to remain restless. They are always running around remaining restless and unable to sit in one place. These behaviours are not in their control, which leads to significant distress. It is a disorder of brain which presents with behavioural symptoms and leads to poor academic performance and social functioning. Children typically develop hyperactivity, do not sit in one place, they're unable to focus their attention on any task. The problem begins much early in the age and significantly reduces by the age of 17 or 18. In about 20% cases the difficulty continues into adulthood, which presents with symptoms of anxiety and depression. It is a disorder with strong genetic component. A small percentage of ADHD problem may be caused by drinking and smoking during pregnancy, complications during pregnancy and labour or any injury to brain after birth and exposure to toxic substances. Although exact cause of the disease is not known, modern methods of scanning the brain has shown some abnormalities between those who ADHD and those who do not.

There are many factors that might contribute to ADHD, these include genes, cigarette smoking/ alcohol intake during pregnancy and low birth weight. The cardinal three symptoms which form a typical constellation of symptom include: inability. To focus attention (Inattention), Hyperactivity and Impulsivity (acting without thinking).

CHAPTER 8
PERSONAL DEVELOPMENT

71. ENHANCING PROTECTIVE MECHANISMS

So far we have seen that mental health problems can be minimised by reducing the risk factors which are involved in perpetuating the mental ill-health. Though some conditions of mental health abnormalities may be prevented by reducing the risk it will not be enough for prevention in long-term course. This is because the risk factors can be of several types, and each one have their own lethality (potential to cause abnormality). These risk factors are not specific. E.g. we cannot say that one has developed depression because of cannabis abuse, and if there was no cannabis abuse depression would not have surfaced. Similarly, if one is having financial issues at home and he fails in the exams, has no funds to pay the following years fees, if such a person develops depression, it cannot be said for sure, which stressful factor is primarily responsible. Moreover, risk factors work in synergy and their compound impact is much larger than expected. Going by the principle of risk reduction, we will have to target risks arising from multiple dimensions of psychological, social or cultural nature. These risk factors are classified into two types. 1. Modifiable and 2. Non-modifiable. For example, risk due to family history, or previous episode of illness, trauma, bereavement, cannot be reduced however, their effect can be reduced to certain extent by building protective mechanisms. Because of these reasons, adopting the strategy of reducing the risk is not a good plan. For effective prevention, both the methods have to be adopted. Building protective factors creates positive environment which improves motivation, self-awareness, self-confidence and ability to look for options. The most common method for development of protective mechanism is to adapt mental health promotion plans or incorporate its strategy in a well-structured plan.

We always talk about strength and weaknesses in our life. It is a popular discussion, whether one is strong or not strong. Virtually the terminology strong or weak is a misnomer. Factually it means that how effectively we can deal with adverse situations or adverse factors. This characteristic is because of protective mechanisms. These mechanisms lie within us. It can be increased or decreased based upon resources and supports available to us and also by changing our methods to deal with adverse situations. Everyone has effective protective mechanism; it may fall short of fighting an unusual situation. Only in some cases people lack the protective mechanism which can lead to psychological abnormalities. Though we may say that since a greater number of people are suffering from stress their ability to protect themselves may be declining, however, this needs to be evaluated in the backdrop of social complexity. There are number of things which are known to increase positivity, mental attitude, personality and grit. A large part of these characteristics come with us since birth. Some of it is nurtured during childhood development and experiences. How protective factors work to prevent mental disorders is a novel area of research. It is worth exploring how cultural, religious and spiritual dimensions are involved in providing strength to human beings.

PERSONAL DEVELOPMENT AND MENTAL HEALTH

Mental health is not the same thing as the absence of a mental illness. Mental health includes emotional, psychological and social well-being. It can influence: How you feel about yourself, your ability to solve problems and overcome challenges, your ability to build relationships with others and contribute to your community and Your ability to achieve your goals.

Personal development is a technique to promote mental health status i.e. means which help you to maintain positive state of mental health and achieve a state of wellness.

Thus, personal development is a process to achieve total healthy state which includes emotional, physical, social, cognitive and spiritual dimensions.

It is a comprehensive set of interventions which allows you to achieve a sense of accomplishment, happiness and satisfaction. It provides emotional stability, a clear thought process to understand the meaning of life – and carry yourself in all possible situations. A stable and organised state improves your involvement in nature, self and others, develops sense of social responsibility and a spiritual mindset. It is a personal journey and process for fulfilment and self-confidence, it facilitates insight into recognising and respecting your own self.

The principle of wellness is based upon managing stress response which leads to physiological changes.

Some of the interventions which are commonly proposed are:

Yoga
Mindfulness
Mood regulation
Social engagement
Stress management
Coping and building resilience

Personality development
Building self-worth and emotional capital
Building resilience
Spiritual mindset
Positivity
Anger management
Physical exercise
Behaviour modification

72. WELLNESS

The practical failure of psychiatry to improve well-being is not surprising because focus of psychiatry has been on mental disorders, not on the understanding or development of positive mental health.[290]

Wellness is a concept which is all about how people can enhance the quality of their lives and avoid serious illness by making simple but sometimes surprisingly difficult changes to their lifestyles. Wellness is a broad topic that includes disease prevention, stress reduction, and even personal, social and spiritual growth.

Our mental health/wellness allows us to realise our potential, cope with stress effectively, bounce back from life challenges and be active, productive members of our communities. It is a conscious pursuit of spiritual growth, life purpose, and self-actualisation. It is attained by those who are motivated by the desire to grow and find meaning in life, rather than by insecurities and an attempt to fit in a state of wellbeing means:[291] knowing yourself better in order to identify what holds you back to become the best you, having ability to be able to fully exploit your talents and capacities to fulfill your potential and find your purpose and meaning. Mental wellness goes hand-in-hand with physical health. When you eat well, get enough sleep and stay active, your emotional health can improve. Following healthy routines can improve your self-esteem, help mental function, and make it easier for you to deal with stress. In turn, feeling mentally well can boost your motivation to stick with healthy habits.

No one experiences perfect mental health or well-being all of the time. We all have to learn how to balance the different aspects of our lives. When things in our life change, we have to re-establish the balance. However, ongoing mental health problems can take a real toll on your well-being and affect

- Relationships with others
- Sleep
- Appetite
- Energy levels
- Ability to think clearly or make decisions
- Physical health
- Life satisfaction and more

How each of us defines our mental health/wellness can be very different and quite individualised. It is important to keep in mind, that good mental health/wellness is not about avoiding problems or having the perfect life. Rather, it is about living well and feeling capable despite life's challenges. Our mental health and our capacity to maintain our mental wellness is based on many factors. Lifestyles that incorporate a holistic approach that focus on our physical, spiritual, emotional, social and intellectual health, place us in the best position to live a healthy, mentally well, life.

Spirituality in a clear, meaningful way that will help you reach your human potential and become the best and happiest. You can realise the effect of spirituality on your physical and mental health, and the way it contributes to your happiness and life satisfaction, Discover the wonderful person you are, with a deepened awareness of your true identity and a desire to return to your authentic self. Identify and honour your vales in your thoughts, words, and actions, forming a solid foundation that will direct you to lasting happiness and a fulfilling life.

Wellness is not a new idea. Objective of health has always been to achieve a happy state of mind rather than just being free from diseases. The western world's healthcare establishment has historically always focused on illness and curing illness. Medical doctors, psychologists and other health professionals are primarily taught categories of disease and how to fix those diseases.[292]

Personal development is an integrative approach to combining biological, psychological, social, and spiritual approaches to mental health. The scientific basis for this science of well-being.[293]

Action can be taken to promote positive mental health for individuals and communities at the individual, community and system level. At the individual and community level, mental health promotion strategies focus on enhancing individuals' empowerment and participation and can target a range of environments or settings, such as the workplace, home, school or community. These strategies primarily seek to strengthen factors that protect positive mental health, lessen risk factors for poor mental health and/or address the social determinants of health. At the system level, strategies focus on addressing the social determinants of health and must involve work across a range of sectors and policy areas, such as housing, employment, social assistance, settlement and others.

Emotional intelligence enables us to monitor our impact on others, manage our own stress, and respond more effectively to others.[294]

Improving our emotional intelligence can help us achieve number of mental attributes and regulate several psychological and physiological functions. It facilitates the process to have insight into our emotional triggers, identify our emotions and the sources of our feelings and reduce the likelihood of making poor choices. It helps in managing conflict more effectively and reduce the intensity of negative emotions. Emotions that are strongly positive or negative can lift or lower the energy of a team. Regulating mood by slowing down breathing, reducing tension and preventing future tension. Putting anger into perspective by challenging angry thoughts and identifying anger as a 'secondary emotion' – meaning that it may be a symptom of an underlying 'primary emotion' that may be hidden or more difficult to deal with. Examining exactly what an emotional response may be and the nature of emotional triggers helps to address different situations. Examining thoughts, which have a direct influence on feelings and understanding barriers is a first step toward being comfortable and effective when dealing with negative emotions. Fulfilling basic human needs is critical for overall life satisfaction. It thus can achieve:

- Reduction in anxiety.
- Improved moods.
- Clearer thinking.
- A greater sense of calm or inner peace.
- Increased self-esteem.
- Reduced risk of depression.
- Improvements in relationships.

Benefits of mental health through physical fitness include, but aren't limited to:

- Sharper memory.
- Clarity in thinking.
- Higher self-esteem.
- Better sleep.
- Increased energy.
- Stronger resilience.
- Increased BDNF (Brain-Derived Neurotrophic Factor), which improves neurotransmission.

The five main aspects of personal health are physical, emotional, social, spiritual, and intellectual. In order to be considered 'well'. it is imperative for none of these areas to be neglected (1) physical, (2) emotional, (3) intellectual and (4) spiritual 5social.[295]

The benefits of intentionally practicing improving mental health are a response to the chronic stress reported at epidemic levels around the world. Chronic stress has been proven to deteriorate the hippocampus.[296] This stress also leads to decreased concentration and memory, confusion, loss of sense of humour, anger, irritability, and fear. Obviously, stress is not good for the brain, and improved mental health practices can reduce the risk. Personal development is not a long-term goal or objective, or even social ambition. It is the continuous assessment along with realigning of essential goals that enables you to properly identify and optimise your functional abilities along with potential. Personal development is a vital part of personal growth. Transformation is continuous and inevitable.[297]

Personal Growth is about evolving and is the continuous process of growing yourself to realistically achieve your greatest ability and is vital to your mental health, success, and happiness.

73. LIFE-STYLE INTERVENTION

Lifestyle treatment – truly called as treatment for illnesses and modern names for ancient therapies.

Significance and merit of lifestyle factors as contributors to and treatments for multiple conditions have been seriously underestimated. It has been ignored and its effectiveness has not been properly explained. In fact, it is a comprehensive treatment regime for health, vitality and mental well-being. It is yet to be recognised for its role in accomplishing individual and social well-being, and for preserving and optimising cognitive brain function. Consequently, lifestyle changes are underutilised despite considerable evidence of their effectiveness in both clinical and normal populations. These treatments are sometimes as effective as either psychotherapy (talk therapy) or medications and can offer significant therapeutic advantages.[298] This includes exercise, nutrition and diet, relationships, recreation, relaxation and stress management, religious or spiritual involvement, and service to others. Lifestyle treatment is a combination of therapeutics which restores health from state of illness. This comprehensive management accomplishes the following:

1. Facilities symptom remission
2. Improves vitality
3. Restores state of health
4. Facilitates transition from state of illness to state of health
5. It may minimise the dosage of medications normally used for treatment of psychiatric disorders.
6. Improve state of general well-being
7. Improve physical health
8. Improves acceptability of treatment
9. Considered as 'real-life treatment'
10. Improves compliance in a treatment programme
11. Improves immune response
12. Safeguards physical health
13. Helps in recovery of many disease like hypertension, heart disease, diabetes etc.
14. Finally, it is useful is reducing risk for a number of physical and mental conditions.

Lifestyle treatment is truly a biological treatment. It leads to changes in the brain and body chemistry and facilities restoration of neurochemical and electrochemical activity in the brain.[299]

Lifestyle management consists of relaxation therapy, physical exercise, nutritional balance, cultural and traditional practices, disciplines for life, time management, self-regulation, yoga therapy and meditation, and Spiritual wellness.

Enough research has been conducted to examine its effectiveness in depression, severe mental disorder, heart conditions, cancer, organ transplant, and chronic medical conditions. It has been found effective in number of such conditions. Lifestyle treatment is being recommended more often now than ever before.[300]

Studies have shown that our diet can influence our mental health, for both good and bad. Fruits and vegetable are associated with better mental well-being. Sugar, of course, should have only a minimal place in your diet. Not only can it spark rapid weight gain and an addictive response in some, it has been linked to higher rates of depression and can make mental health symptoms worse. Research data showing that engaging in sports or moderate to rigorous physical activity[301] partaking in cultural or mental activities are valuable methods. It doesn't matter what type of activity—is selected, what matters is to do it. Studies have shown that exercise can reduce anxiety and depression and improve mood, self-esteem and cognitive function from swimming, to jogging, to lifting weights, or playing sport all have their merits.

74. WHAT DOES PERSONALITY INDICATE?

There are billions of people in this world but not any two are alike – in all respect. What makes them different, is their personality. That does not pertain to how they look but like how they behave.

Personality makes people unique. It has hundreds of characteristics or traits.

In general and conventional terms these traits often represent the state of mood, thought, behaviour, mindset, intellectual ability, spiritual characteristic, belief system, value system and many other physical and mental qualities.[302]

Personality is constituted by three factors

1. Genetics – the feature which we get from our parents
2. Environment – where we live, and
3. Experiences during the early course of life.

Many times our behaviour which is also part of personality reflects our experience.

It is common knowledge that confident people are more likely to succeed. Often the question arises that can level of confidence be improved?

Confidence is expression of the characteristics like social skills and cognitive features. The number of factors discussed here contribute building one's confidence. One of the important aspect is the personality. Personality is the most important and fundamental psychological feature which has inputs from thoughts, emotions, and ability to judge a situation along with intelligence and social skills. Personality has several characteristics and not all of them are obvious. Many times certain features may lead to psychological problems. E.g. sometimes what can be impulsive or hyperactive or anxious or restless. Personality characteristics are difficult to change however it can be discussed how to minimise negative psychological impact. Broadly speaking personality factors are positive and contribute to a great deal in accomplishing success.

Personality refers to individual differences in characteristic patterns of thinking, feeling and behaving. The study of personality focuses on two broad areas:

One is understanding individual differences in particular personality characteristics, such as sociability or irritability.

The other is understanding how the various parts of a person come together as a whole.

Personality begins to shape after birth, matures and continues to develop until teenage/early adulthood.

Personality is also associated with certain brain changes. It is observed that damage or dysfunction of the brain causes a definite change in personality. We often see this in the elderly population who develop brain disorders like dementia.

Personality is a relatively stable construct like any other part of our physical body, once it completes its growth, little changes. All the shades and traits remain, some may be obvious others may not, under circumstances of stress we may see traits which were not seen so far have now become obvious or obvious traits have increased in their severity of degree.[303]

Personality has a close relationship with a psychiatric disorder. Personality disorder by itself is a valid psychiatric diagnosis and personality goes through a definite change in most of the psychiatric conditions. It's like a ground on which a tree of all mental faculties grows and therefore all mental disorders will have shades of change in personality.

The personality function is a stable construct, it neither increases nor decreases in normal conditions, any change in personality is always a matter of concern. It suggests that something in the life of the person is certainly changing.

Normal personality change is a part of the process of transition from adolescence to teenage.

75. PERSONALITY TRAITS

Traits are the building blocks of personality. So what is a trait? In short, it's a relatively stable way of thinking and behaving that can be used to describe a person and compare and contrast that person with others.[304]

Traits can be cast in very broad terms, such as how positively disposed a person generally is toward other people, or in more specific ones, such as how much that person tends to trust other people. These more specific aspects of personality are sometimes referred to as 'facets'. Personality traits are usually considered distinct from mental abilities (including general intelligence) that are assessed based on how well one responds to problems or questions.

A personality trait is a characteristic pattern of thinking, feeling, or behaving that tends to be consistent over time and across relevant situations.

There are billions of people in this world but not any two are alike – in all respect. What makes them different, is their personality. That's not who they look but like how they behave and have many other characteristics.

Personality makes people unique.

It has hundreds of characteristics or traits

In general and conventional terms these traits can often represent the mood, thought, behaviour, mindset, intellectual ability, spiritual characteristic, belief system, value system and many other physical and mental qualities.

Personality is constituted by three factors 1-genetics – the feature which we get from our parents 20 environmentwhere we live and 3 experiences during the early course of life.[305] Many times our behaviour which is also part of personality reflects our experience.

Personality begins to shape after birth, matures and continues to develop until adolescence or early teenage.

Personality as 'individual differences in characteristic patterns of thinking, feeling and behaving'.[306]

However you define personality, it's an important part of who you are. Personality shows a positive correlation with life satisfaction.[307] With personality having such a large impact on our lives, it's important to have a reliable way to conceptualise and measure it.

Personality approaches describe a youth's characteristics that are considered relatively stable across time and situations and include regulatory abilities, such as cognition, emotions, and behaviours that serve as primary targets of intervention programmes.[308]

Personality is also associated with certain brain changes. It is observed that damage or dysfunction of the brain causes a definite change in personality, we often see this in the elderly population who develop brain disorders like dementia.

Personality is a relatively stable construct like any other part of our physical body, once it completes its growth, little changes. All the shades and traits remain, some may be obvious others may not, under circumstances of stress we may see traits which were not seen have become obvious or obvious traits have increased in their severity of degree.

Personality has a close relationship with a psychiatric disorder. personality disorder by itself is a valid psychiatric diagnosis and personality goes through a definite change in most of the psychiatric conditions. It's like aground on which a tree of all mental faculties grows and therefore all mental disorders will have shades of change in personality.

The personality functions is a stable construct, it neither increases nor decreases in normal conditions, any change in personality is always a matter of concern, it suggests that something life of the person is certainly changing.

Normal personality change is part of the process of transition from adolescence to teenage.

76. SIGNIFICANCE OF KNOWING PERSONALITY TYPE

To know yourself generally, people become aware of it after a long time in life, but everyone should understand the nature and type of a person. Knowing one's personality will help in understanding of:

a. Cognitive ability
b. Functional capacity
c. Performance in job, education
d. Risk factors for health
e. Social characteristics
f. Serious limitations or caution
g. Possibility of mental illness and physical illness

It is possible to get this information because personality is a collective reflection of many mental characteristics e.g. mood state, intellectual capacity, thought process, the field of interest, the field of excellence etc. Personality type also reflects the biochemical aspect of life and it can predict the possibility of physical abnormality e.g. behavioural traits related to cardiac disease or diabetes. Thus one can have some idea to predict:

- Performance
- Health risk
- Cautions for risky behaviour

Since personality type does not change, to a large extent, and remains stable prediction of various features becomes possible with some degree of reliability.

Personality traits which are reliable to indicate the likelihood of future behaviour, abilities or a psychiatric disorder are:

1. Limitation in intellectual ability
2. Field of exceptional qualities
3. Academic achievement
4. Ability to form a relationship with people in society, known or unknown.
5. Ability to form a romantic relationship
6. Ability to sustain a relationship or frequently get bored with a relationship
7. Avoid interaction
8. Inability to take responsibility

Common traits of significance

1. Excessive Anxious behaviours
2. Aggressive behaviour
3. Depressed in mood
4. Overjoyed in behaviours
5. Suspicious in the thought process
6. Obsessive in thoughts
7. Compulsive in behaviour
8. Organised in behaviour or doing activities
9. Concentration or inability to focus
10. Attention seeking
11. Avoiding others
12. Impulsive
13. Inability to take responsibility
14. Shallow emotion
15. Inability to relate or connect emotionally
16. Inadequate in functioning
17. Remaining insight less

Personality traits significantly indicate:

a. Behavioural traits of a psychiatric disorder are seen in personality before the onset of an illness.
b. People are more likely to develop a psychiatric disorder according to the personality type e.g. if a person is suspicious, he/she is more likely to develop a disorder of thought like paranoia, delusions, paranoid schizophrenia etc. while. An obsessive person is likely to develop problems like an obsessive-compulsive disorder
c. Change in personality type is reliable to the marker of psychiatric or neurological disease.
d. Personality traits can be defined as normal and abnormal depending upon the natural consequences. if a personality trait starts interfering in daily life to a significant degree in any of eh social, mental or physical areas it can be called abnormal e.g. if a person who is obsessive and likely to keep his study room excessively clean, starts becoming mentally preoccupied with thoughts and activity cleaning a depends more than the usual amount of time in keeping the room clean, his behaviour warrants the possibility of an obsessive-compulsive disorder. Similarly, if a person is depressive and feeling low in mood is part of his 'persona', generally spends

> time alone a withdrawn starts seclusion and remaining absent from job because of changes in his mood, a possibility of moor disorder must be considered.

It is extremely difficult to determine abnormality from normality much before significant deterioration has taken place or any risk behaviour has developed. This is a clinical skill which mental health professional learn during their training. However, everyone in the family needs to be aware of what is the nature of normal personality and when it is becoming abnormal. Information about such change becomes available after an illness has developed.

77. BELIEVE THAT SITUATION CAN CHANGE

She was of age 20 years, shy, thin, never did she interact with anyone with confidence or command, always a victim of her father's criticism and humiliation for being so unattractive. It was repeatedly imbibed on her that no one could be interested in her because she was not charming. She and her father the two members in the household, lived in a village which by a river separated from the mainland. The father was out of job, shameless and lazy, his wife was no more. This man had lost 3 of his sons to infectious disease and was now leading his frustrating and hopeless life with his unattractive daughter. He could no more appreciate the normal things happening around him, his only daughter was a subject of his anger and he tried to be critical so that she could change and present herself better. But the poor girl was so down with guilt that she let a life with downcast eyes filled with hopelessness and dried up tears. She was listless and without any vigour or energy. The girl who lived with her father was always a victim of the morale of her father who said that no one would come and he will not find a single cow in rerun of her marriage (this was accustom in that village that the bridegroom would present few cows to the father while asking hand of his daughter to marry)

One day came a young man from a nearby village and met the father of the girl who was surprised that anyone would want to marry this girl. The father was sure there was some kind of misunderstanding and he was not at all sure of the intentions of the boy who was asking his daughter's hand in marriage. He raised his demand and said he would take three cows right away and two after the marriage was ceremonies. The young man went away after making note of the demand. The father was sure that the boy was never going to return because he was not genuinely interested in her.

The young man came back and he said he would get married and offered 11 cows, and not just 5 as per the demand. He had an inkling that this father was greedy, but he wanted to marry this girl because he had liked her. Both were married the following Sunday. After one year she returned to her father's house.

The father was amazed to see a beautiful and charming daughter full of confidence and not just the father but all the neighbours were surprised at such a transformation in an years time. The story is simple. it's about the psychological qualities, the environment has a lot of influence. Whenever it is a positive environment which can increase the morale of the human being everything changes. She changed because she was in a loving environment with a confident person and he could infuse the same in her mindset. It's never late and it is possible.

People are born with one set of characters and they learn the other set of characteristics from the environment. What does the environment consist of, it is not constructed without people who are living in your proximity? Depending on one's ability to grasp the influences of another one can bring positive changes

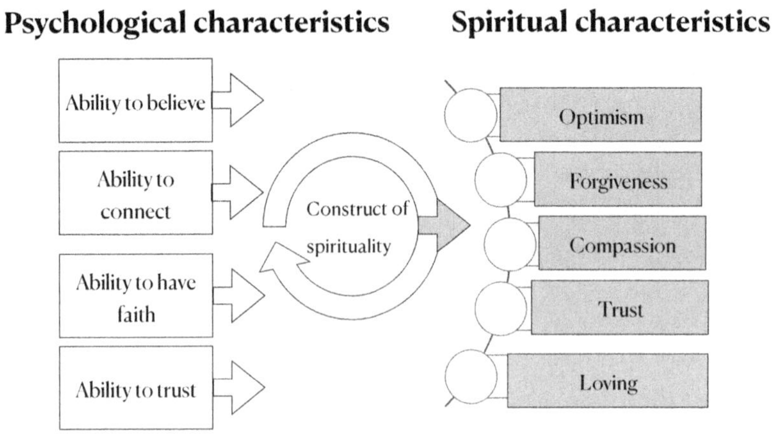
Psychological characteristics
Spiritual characteristics
Ability to believe
Ability to connect
Ability to have faith
Ability to trust
Construct of spirituality
Optimism
Forgiveness
Compassion
Trust
Loving

Spirituality enhances ability to deal with stress and trauma-1

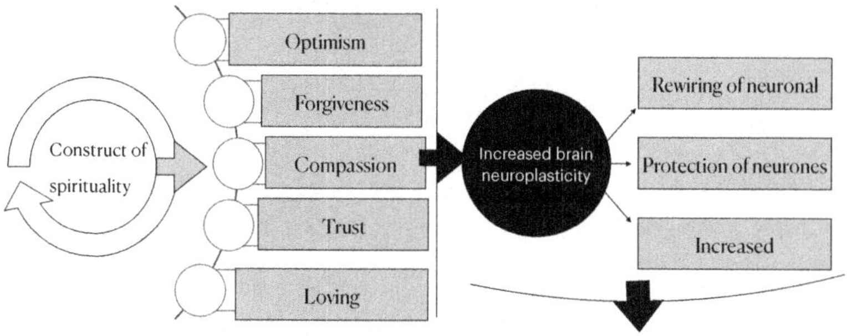

Spirituality enhances ability to deal with stress and trauma- 2

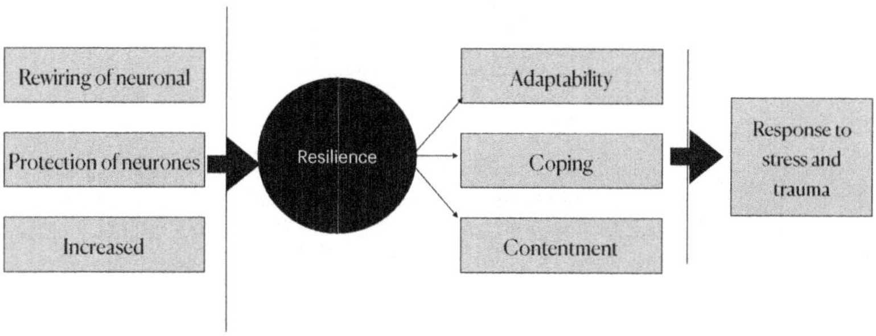

Spirituality modulates learning

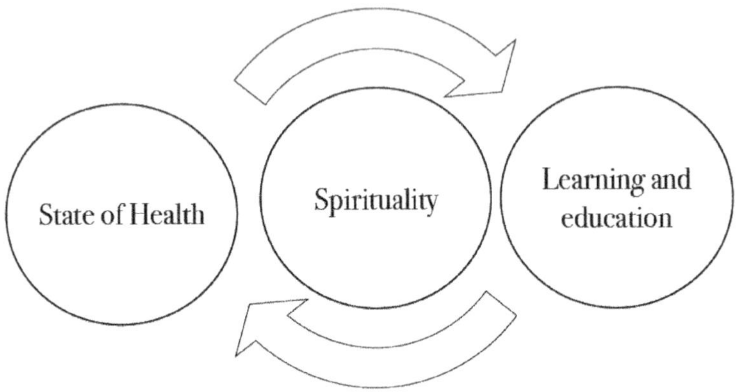

CHAPTER 9
SPIRITUAL MENTAL HEALTH AND SUCCESS

78. SPIRITUALITY, YOGA AND LESSONS FROM BHAGVAD GITA

INTRODUCTION
The idea of success is always changing. In the past, success was seen as achieving only material items. Then, came the onslaught of people feeling both empty and lost. Turning to **Spirituality** to void the feelings of emptiness. Success is many things, in fact, these factors are the basic spin-off for securing monetary success. Only when we have sound health, innate happiness, a passion for life and our career do we really achieve the big stakes when it comes to financial success.[309]

Spirituality has direct effects on purpose in life but had only indirect effects on academic engagement and academic success. Purpose in life had direct effects on academic engagement but only indirect effects on academic success.[310]

Spiritual experience, mindset and practice facilitate the process of success and achievement.

79. UNDERSTANDING SPIRITUALITY

Spiritualism is a part of Indian civilization ever since its existence.

It occupies a highly valuable and respectable position due to its relationship with mind and soul. Spiritualism in India and many eastern countries is recognised as a way of life which provides eternal joy. The spiritual joy is considered superior to the intellectual joy and provides ultimate satisfaction. It is identified with something superconscious and closer to divinity. The spiritual experience brings the knowledge of super consciousness and spiritual individuals experience ultimate satisfaction lesser degree of frustration & disappointment but.

Spirituality is considered a broader concept than religion. The concepts of spirituality are varied, but by and large each school of spirituality considers that religion is a subset of spirituality which encompasses a system of beliefs and practices observed by a community, supported by rituals that acknowledge, worship, or communicate, these may be the Sacred, the Divine, God or Ultimate Truth, Reality or Nirvana. Thus, religion is one way for spiritual people to express their spirituality. It also clarifies that religious people, by definition, are spiritual people, but not all spiritual people have to be religious. These beliefs and goals help us find meaning and purpose in life and a sense that we are connected to something of greater significance than us.

Spirituality is experienced by everyone. Some people believe in it and others do not. Spirituality is now included in the field of medicine. While examining a patient if we pose questions about their spiritual attitude and beliefs, it is not a surprise that more than half of the patient population unhesitantly admit about their belief in a superpower and belief in God. It is believed that doctor's faith or spiritualism may also be influencing the patients' treatment. Studies have tried to examine this issue and it is found that about 20% of doctors are found to be believers in spiritualism and faith.

80. SPIRITUALITY IS THE 4TH DIMENSION OF HEALTH

Clinical position of spirituality in mental health as well as in physical health is firmly rooted in the knowledge base of medicine and wisdom of physicians since historical times. The premise for discussion about spiritualism is that health and disease also have a dimension of spirituality and spiritual practices are remarkably effective as an intervention for psychiatric problems on their own and much better in combination with other well-known treatments. If that's the case, as it is, prevention of psychiatric diseases is not unlikely by enhancing the individual's 'SPIRITUAL WORTH'.

The special group of WHO executive board (1998) proposed that the amendment is required in the preamble of its constitution. They proposed a new definition of health as: 'Health is a dynamic state of complete physical, mental, spiritual and social wellbeing and not merely the absence of disease or infirmity.' The board rejected the proposal, but it hardly made any difference to the growth of this speciality. Experts in research continued to consider spirituality as necessary dimension of health.

Spirituality has been considered as one of the determinants of mental health since a long time. Several organisations considered spirituality related to mental health and mental disorders. World Health Organization develops International Classification of Diseases (ICD) to define all medical conditions. which is used all over the world. American Psychiatric Association conducts the research and defines all the disease to develop a system is known as 'Diagnostic and Statistical Manual' (DSM). These are quite popular and used in routine clinical work in several countries. In both the systems religion, spirituality, and psychiatric illnesses share a complex relationship in the realm of diagnosis. Historically, however, these three constructs have existed in a understanding of health related abnormalities.[311] The DSM-5 includes religion and spirituality as part of pathology or culture. Religion as a cultural derivative only reflects the human aspect of religion.[312,313] Spirituality provides a systematic outline for incorporating culturally relevant information when conducting an examination of a patient and formulating multiaxial diagnosis. [314,315]

Spirituality appears to be an independent internal construct of human being's psyche, which offers a protective network for everyone. It protects moral, ethical values, social norms, regulates brain-mind functions, and overall contributes towards the development of orderly personality with high self-worth. It is a part of medical assessment, a stand-alone treatment as well. It is the most sought after therapy for end of life support for terminal or chronic severely ill patients to make the difficult journey of life easy.

81. SPIRITUAL HEALTH

Spiritual health is that dimension of health which deals with the everyday problems, facilitating the utilisation of one's full potential. It entails a condition of spiritual well-being which include a range of determinants like personal, social, economic and environmental factors.[316,317]

> *"Ayurveda is a knowledge which indicates the appropriate and inappropriate, happy and sorrowful conditions of living, which is auspicious or inauspicious for longevity, as well as the measure of life itself"*
>
> – *Charak Sanhita 1.41*

Confluence of spirituality and health has been known since the time of Vedic sciences. Ayurveda is the fourth branch of Vedic sciences. Yoga Meditation and Astrology are the first three and Ayurveda is its branch for dealing with physical body. According to Ayurveda a disease is viewed as lack of proper cellular function due to an excess or deficiency of Vata, Pitta or Kapha. Disease can also be caused by presence of toxins. In Ayurveda, body, mind and consciousness work together in maintaining balance.

According to Vedic sciences Ayurveda is 'an integral spiritual science devised to give a comprehensive understanding of all universe.' Ayurveda includes herbal medicine, dietic, body work, surgery, psychology and spirituality. Spirituality thus is the core feature of health and psychology.

The practice of medicine was originally based on spiritual sciences. The physicians were trained with spiritual knowledge. The medications used were substances to regulate the disease components. The advancement of modern medicine during the past 200 years focussed its attention on disease, rather than health. It believed in cellular and molecular level of pathology and for unknown reasons neglected the science which involved genesis of fundamental material for life. As time passed by, we learned more about illnesses and less about prevention and well-being. In last 30-40 years it was realised that the large number of patients were not improving beyond symptomatic remission. Their sense of pleasure and happiness did not return and in many treatments, patients did not gain psychological improvement. Obviously, despite revolutionary advances in treatment and a better understanding of the causes of illness, something was missing in therapeutics. At this juncture it did not take much to realise that the entire concept of health was erroneous. Thus, contribution of social factors and mental health was incorporated in definition of health. This solved the problem of achieving desired outcome to some extent. It is only after the physicians started thinking about health conditions and prevention of diseases that spiritual component was brought in as an integral part of health. Today there is a strong movement to understand illnesses from a spiritual perspective to find out more about the abnormalities in the spiritual health and to design treatments based on the theory that increasing spiritualism will improve the outcome of treatment in a patient.

In ancient times medicine was considered abnormality of a spiritual and religious causes of physical or mental illness. However modern medicine explicitly moved away from any role of religion or spirituality in medicine.[318] Which is now showing a trend of re-appearance supported by research findings.

A recent survey endorses the facts about spirituality among patients as well as among doctors. The study was conducted in the United States, it highlighted that,[319] 76.5% of Americans consider themselves to belong to a faith, 37% described themselves as spiritual, but not religious and the remaining 42% said they were neither.[320]

A study on "Spirituality and health: a knowledge, attitude and practice study among doctors of North India", found that 65.65% had a strong or very strong belief in the spiritual dimension of health; 55.22% believed in the preventive role of spirituality; 80% believed in the curative role of spirituality and a similar proportion held the view that spirituality has an important role in day-to-day patient care. The most significant finding was that 93.48% of the doctors believe that a spiritual person deals better with stress.[321]

In last two decades there have been rapid advances in this field. While this change was occurring the concept of mental health was also undergoing an evolution. As a result, spirituality became a part of mental health care.[322]

Origin of this bidirectional relationship lies in the roots of the concept of health, based upon multiple theories primarily from Vedic sciences, the Ayurveda and the concept of spirituality in modern medicine- the WHO definition. Similarly, almost all religions have described spiritual health and mental health as complementary to each other. They have defined that this intricate relationship attains good mental health and spiritual mindset and vice-versa. There is no doubt that spirituality and mental health is intricately related. Those showing poorer spirituality have poor mental health and more incidence of, mental health challenges, e.g., presence of substance abuse disorder or addiction. Some groups of patients may be more vulnerable for mental illnesses, possibly because of several risk factors, like genetics, childhood abuse etc. these may be responsible for such pathology. We need more research into this area to carry out studies of risk factors and psychopathology among people with spirituality and religious group and those without a mental disorder.

Further, the Spirituality specialist is a member of the multidisciplinary team which undertakes the planning of treatment and care. It is now slowly getting into the field of training and education in medical institutions. It is well established now that spirituality is an independent paradigm of health. By and large, the relationship between spirituality and mental health works towards the advantage of a person.

Concept of spirituality and its relevance to mental health has been aptly described by the Royal College of psychiatrists, UK.[323] It says that 'spirituality is something everyone can experience, helps us to find meaning and purpose in the things we value, can bring hope and healing in times of suffering and loss, encourages us to seek the best relationship with our-selves, others and what lies beyond.'

It was well known that spirituality is close to mind. There are certain biological changes in brain and related biochemical parameters which increase the vulnerability for developing mental disorder. Number of findings from a modern method like neurochemistry, immunology, electrophysiology and brain imaging brought in convincing evidence that spirituality was a dominant determinant of health and disease.

In majority of studies, the results, which have been thoroughly analysed, showed significant improvement due to spiritual intervention. Number of specific treatments were developed for several diseases. Now it is practised in a clinical setting, many hospitals have programs for hospitalized as well as out-patient's treatments, priests and chapels have found places in hospital premises.

"Individual's spiritual health can deal with day-to-day life in a manner which leads to the realization of one's full potential, meaning and purpose of life and happiness from within".[324]

Those who have faith and trust can establish a better relationship with doctors and caregivers. Likewise, there are other human qualities which are not well-defined in 'illness' model, though they significantly affect life of those who are suffering. The attributes like resilience, optimism, trust or faith and capacity of being connected to any superpower constitute the spiritual qualities. Spiritualism is widespread in everyone's life, in fact there is no one without it.

During the practice of medicine, it was observed that several qualities of human beings are related to the health status. It is a general observation that spiritually minded people generally maintain healthier life than those who are not. Their overall well-being and happiness gave them greater confidence. It is generally noted that people with incurable diseases or chronic resistant conditions turn to 'spiritual healers' or temples or priests to seek relief from pain and sufferings. They seem to experience relief in the comfort zone and are satisfied that they have done their best, or all that can be done. Many would term it as religiosity, not spirituality.[325] Though the two are different there is a significant overlap in terms of practices and outcomes. Moreover, religiosity by itself is helpful for reducing the sufferings of people with physical as well as mental disorders. Millions flock around temples to 'seek blessings' for health and wealth. The concept was seen as positive while many would consider it as 'superstition' implying that spiritual recourse is devoid of any scientific evidence. Of course, in several conditions where relatives take their patient in hope of 'cure' from curse of the evil which resides within or around the affected person is a superstition, and the difference between the two is obvious.

One study demonstrated that psychiatrists had lower levels of beliefs and practices than did patients and the general population. In both groups, 47% felt there was "often or always" a place to include spirituality in psychiatric assessment, although the perceived importance differed. Among patients, 53% felt it important to have this issue addressed, and 24% considered the psychiatrist's spiritual interest is important in their choice of the treating psychiatrist. Barriers to addressing the issue of spirituality and mental health-related to psychiatrists' concern regarding its appropriateness and patients' perception that interest is lacking. Psychiatrists' own beliefs and practices were strong predictors of spiritual inquiry.[326]

Advancement of spiritualism brings hope for healing in the times of distress and suffering. It encourages to establish a relationship with oneself. The spiritual experiences are part of human life, these are important for everybody irrespective of their intellectual or emotional ability of strength.

Spirituality is closer to mind and soul and it is examined in that perspective. Scientific studies show several changes in biological parameters like neurochemistry, immunology, electrophysiology and brain imaging brought in convincing evidence that spirituality was a dominant determinant of health and disease. Further number of specific treatments have also developed. Now it is practiced in clinical setting, many hospitals have programs for hospitalized as well as out-patients' treatments, priests and chapels have found places in hospital premises. Spirituality specialist is a member of multidisciplinary team which undertakes planning of treatment and care.[327]

The field of spiritual health made significant progress and following key points are the leading findings:

- Spirituality can now be quantified, this allows comparison of one treatment to another.
- There are clinical conditions which are described as 'Abnormality of spirituality'.

- Spirituality leads to reduced severity of an illness and reduced incidence of mental disorder. It promotes psychological health. It can help prevent mental disorder.
- Yoga is a popular spiritual intervention. It has been tried and was found to be effective, similarly, principles of Bhagvad Gita have also been useful in dealing with psychological disorders.
- Spiritual people are more likely to volunteer or donate to the poor; regular community service can serve as a buffer against the effects of stress, thus leading to longer life. In several mental disorders spirituality is found to be closely related to health conditions such as alcohol and illicit drug dependence.
- A spirituality based intervention is generally helpful as:
- A stand-alone treatment for clinical condition e.g. psychological distress or psychosomatic illness
- As an adjunct treatment along with other treatments in complex mental disorders, e.g. schizophrenia
- A primary treatment for conditions like depression, in crisis as well as in regular situations
- As a palliative treatment for chronic, debilitating conditions like cancer
- Some of the more common themes in the literature describe it using one or more of the following elements:
    - a sense of purpose
    - a sense of 'connectedness' – to self, others, nature, 'God' or Other
    - a quest for wholeness,
    - a search for hope or harmony
    - a belief in a higher being or beings
    - some level of transcendence, or the sense that there is more to life than the material or practical and those activities that give meaning and value to people's lives.[328,329,330]

In the field of patient care several recommendations have been made from organization like WHO or American Medical Association. Broadly people follow WHO recommendations which is from the 67th World health Assembly agenda item. The care of patients has been: "Strengthening of palliative care as a component of comprehensive care throughout the life course," to enhance the training of health care professionals in spiritual needs.[331]

With advent of spiritual medicine, spiritual care has been designed which is being practiced in several settings (mainly in western countries). Integrating this care into routine patient management improve treatment outcome and level of satisfaction.

A study of nearly 9,000 patients found that chaplaincy visits increase patients' willingness to recommend the hospital and are more satisfied with their overall care.[332]

Another study demonstrated that cancer patients demonstrated significant effects on several end-of-life experiences.[333] Greater spiritual support from the health care team was associate with substantial increase in quality-of-life scores near death, as reported by patients' caregivers.[334] Patients who reported a high level of spiritual support were more likely to receive care outside the hospital and less likely to die in an intensive care unit, which were in turn associated with significantly lower health care costs.[335]

Spirituality is an experience which gives you a sense of inner peace, comfort, strength, love, and connection. Spirituality can be defined as the subjective feelings, thoughts, experiences, and behaviours that arise from a search or quest for the sacred. Without spiritual awareness a human being is no better than an animal. It is spiritual understanding that makes a human a human, not the advancement of technology, or even the ability to read and write. Spirituality is the way you find meaning, hope, comfort and inner peace in your life. Many people find spirituality through religion. Some find it through music, art or connecting with nature, others find it in their values and principles.[336]

82. SPIRITUALITY – UNIQUE IN EVERYONE

Characteristics of Spiritual Health include three components.[337] first is self-evolution where the individual is analyzing and applying the self in terms of thoughts and actions with respect to the wider perspective and nurturance-art. The second is Self-evolution has been defined as a state of BEING where the individual is consciously aware and responds to the situation, events, people and environment with engineering from within and Deeper Meaning-Purpose of Life. The third is Transcendence which is defined as a state of inner happiness and behaving accordingly through universal love-sublimating jealousy and considering oneself as a part of the supreme (beyond self).

Spirituality holds that all life is interconnected. There is a unity of body, mind, and spirit, and, indeed, of everything living on this planet. Spirituality involves relationship, a relationship with someone or something beyond us, someone or something that sustains and comforts us, guiding our decision making, forgiving our imperfections, and celebrating our journey through life. This someone or something can be another person, a spiritual guide, a belief in the goodness of human nature or a belief in God. Trauma, loss, and illness challenge what anchors us. The onset of a psychiatric disability is one such traumatic experience.[338] Spirituality is a feeling of connection to something greater, or simply, Connectedness, which is inherently desired and experienced by cultivating a relationship with oneself, one's community, one's environment, and one's orientation with the transcendent

Spirituality is a feeling of connection to something greater, or simply, Connectedness, which is inherently desired and experienced by cultivating a relationship with oneself, one's community, one's environment, and one's orientation with the transcendent.[339]

Spirituality involves exploring certain universal themes – love, compassion, altruism, life after death, wisdom and truth, with the knowledge that some people such as saints or enlightened individuals have achieved and manifested higher levels of development than the ordinary person. Aspiring to manifest the attributes of such inspirational examples often becomes an important part of the journey through life for spiritually inclined people.

Spirituality is a part of cognitive/intellectual & emotional life. Its expression involves behavioural, interpersonal and psychological changes that make up a human being. A connection between spirituality and mental health has been recognised in Eastern as well as Western ideologies for many centuries.

All living entities are spiritual in essence, for the soul in all living entities is a minute, spiritual spark of the consciousness of the Supreme. By far, most living beings are not aware of their spiritual essence. In the lower species, for instance, there is no awareness of the soul. In the animal species there is merely total absorption of the consciousness in eating, sleeping, mating, and defending.[340]

One of the important content/dimension of spirituality is the 'soul' (emotional or intellectual energy or intensity). It refers to an energy which is within us; it never dies, is never destroyed, and transmigrates from one human body to another after death. It has been of significance for both health and disease and people lived a 'spiritual-way of life'. It has a pronounced impact on education as well.

Everyone has a unique and specific type of spirituality; no two people have a similar dimension of spirituality. Some will know, understand, and believe in it; others may know, understand, but not believe in it.

There remains perceptible gap in theory and practice of spirituality in medicine. Some of the possible barriers which curtail a discussion:

- Inadequate educational preparation and lack of competence in spiritual care.
- Emphasis may be placed only on biopsychosocial issues
- Spiritual care has been described as lacking a scientific base, compounded by the associated problems of time constraints and shortage of human resources.
- Lack of clarity of the concept.
- Religion is taken to be synonymous with spirituality.
- There are conflicts in belief and value systems among mental health professionals,
- Spiritual care can be personally challenging to most mental health practitioners and the practice setting or institution may be a barrier.
- There is an absence of the right kind of relationship between the clients and the practitioners (it has been described as the 'it and thou mentality'), reflecting a rigid model of care.[341]

83. MOST PEOPLE ARE SPIRITUAL

Spiritualityispresentineveryoneinallstagesoflife,perhapsit'satitshighest soon after birth and gradually declines, to the extent that as we grow older our need for seeking spiritual experiences and solace becomes higher. Healthy people have higher spiritual self-worth than those who are the victims of illnesses.

Most individuals are spiritual, they can use spirituality to cope with distress, and may also wish to address spirituality in treatment. Spirituality could, therefore, play a pivotal role in disseminating evidence-based treatments, while providing newer vistas to enhance our understanding of the human beings.[342]

It is not quite clear if spirituality is present since birth or it is a characteristic which people develop during the period of growth. It is less likely that a person is born without an element of spirituality. Spirituality in childhood does influence health of children in the same way it affects adults.

It is possible to say that spirituality begins at birth, grows slowly, it's nurtured through connectedness with people. It reflects thoughts, intellect and hope. It regulates mood, generates energy and connectedness with nature. It constitutes trust, faith and wisdom. It reflects the light of supreme and connection with people.

People wrongly feel that spirituality is meant for old age. Spiritualism is at its highest or best at birth, and it begins in the mother's womb and lasts a lifetime.[343] If not practised it may be dormant, may appear to be absent, but, it is there in every breath of your life. It can re-emerge whenever our self-worth and ability to submit to 'the Supreme' enhances. There is some evidence from research and opinion of scholars:

Spiritualty can transform people which changes its effects on health as well. For example in people who are unwell, once they start practicing methods to enhance spirituality, some of them recover from the illness, and also achieve certain human characteristics which were not present before they became ill. The state of recovery is likely to be effective for longer period. People may develop behavioural traits of thought process like becoming more compassionate and loving after practice of spirituality. Many times the person acquires a totally reformed personality, improvised way of thinking and behaving, they care better for themselves and others, and also for the nature, which may include stopping harmful activities or habits which may affect the environment.

However from mental health and therapeutics point of view other questions are more important e.g.

- What are the characteristics of person who has high spirituality,
- Who is the right candidate for spiritual interventions, and
- Who are the people where spiritual intervention is not likely to work?

Several characteristics have been isolated based upon number of studies; e.g.

- Experiencing compassion towards others is one the strongest correlates of living a spiritual life.
- Spirituality is linked to many important aspects of human functioning—spiritual people have positive relationships, high self-esteem, optimism, and a meaning and purpose in life.
- Spiritual individuals strive towards a better life and consider personal growth and fulfilment as a central theme for their life.
- Benefits of spirituality include taking responsibility for one's actions, acceptance of uncertainty, courage to take risks, courage to change things and establish harmonious relationship with self and others.

Studies suggest that:[344,345]

- Spiritual people are gracious.
- Expressing gratitude is associated with many positive emotions such as optimism and overall vitality.
- Spiritual people are compassionate.
- Spiritual people flourish.
- Spiritual people take time to savour life experiences.

People who report having a spiritual practice are more likely to

- Live longer;
- Report higher levels of happiness;
- Experience more commitment to their romantic partners;
- Promote the healthy development of their children;
- Cope better with the death of a loved one;
- Have a lower risk of depression and suicide.

Spiritual people engage in practices known to reduce levels of stress.

- Spiritual individuals are more likely to volunteer or donate to the poor; according to research, regular community service can serve as a buffer against the effects of stress, thus leading to a longer life span .

Some of the characteristics possessed by spiritual people are:

- Belief that all living creatures deserve respect,
- Maintaining and nurturing relationship with others,
- Nature should be respected,
- Relationship with a higher power/universal intelligence,
- Spirituality gives them inner strength,
- Faith as a higher power,
- To strive to correct the excess in own life-style patterns/practices,
- Prayer as part of the spiritual nature,
- Making life choices as a way of keeping their spirituality alive.

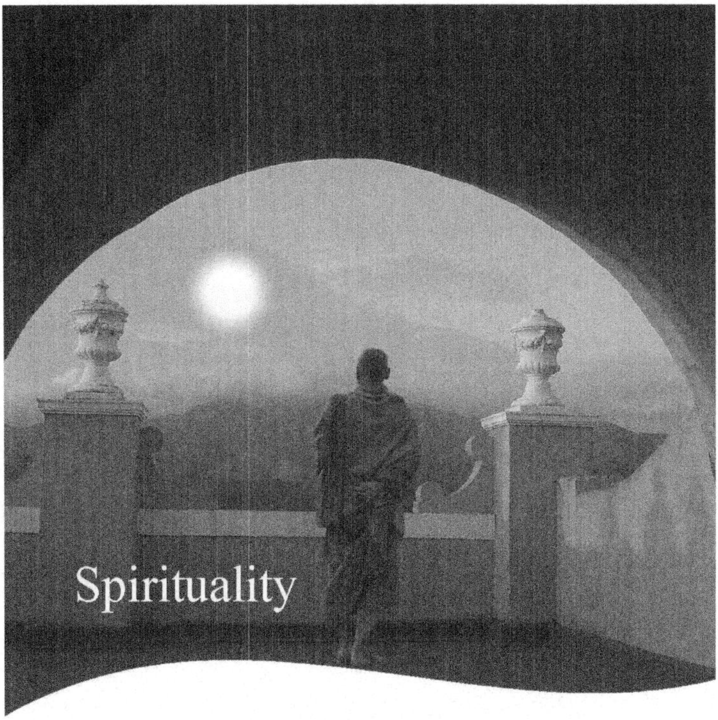

The 4th dimension of health

Spiritual health

Spiritual mental health

Spirituality and intelligence

Spirituality and educational attainment

Spirituality is unique in everyone

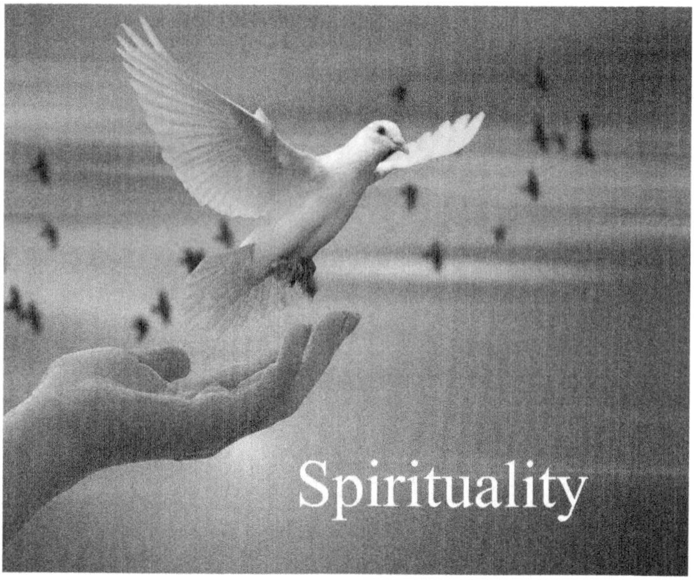

Presence of mental disorder leads to lower spirituality

Spiritual people are less likely to develop a mental disorder and improve better with treatment

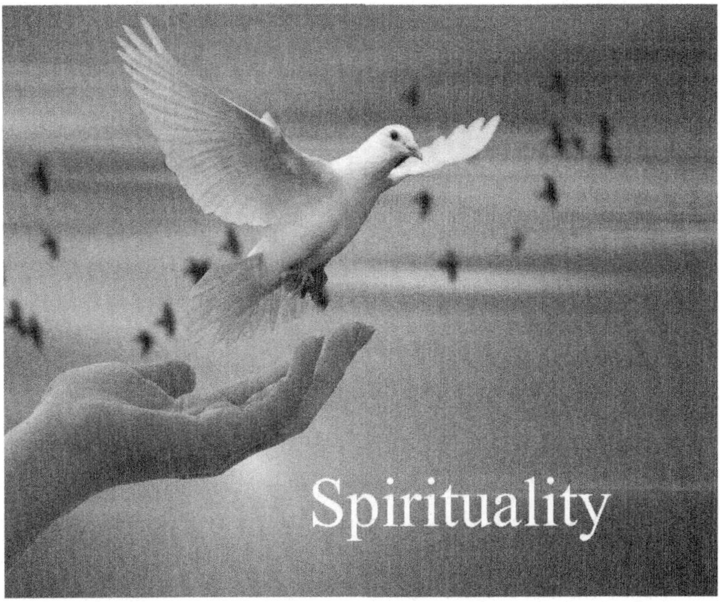

Improves problem solving, mechanism of learning, threshold for stress tolerance and response to adverse psychological events

84. RELIGION AND SPIRITUALITY

Spirituality and religion are not the same, and these two terms cannot be used interchangeably. Both are related and are a construct of mind and body. Spirituality, as well as religion, affect the mind and brain, determine the quality of life and influence various functions of day to day living. Spirituality without religion is a sustainable reality. Its benefits are possible without religion.

There are three categories of people in context when we talk about spirituality and religion:

Those who are spiritual minded and do not believe in religion.

Those who are religious as well as spiritual in the mindset.

Those who are knowledgeable about spirituality, as well as religion, but have no belief in either.

A religious person always believes in spirituality. For may be the two are inseparable and perhaps religiosity is the pathway for spirituality.

The merits of spirituality are almost the same with or without religiosity.

The issue of spirituality and religion not only appear closely associated by popular perception but these are quite intermingled on many occasion. Though spirituality is by and large culture free religion is not an therefore this association become complex in wider international and geo-cultural perspective. In Indian ethos spirituality is essentially ingrained in religious beliefs, thoughts and practices.

Though religion is therapeutic, there is enough evidence of religiosity being an effective measure to reduce distress of a mental illness, it is impossible to state that religiousness alone has been responsible for escalation of mental pain. Much of the difficulties lie in the fact that not much research data is available.

'In western countries until the early 19th century, psychiatry and religion were closely connected. Religious institutions were responsible for the care of the mentally ill. Psychiatry has a long tradition of dismissing and attacking religious experience. Religion was once seen by mental health professionals in Western societies as irrational and outdated, it was and is viewed as a result in emotional instability.'[346] Much has changed now and there is more acceptance of religion in the academic as well in medical culture.

The spirituality as well as religiosity, enhance individual experience to further adaptive capacity in order to build a mechanism for protection against the illnesses.

Religiosity is especially important in times of heightened stress and vulnerability, for example, when experiencing a life-changing event such as divorce or bereavement. In these cases, religiosity is a resource that can help people mentally to adjust to a new reality.[347]

Stresses and strains as well as uncertainties of life, can be tolerated more easily by the believers. Research indicates that religiosity or religious beliefs and values can enhance recovery from mental illness aiding in the healing process. Majority of well-conducted studies found that higher levels of religious involvement are positively associated with indicators of psychological well-being (life satisfaction, happiness, positive affect, and higher morale) and with less depression, suicidal thoughts and behaviour, drug/alcohol use/abuse. Usually, the positive impact of religious involvement on mental health is more robust among people under stressful circumstances.[348]

I can state with fair degree of confidence that R-S theme i.e. 'religious-spiritual factors' are most relevant while explaining how patients suffering from mental disorders experience peace and happiness whenever they start having some insight into their problem.

Religion and spirituality can promote mental health through positive religious coping, community and support, and positive beliefs.[349]

85. OPTIMISM AND RESILEINCE

Optimism is defined as the degree to which one expects positive experiences in the future.[350,351] It is positively associated with psychological well-being both in the general population and among medically ill patients.[352] This relationship holds for patients with cancer, among whom optimism is positively associated with psychological well-being and negatively associated with distress and depression,[353,354] and pessimism is positively associated with poorer health-related Quality of life (HRQOL)[351] and increased anxiety and depression[355] Several mechanisms driving the relationship between optimism and psychological wellbeing have been suggested, including higher expectations of the results of health related behaviors and the use of more adaptive coping strategies[356]

Spirituality and optimism are essential factors of health and well-being.[357]

Specifically, recent studies found that spirituality and optimism are associated with an improvement in immunological markers and also contribute to slowing disease progression.

86. MENTAL DISORDERS AND 'SPIRITUAL ABNORMALITIES'

Since spirituality is a dimension of health it is not unlikely to find abnormalities arising due to deficiencies in the spiritual worth of an individual. These have been named as spiritual diagnosis or abnormalities, rightly so, it is very difficult to elucidate the position of spirituality and the cycle of cause and consequences.

Scholars have conducted many studies and literature reviews on the relationship between religion/spirituality and a wide range of physical and mental health conditions, including high blood pressure, cerebrovascular disease, or heart disease. Further there are also other findings available e.g.

immune system dysfunction,
improved ability to cope with cancer,
chronic illness,
longevity,
health behaviours such as in living with pain and disability, and smoking cessation /prevention.

Thus, spirituality may be responsible for symptoms of an illness. Low spirituality may lead to psychiatric ill-health and those who are suffering from a dullness possess lower spirituality. A treatment leading to successful recovery also enhances spirituality.

Moreover, spirituality has received much interest in health-care services, in which spiritual care has been considered as inseparable from physical, social and psychological care because together they form the whole range of treatment.

At the same time stress and anxiety can have spiritual symptoms, including:

a loss of meaning in life
obsessional religious thoughts and actions
feelings of alienation and indifference
loss of previous spiritual belief
no sense of the future
fear of death
fear of the consequences of 'sins' or religiously-defined 'bad' behaviour and/or an inability to focus on 'God' or to meditate.

Reduction in symptoms of mental disorders have been reported by spiritual interventions, e.g. one spiritual pathway that has shown to reduce stress and related symptoms in war survivors is meditation on a word or phrase with spiritual significance (called a mantra) repetition recitation of mantra significantly reduces symptoms of stress, anxiety and anger, as well as improves quality of life and spiritual wellbeing.[358]

Effects of trauma on mental health may be better understood by taking a broader perspective that includes resilience and recovery as well as damage and symptomatology.[359]

Spirituality in relation to several disease conditions is well studied. About half of cancer patients and others with chronic diseases experience some spiritual struggle.[360] Spirituality plays significant role in keeping up the morale of patients suffering from chronic debilitating illness or a condition with no cure and control. This fact has recently been recognized as a priority in palliative care practice and research.[361] Spiritual distress has been observed in palliative patients.[362] Spirituality has been studied and practiced for management in hospital as well as in the community for a number of disorders, in addition to patients with cancer[363] e.g.

heart failure[364]
respiratory insufficiency
kidney failure[365]
mental illness[366]

Is it likely that people with high spiritual worth or those who have been practicing methods of spirituality, are able to handle stress-induced crisis in a better manner?

Modern research is increasing and many researchers in several institutes are involved in studying the question about how spirituality brings about changes in human-beings.

Effectiveness of spirituality is beyond need of any evidence, however in order to demonstrate it, we will have to develop the hypothesis for intervention as well as for prevention.

Some such experiments are available, specifically for yoga, meditation, theory of Gautam buddha, mindfulness, relaxation, theory of Dalai Lama etc.

Most ancient civilisations have had some of the other kind or concept which reflects spirituality or spiritual-like-thinking. The emerging evidence generally supports this shift in perspective and points towards a protective or beneficial effect of religious or spiritual activity for mental health.[367, 368] Although this relationship changes depending on how spirituality is expressed or which aspects of it are measured, positive associations have been found between some styles of religion/spirituality and general wellbeing, marital satisfaction and general psychological functioning.[369] Similarly, some research shows that certain spiritual or religious activity can have an effect on the mental health of those experiencing depression, anxiety, post-traumatic stress or schizophrenia and it is to that research that we now turn.

With increasing understanding of spirituality as a dimension of health, mental disorders have also been studied, not surprisingly the findings do support:

A spirituality based intervention is generally helpful as

1. A stand-alone treatment for clinical condition e.g. psychological distress or psychosomatic illness
2. As an adjunct treatment along with other treatments in complex mental disorders e.g. schizophrenia
3. A primary treatment for conditions like depression , in crisis as well as in regular situations
4. As a palliative treatment for chronic, debilitating conditions like cancer.

87. MENTAL MECHANISM AND SPIRITUALITY: VARIOUS VIEWPOINTS

The Indian Vedanta philosophy describes four approaches for making an advance in the spiritual life namely Karma Yoga, Raja Yoga, Bhakti Yoga & Jnana Yoga. These principles have been extensively researched in social philosophical and biological sciences.

Patanjali, the great sage, was the chief exponent of this (Ashtang) yoga who has contributed to our work on spirituality. We can no longer look at the mind and body as separate entities. It is probably safe to say that by 2050 a sufficient knowledge of biological phenomena will have wiped out the traditional dualistic approach of body/brain, body/mind and brain/mind.[370]

Similarly, Vipassana has been popular intervention for people in stress or for those who wanted a spiritual 'experience'.' is not a simple undertaking. It is a deep journey into the mind that can be at times distressing, but the gains are proportionate to the effort, time and dedication gave. Change does not come by accident or miracles.

Vipassana works based on the scientific principle of cause and effect. One has to work hard at one's past conditioning to experience the higher and subtler forms of realities hidden inside the deeper reaches of the mind. On this path, one learns after a while that the peace which comes from within is much more enjoyable than the transient excitements and happiness which can be obtained from without.[371]

88. SPIRITUALITY IN DEPRESSIVE DISORDER

Depressive disorder has an enormous impact on a person's ability to function at work, in relationships, and in other areas of life. The World Health Organization projects that, by the year 2020, major depression will be the world's second most debilitating condition; only cardiovascular disease will cause more disability

Those parents who had severe depression had low spirituality. One study found a positive correlation between spirituality and mental health Various aspects of spirituality have been associated with a lower prevalence of depression in a wide variety of specific populations, including college students, the elderly,[372, 373] disabled veterans, and women recovering from hip fractures.[374, 375]

89. CHARACTERISTICS AND REFLECTION OF SPIRITUALITY

Sense of identity
Self-awareness
Joy of life
Inner peace
Meaning in life
Connection with the nature
Awe at a breathtaking view
Oneness with nature
Hormone with environment
Sense of magic in environment
Love of other people,
Forgiveness towards others
Trust between individuals
Respect for others,
Kindness towards other people
Transcendental
Personal relationship with God/divine
Worship of the creator
Oneness with God
Peace with God
Prayer life

90. SPIRITUATILITY AND DISTRESS

Spirituality reduces stress and distress caused due to trauma. Since normally some types of stress or trauma are known to precede most psychiatric disorders, the trauma can be identified as a precursor and spirituality play a significant role in the prevention of mental disorders. It has been evaluated in several medical and psychiatric conditions with high rates of success. Healthy people have higher spiritual self-worth than those who are the victims of illnesses. How spirituality is related to an abnormality in the mental mechanism? Spirituality is present in everyone in all stages of life, perhaps it is at its highest soon after birth and gradually declines, to the extent that as we grow older our need for seeking spiritual experiences and solace becomes higher. Healthy people have higher spiritual self-worth than those who are the victims of illnesses.

Psychiatric treatments offer properties to prevent future episodes of illness. These can also prevent future illness when given if someone has only non-specific symptoms. Since spirituality is also an active treatment, it is expected to yield a similar outcome for prevention as well.

It reduces the risk as well as enhances the protective factors.

Positive beliefs, comfort and strength gained from religion, meditation and prayer can contribute to healing and a sense of well-being. Improving spiritual health may not cure an illness, but it may help you to feel better, to prevent certain illnesses and to cope with illness or death. Everyone is different, so what works for others may not work for you.

Mental health promotion is the most effective measure of minimizing the chances of developing a mental illness. We can enhance our efforts to identify mental health issues at the earliest. We can help prevent future episodes and reduce the burden of mental disorders.

I believe that there are methods which can enhance spirituality in an individual. Spirituality promoting interventions are well known and tried in various medical conditions, e.g. yogic practices are effective for intervention and prevention.

Since normally some types of stress or trauma are known to precede most psychiatric disorders, the trauma can be identified as a precursor and spirituality play a significant role in the prevention of mental disorders. It has been evaluated in several medical and psychiatric conditions with high rates of success.

91. SPIRITUAL TREATMENTS ARE EFFECTIVE

- Reduces stress.
- Reduce symptoms.
- Improves tolerance and coping.
- Biological changes are correlated.
- Improves sense of well-being, positivity, hope and satisfaction.

Treatments based upon principles of spirituality as well as religion have been used in depression and other mental disorders since long time. The studies used qualitative analysis to examine different dimensions representing spirituality. Commonly the treatments are called 'Spiritual-Religious' (S-R), researchers have identified several conditions of physical health, mental illness as well as patients with both mental and physical illness benefiting from the treatment. Further the treatment has been studied in general stress condition and several parameters of intellectual and cognitive conditions, personality etc.

The treatments have been studied among adults and elderly people, only occasionally children have been the subject of such studies.

In a number of situations, spiritualism works for intervention or coping. One of the ways is to enhance the spiritual capacity so that one can deal with adverse situations in a better manner. Enhanced cognitive ability and resilience are the main features which directly affect the impact of an adverse event or level of stress. Religious involvement and spirituality are associated with better health outcomes, including greater longevity, coping skills, and health-related quality of life (even during terminal illness) also less anxiety, depression, and suicide. Addressing the spiritual needs of the patients may enhance the recovery from illness.

Spiritual interventions by themselves can be designed, measured and administered. The host of evidence exerts where such treatments are effective and generally used either in the acute state, in a crisis or while dealing with unresponsive or chronic conditions. It is not well determined though what type of interventions are effective or if all spiritual interventions are equally effective.

Spirituality promotes psychological health, reduces distress caused by any abnormalities and at the same time improves learning capacity and acquisition of knowledge. Spirituality is by itself a cognitive process which allows better perception and organised thinking, problem solving, attention and concentration. Thus, individual is in a better position to identify psychological threat and to respond. Spiritualism and cognition enhance resilience which leads to adaptability to stress factors. It is known that most of the psychiatric disorders are followed by an experience of trauma or stress. This explains how improved learning and cognition reduces stress and improves psychological health.

Some forms of religious and spiritual coping can be more problematic. Life events can shake and shatter people spiritually as well as psychologically, socially and physically. People may struggle spiritually with their understanding of God, with inner conflicts or with other people. A growing body of research has linked these spiritual struggles to higher levels of psychological distress, decline in physical health and even greater risk of mortality. Thus, it is important for psychologists and other health care providers to be aware of the dual nature of religion and spirituality; they can be vital resources for health and well-being, but they can also be sources of distress.

Psychiatric treatments offer opportunity for prevention of future episodes of illness. Since spirituality is also an active treatment, it is expected to yield similar outcome for prevention as well. It reduces the risk as well as enhances the protective factors.

Positive beliefs, comfort and strength gained from religion, meditation and prayer can contribute to healing and a sense of well-being. Improving spiritual health may not cure an illness, but it may help you feel better, to prevent certain illnesses and to cope with illness or death. Everyone is different, so what works for others may not work for you.

Mental health promotion is the most effective measure of minimizing the chances of developing a mental illness. We can enhance our efforts to identify mental health issues at the earliest. We can help prevent future episodes and reduce the burden of mental disorders.

I believe that there are methods which can enhance spirituality in an individual. Spirituality promoting interventions are well known and tried in various medical conditions, e.g. yogic practices are effective for intervention and prevention.

92. CAN SPIRITUALITY BE ENHANCED?

Once a clinician identifies a person having an illness they can be benefited with spirituality and a suitable intervention is necessary. Such interventions are often required in a number of conditions. Some of the common conditions are described here:

1. Spiritual intervention will help even for a short period during illness.
2. During a crisis like situation, either due to physical or mental condition, e.g. trauma or severe stress.
3. Long-term spiritual intervention is required for a person who has chronic long-term illness of either physical or mental illness.
4. Many patients suffer from terminal illness where their hope for life is considerably diminished and they find it extremely distressing to live with such conditions e.g. cancer, or intolerable pain in cancer. Spiritual intervening is required for making life easy for this condition-palliative treatment.
5. In some countries patients can choose to pass on or die due to intractable conditions, spiritual intervention is advisable for 'end-of-life' support.

There are several ways to strengthen spirituality. Spirituality gives you a sense of inner peace, comfort, strength, love and connection with supreme. The treatments can be in form of community service, volunteer work, prayer, meditation, devotional singing, reading inspirational books, nature walks, quiet time for thinking, yoga, playing a sport or attending religious services.

I have seen it in several psychiatric hospitals and worked together with spiritual healers who remain available to help in complex cases in a psychiatric institute. Most of the advocacy groups, mental health professional organizations and non-governmental agencies are promoting spirituality for the welfare of the patients.

93. CLINICAL AND BIOLOGICAL FINDINGS

Experiences of researchers- (findings from selected studies have been quoted)
'The research show that the religious beliefs and spiritual practices prevent the spiritual and physical, as well as mental, illnesses and, at the same time, reduce the recurrence of the diseases and their symptoms. On the other hand, it accelerates the recovery rate and increases the probability of returning to the initial state'.[376]
'Forgiveness, negative religious coping, daily spiritual experiences, religious support, and self-rankings of religious/spiritual intensity significantly predicted mental health status. Religion/spirituality was unrelated to pain intensity and life interference due to pain. This study establishes relationships between religion/spirituality and health in a chronic pain population and emphasizes that religion/spirituality may have both costs and benefits for the health of those with chronic pain'.[377]
'The findings of this project indicate that specific facets of religious and spiritual belief systems do play direct and unique roles in predicting rehabilitation outcomes whereas religious activity does not. Notably, a self-reported individual connection to a higher power was an extremely robust predictor of both subjective and objective outcome'.[378]
'Religion is relevant for the treatment of people with schizophrenia in that it may help to reduce pathology, to enhance coping and to foster recovery. In the treatment of these patients, it appears useful to tolerate diversity, to respect other beliefs, to ban proselytism and to have a good knowledge of one's own spiritual identity'.[379]
Religion had a positive effect for 71% and a negative effect for 14% of the 115 patients interviewed. Religion influences the sense of self, symptoms, social functioning, the comorbidity of substance abuse, suicidal attempts and adherence to treatment. Then religion is relevant for treatment and should be evaluated systematically. The aforementioned clinical grid is suitable for this purpose. It proved its applicability to a broad diversity of religious beliefs, even pathological ones. Inter-judge reliability and construct validity were high and specific training is not required.[380]

94. CHANGES IN THE BRAIN AMONG PEOPLE WITH SPIRITUALITY

While discussing the relationship between spirituality and mind, the obvious question is 'how does it work?' 'The psychic system, no doubt, works through the equilibrium of mind and brain where the brain is the seat of the mind, power of the mind is potentiality unlimited and its exanpse is infenite. It is not possible to draw a structure that can describe all its attributes. The relationship of mind and brain that affects human behaviour, thinking. Mood and intellect are likely to be essentially biological, however the evidence of such a phenomenon in terms of biology, including bio-electrophysiology and neurobiology or cell biology, is missing.

Since we don't know the biological process of brain-mind equilibrium, there is a scope for thought about the other theories, though the possibility of other theories exist anyway. There comes a role which a supreme mechanism usually terms 'spiritualism' comes in' thus a gap exists.

Concepts of spirituality have tried to fill this gap. Spirituality being a mental mechanism is most likely to have some biological connotation, with origin or consequence of brain mechanism.

This aspect is under investigation as there is a need for more specific evidence to address the question of changes in the structure and function of the brain.

Study of the effect of spirituality on changes in brain function has been a topic of interest for more than five decades. The interest has become more pronounced after technology made it possible to visualise brain activity.[381] The primary investigation has been the study of structural and functional changes in the brain. The study of electrical or electrophysiological processes, brainwaves and neurochemistry provides information about the state of health and well-being of a truly spiritual person. The main symptom of biological influence of spirituality appears to be on neuropsychological or cognitive feature, that is, the features which connect thought, mood and intellect to traits like faith, believe and trust.

The effect of spirituality has been studied through the mechanism which creates spiritual experience in human beings. This has been though study of cognition, neuroimaging, neurochemistry and genetics.

Researchers have tried to re structure the information to develop a biological construct, but so far the attempt has not been successful.

Modern instruments have provided access to brain for observation. The easiest one is to examine the tools which directly enhance the spirituality, and it works by improving resilience, cognition, tolerance and psychophysiological states. It harmonises mental activities, for example, there is a close and natural association between cognition resistance, and positive psychological characteristics. Everything that will boost these three parameters shall enhance spirituality and the critical mass of spiritual worth.[382] For example, early studies of meditation practice often used electroencephalography (EEG), which measures the electrical activity in the brain.[383, 384] Neurobiological investigations have potential to provide exciting information which can explain the experience of spirituality.

Several studies have revealed changes in blood pressure and heart rate associated practices with meditation,[385] changes in the activity of the nervous system, respiratory rate and decreased oxygen metabolism.[386] Measures of hormone and immune functions have also been explored, especially as an adjunct measure to various clinical conditions. Hormonal changes associated with spiritual practices include cortisol, noradrenaline, endorphins, sex hormones and growth.[387, 388]

Of late, there are some reports which suggest that some areas of the brain, mainly the non-dominant ones, are involved in the appreciation and fulfilments of spiritual values and experiences.[389]

Functional neuroimaging studies of religious and spiritual practices have utilised PET, single-photon emission computed tomography (SPECT) and functional magnetic resonance imaging (fMRI). Functional MRI primarily measures changes in cerebral blood flow in brain structures during a specific task.[390,391,392] The ability to measure neurotransmitter systems is unique to PET, and SPECT imaging at present.

Structural, functional and neural network brain imaging research provides new insights into the neurobiology of mindfulness, meditation and spirituality.[393]

Meta-analysis of 21 morphometric human brain studies with 300 subjects identify consistent alterations of eight brain regions that impact meta-awareness, exteroceptive and interoceptive body awareness memory, and emotional regulation.[394]

Recent meta-analytic reviews of MRI studies suggest that meditation reduces default mode network activity with enhancement of focus and attention.

Meta-analytic assessment of MRI studies indicate that meditation improves working memory, attention and emotional regulation through functional activation of a wide network that includes bilateral middle frontal cortex and cingulate and insular cortices among others.[395]

Frontal, insular and temporal cortices have been reported as altered by meditation and mindfulness meditation with the hypothesis that these mental activities may cause 'neuroplastic changes' in the structure and function of brain regions involved with regulation of emotion, attention and self-awareness.[396]

Limited data on the neurobiology of religious/spiritual practices as compared to meditation suggest differences in the balance between prefrontal and parietal cortex activation although numerous similarities also occur.[397]

The identified neuroanatomical regions correlated with components of spiritual thought or experience including a sense of self (insular regions), emotional modulation (frontal and cingulate regions) and executive planning (prefrontal cortex).

There is clear evidence from neuroscience that yoga, which symbolises spirituality, shows specific changes in the brain. It improves psychological and spiritual characteristics of an individual and shows improvement in various conditions to good health.

It facilitates progress from disease to a healthy state. Yoga is perceived as a form of intelligence, considering it integrates abilities which establish a balance between physiological, emotional, cognitive and motivational processes. Yoga involves different techniques such as physical postures (asanas), controlled breathing (pranayama's), deep relaxation and meditation.

Some of the research explores the association between spirituality and mental health attempts to understand the mechanisms through which potential benefits may occur.[398]

95. SPIRITUALITY AND MENTAL HEALTH

It was a general observation that those who practice spirituality generally maintain a healthier life than those who did not. They are overall satisfied and happy. Spirituality gives them positive sense of attitude and a high level of confidence. It was a general sight that several people with incurable diseases or chronic resistant conditions turned up to 'healers' or temples or priests to seek relief from pain and sufferings and they do get into a comfort zone and feel satisfaction of doing enough.

Mental health promotion is the most effective aspect for minimising the chances of mental illness. We need to enhance our efforts to identify mental health issues at the earliest.

We can help prevent future episodes and reduce the burden of mental disorders.[399]

Another significance of mental health promotion entails full utilisation of their potential and possesses ability to solve problems of a human being in a better and comprehensive manner. It improves intellect, wisdom and resilience. It enhances cognition. People can promote mental health by reducing the chances of mental disorder, develop cognitive well-being, and achieve better spiritual credits, happiness, pleasure and satisfaction. They can also function better, contribute to society and maintain robust physical health. Improving spirituality has multiple advantages, for example,

Mental health promotion
Spiritual well-being
Cognition, intellect and wisdom
Prevention of mental illness
Utilisation of full potential of individuals
Better physical health

I believe that there are methods which can enhance spirituality in an individual. Spirituality promoting interventions are well known and tried in various medical conditions. Similarly, it can also prevent mental disorders by increasing an individual's protective factors. Yogic practices are effective for intervention and prevention.

It produces qualities such as love, honesty, patience, tolerance, compassion, a sense of detachment, faith and hope. Of late, there are some reports which suggest that some areas of the brain, mainly the non-dominant ones, are involved in the appreciation and fulfilment of spiritual values and experiences[400,401]

96. SPIRITUALITY AFFECTS GENERAL WELL-BEING

Although this relationship changes depending on how spirituality is expressed or which aspects of it are measured, positive associations have been found between some styles of religion/spirituality and general well-being, marital satisfaction and general psychological functioning.[402] Similarly, some research shows that certain spiritual or religious activity can have an effect on the mental health of those experiencing depression, anxiety, post-traumatic stress or schizophrenia, and it is to that research that we now turn to.

With increasing understanding of spirituality as a dimension of health, mental disorders have also been studied, and not surprisingly the findings support the following:

1. Severely ill people have very low spirituality.
2. When individuals possess high spirituality, even when they develop disorders the intensity is low, their stress level is also low and the distress due to illness is much lesser. They are even at peace with their problems.
3. Regular practitioners or teachers of spirituality, in theory, are not free from diseases in their life but their coping with medical conditions are relatively better.
4. Patients with higher spirituality respond better to treatment.

Decreased rates of mental disorder

Religion and spirituality are associated with decreased rates of mental illnesses. Some studies show decreased rates of suicide in religious populations, but the association between religion, spirituality and suicidal behaviours in people with mental illness are understudied.[403] Several studies have been assessing the role of spirituality and religiousness (S/R) on well-being, quality of life, physical and mental health worldwide.[404] Likewise, there is promising evidence that spiritual worth may enhance positive clinical outcomes in clinical practice.[405]

Spiritual people have better tolerance of stress

Stress and strain as well as uncertainties of life can be tolerated more easily by the believers.

Research indicates that religiosity or religious beliefs and values can enhance recovery from mental illness aiding in the healing process. Majority of well-conducted studies found that higher levels of religious involvement are positively associated with indicators of psychological well-being (life satisfaction, happiness, positive affect and higher morale) and with less depression, suicidal thoughts and behaviour, drug/alcohol use/abuse. Usually, the positive impact of religious involvement on mental health is more robust among people under stressful circumstances.[406]

1. Spirituality builds of psychological defence and reduces stress related to trauma or anxiety. Generally, stress is a precursor with high predictability of future illness, in other words most of the psychiatric disorders have stressful conditions preceding the illness. Spirituality increases resilience to deal with it.
2. Spirituality works at the cognitive, behavioural and affective system, as explained earlier. Psychiatric disorders consistently show abnormalities in these three mental attributes.
3. In presence of spiritual characteristics, neuroprotection of brain cells is taking place with rapid pace which in turn strengthen biological mechanism to minimise the adverse effect of psychological trauma.
4. People experience satisfaction and have better tolerance; their sense of well-being is high which significantly reduces distress.

Spiritualism is a protective factor. Spiritualism will enhance connectedness, interpersonal skills, contentment and will lead to emotional maturity.

The positive relationship of spirituality to mental health in a number of mental health problems has been encouraging. This has been observed across several psychiatric condition, for example, depression, anxiety, trauma and schizophrenia as well.

Spiritual involvement is usually associated with lower levels of depression, substance use/abuse, lesser cognitive declining, better quality of life, well-being, and functional status in older persons. Despite the number of studies showing this relationship, few have yet investigated the effect so fad dressing spiritual needs or carrying out religious-spiritual interventions.[407]

97. SPIRITUALITY FOR ACADEMIC EXCELLENCE

Spirituality is a protective mechanism for the younger generation. Student life is most precious because at this age they are developing skills and knowledge bases. They are preparing themselves for a larger goal. The world has been watching over the life of adolescents and students in colleges and universities. Since quite some time student life has come under considerable psychological pressure. The psychological problems of students are compelling and we find that with every passing day an increasing number of students attempt suicide, get sucked in the whirlpool of alcohol and drug abuse, develop delinquent behaviour, violence, and expose themselves to the risk of HIV and AIDS. Most young people in the age range of 15 to 25 years die due to motor vehicle accidents and suicide.

In colleges in India, the situation is no different. One of the reports showed that more than 50% of students in high school have abused alcohol, hard drugs, cannabis and sleeping pills.[408] Further, one in seven students suffers from a psychiatric disorder. Are they biologically challenged? Are they genetically at higher risk or facing insurmountable psychological stress? If that is the case, where is this stress arising from? Are they feeling extreme social stress? It is indeed a question for everyone related to students, family, teachers and doctors. Why is it that young students are in trouble?

One possible answers are their lack of resilience, their mistrust in the support system around them, their perception of uncertainties in life and a culture driven towards consumerism. They are facing irreversible social, economic and cultural transformations which is one potential cause for a mental health problems. There exists a strong evidence for social determinants of mental health, family-related problems and economic changes as possible causes for mental disorders. This offers some answers to the question 'Why are students under pressure?' It is not only parental pressure, but also increased expectation or uncertain future or unemployment. The cause is partially within. No doubt, behavioural and psychiatric problems arise from social and psychological stressors, and there is no denying that some people are at a higher risk and respond adversely to stress and trauma. Their poor coping ability, low resilience and high vulnerability finally lead to a psychiatric disorder. These causes are 'non-modifiable', but what is possible to change is the 'person human being within'.

We are at a crossroad to find the answers to minimise the vulnerability which can offer safety for the life of the young generation. The argument to rethink about bringing spirituality in their lives is not these deficiencies alone but the merits of spirituality to shield the psyche.

In India, there has been a tradition of spirituality-oriented education since the Vedic period. The system of education in Gurukul offered comprehensive development of spiritual, emotional and cognitive development. The style of teaching or teaching methods, curriculum as well as the teaching setting were spiritually designed. The students were living in these schools along with their teachers, and they participated in all possible activities with a sense of responsibility. This established a unique bond between the teacher and student (not disciples). It is acknowledged that this spiritual bonding provided learning with great holistic virtues. College campuses appear to provide many outlets for students interested in spirituality, from loosely organised gatherings to intentional and focused meetings, structured religious groups and other organisations.[409]

98. SPIRITUALITY IN STUDENTS

Spirituality has occupied a central place in growth and development. There exists a culture of spirituality since ancient times. However, the social values and culture of education has gradually started changing. As education became more consumer-driven, the curriculum and teaching methods drifted away from their objectives.

Researchers found that university and college students who can develop a spiritual life are more likely to be both peaceful and successful. University and colleges could be more proactive about helping students develop a spiritual attitude in the broad sense, whether that includes meditation, self-reflection or meeting people of diverse faiths.[410]

Spirituality can enhance academic achievement.

Higher education has the potential and responsibility[411] to develop students holistically, encompassing not only the capacities of their mind but all the elements involved in the journey to mature adulthood.[412] The role and effects of people's spiritual well-being have received more attention in recent years.[413]

One study demonstrated that 80% of college students are interested in spirituality.[414] Also, the study showed that spirituality is positively correlated with tolerance, academic performance and overall well-being.[415, 416] Religion and spirituality are very impactful in students' lives. This is especially true in the college settings. Colleges and universities provide an opportune environment and time for students to explore, dig deeper, question, learn and grow in the realm of religion and spirituality.[417]

In another study, out of 105 respondents to the survey, 81 individuals (77%) responded affirmatively to the question with, 'Yes, I consider myself spiritual.' More women than men responded positively.[418]

Considering the importance of spirituality in well-being, spirituality fits well into medical wellness models.[419]

The new initiative is to find out how to implement and bring spirituality in the curriculum as well as in the institution to frame policy and programmes. However, recently spirituality in students has become an interesting area of research. People are trying to find the answer for all the questions to better the quality of life of students.

Spiritual people engage in practices known to **reduce levels of stress,** for example, spiritual people are more likely to volunteer or donate to the poor; according to research, regular community service can serve as a buffer against the effects of stress, thus leading to longer life. Common characteristics of spirituality has been defined in several ways.

Spirituality/religion is relevant to most human beings; 84% of world's population reports a religious affiliation. Systematic reviews of the academic literature have identified literally thousands of empirical studies showing the relationship (usually positive but also negative) between spirituality/religion and health. However, there has been a huge gap worldwide between knowledge available about the impact of spirituality/religion to health and the translation of this knowledge to the actual clinical practice and public health policies. Spirituality is an integral constituent of mental health, and its dysfunction leads to mental disorders (World Psychiatric Association Section on spirituality and mental health). Abnormality in spirituality is correlated with development and deterioration of illness which leads to poor state of well-being and self-worth. Course of the illness leads to reduced well-being and poor 'self-worth'. Spirituality treatments can improve overall quality of life, reduce distress and restore living for a larger goal in life.

99. SPIRITUAL LEARNING

Learning and attainment of knowledge has been an age old tradition in India. Though it has been so in other civilisation, its position in India is unique. It is one place where health and education both were practised in the crucible of spirituality. Spirituality provided a solid ground to lay the foundation of learning how a cognitive process nurtures in spiritualism. The importance of brain mechanism and functioning was obvious based upon the nature, style and content of teaching and learning. It offered a comprehensive, all-round development (not merely growth) of human intellect and wisdom. Education was enveloped in daily living practices as well as in a specific cultural context, and it is because of spirituality as a method of learning that students grasped a sense of connectedness and believed with extreme confidence and humility.

Process of learning and development of spirituality are closely related. Spirituality provides a foundation for learning. When a child is growing, his spirituality is also growing as the process of learning is progressing. When brain structures are developing, factors like hope, faith and peace create a conducive environment for learning. Both the processes, learning and spirituality, are core features of mental health as well as mental disorder.

Spirituality is indeed an aspect of human development vital to overall health. Positive spiritual coping involves taking cognitive and behavioural efforts aimed at solving a situation, which (depending upon the domain) are manifested in: pursuing a goal, sense and meaning; attempting to focus on inner weaknesses and bring out strength and will power; seeking self-knowledge and thereby inner peace; establishing and maintaining deep and valuable relations, heeding moral values; concentrating on the sense of attachment and oneness with nature, and finding harmony and balance within it, openness to notice miracles in nature; and maintaining a relationship with higher power/God based on the sense of love and trust.

Negative spiritual coping makes it impossible for an individual to draw strength from spiritual resources and blocks the pursuit of sense and meaning in life and hinders its growth in 'upward movement'.

Development and learning proceed at varying rates. Development and learning result from an interaction of maturation and experience. Early experiences have profound effects on development and learning.[420]

The cognitive skills manifested by children are those which are necessary preconditions for spirituality.

Theories of children's spirituality have foundered in their ability to appreciate that children's cognition is organised through structures that are quintessential to spirituality. Thus, cognition and spirituality, which are closely related, together promote learning process.

The interface of academics and spirituality in today's context ranges from research on brain mechanism for understanding biological underpinning to developing online training modules for providing training to enhance spirituality.

High spirituality enhances academic performance.

Strong association of like-minded teacher and students further enhances spirituality.

Spirituality can be enhanced by using several methods including training and training courses.

Students' spirituality can be optimised for better health and wellness, and this is the reason that there is a growing popularity of wellness centres in the universities where learners seek involvement to feel emotionally empowered.

Students react on their experiences sharing and exploring religious and spiritual beliefs on campuses.

Education, influenced by the market, neglects a comprehensive approach to students' intellectual, physical and cultural needs. Market's preference for the technical and natural sciences contribute towards the creation of the mechanical conception of education. These challenges raise questions about outcomes of modern education. Since such education could not balance and fulfil students' material, intellectual and cultural needs, more severe thinking is required about how holistic learning and teaching can pave the way towards a progressive educational model. A growing number of experts are proposing that spirituality be incorporated within the curricula of schools. Many of these are responding to what they perceive as crises in public education caused at least in part by the exclusion of genuine spirituality from elementary and secondary classrooms.

One of the goals in conducting the *Spirituality in Higher Education* study was to develop measures that address various dimensions of spirituality and religiousness[1]. Higher education should attend more purposefully to students' spiritual development.

Some proponents of spirituality in schools argue that the boredom and meaninglessness students' experience nudge them to seek excitement in danger or an outlet for their frustration in aggressive behaviour.[421] For example, claims that drugs, sex, violence and even suicide may be both a search for connection and meaning and an escape from the pain of lacking a genuine source of spiritual fulfilment.

100. SPIRITUAL INTELLIGENCE

Spiritual intelligence is most broadly known as the intelligence with which we access our deepest meanings, values, purposes and highest motivations.[422] It is the intelligence that makes us whole and gives us our integrity.

Spiritual intelligence is the soul's intelligence, the intelligence of the deep self. It is the intelligence with which we ask fundamental questions and with which we reframe our answers.[423] Spiritual intelligence is one of the several types of intelligence, and it can be developed relatively independently. So, spiritual intelligence is a learned behaviour and can be enhanced.

The tools of spiritual intelligence include prayer, meditation, contemplation, conscious awareness of one's tendencies towards fear or anger, shifting one's emotional state away from fear and the ongoing daily practice of staying conscious of one's thoughts, emotions and behaviours.[424]

Spiritual intelligence is 'the capacity of an individual to possess a socially relevant purpose in life by understanding "self" and having a high degree of conscience, compassion and commitment to human values'.[425]

Self-awareness: Knowing what I believe in and value, and what deeply motivates me

Spontaneity: Living in and being responsive to the moment

Being vision- and value-led: Acting from principles and deep beliefs and living accordingly

Seeing larger patterns, relationships and connections; having a sense of belonging

Compassion: Having the quality of 'feeling-with' and deep empathy

Celebration of diversity: Valuing other people for their differences, not despite them

Field independence: Standing against the crowd and having one's own convictions

Humility: Having the sense of being a player in a larger drama of one's true place in the world

Tendency to ask fundamental 'Why?' questions: Needing to understand things and get to the bottom of them

Ability to reframe: Standing back from a situation or problem and seeing the bigger picture or wider context

Positive use of adversity: Learning and growing from mistakes, setbacks and sufferings

Sense of vocation: Feeling called upon to serve, to give something back

101. SPIRITUAL MINDSET

People with spiritual understanding are less vulnerable to mental disorders. Spirituality is not limited to only health-related aspect. A spiritual journey is, in fact, a spiritual development throughout our lives. Young children retain a strong capacity for spiritual awareness. It consists of dimensions such as belief, faith and conviction. People with childhood traumatic events show lesser spirituality. Personal spirituality may be neuroprotective against depression.[426,427] People with high spirituality can manage stress better. Spirituality may develop individually or in communities and traditions.

Nowadays, there is more awareness about religion and spirituality because it constitutes an inseparable part of health and well-being. Research suggests that it has implication on mental health. People with spiritual mindset cope with stress and expression much better, and they are less likely to develop mental health problems. It is therefore possible to use the lessons for prevention of mental health problems, providing relief and facilitating their coping ability.[428]

Many people think that **spirituality** and **religion** are the **same** thing, and so they bring their beliefs and prejudices about **religion** to discussions about **spirituality**. Though all **religions** emphasise spiritualism as being part of faith, you can be **spiritual** without being **religious** or a member of an organised **religion.**

Religion and spirituality are important concepts for every person. He may be a believer or non-believer, but certain facts prevailing in the culture always affect people. Both these terms are closely related to mind-body and brain regulation and therefore gain significance regarding psychological functions as well as abnormal psychological conditions.[429] The basic characteristics of all religions are similar. Religious people generally believe in a higher, unseen power which can control and regulate life. Religion usually refers to socially based beliefs and traditions, often associated with ritual and ceremony, whereas spirituality generally refers to a deep-seated individual sense of connection through which each person's life is experienced as contributing to a valued and greater 'whole', together with a sense of belonging and acceptance. Religiosity can be of two types; (1) public religiosity refers to active participation in a religious congregation, and (2) private religiosity refers to religious belief and practice that occurs less ostensibly, often at home or simply deep in the individual mind. Both forms of religiosity have shown to promote mental health. Everyone is different, so what works for others may not work for you. Do what is comfortable for you.

Certainly, think about the things in your life that give you a sense of inner peace, comfort, strength, love and connection. Set aside time every day to do the things that help you spiritually. These may include community service, volunteer work, prayer, meditation, devotional singing, reading inspirational books, nature walks, quiet time for thinking, yoga, playing a sport or attending religious services.[430]

102. SPIRITUAL COPING

Those children have the innate spiritual capacity and a desire to know more about the mental world, and the spiritual experiences and abilities. Childhoods spiritual coping with stress can be defined as attempts to overcome the stressor based on what is transcendent. Spirituality is indeed an aspect of human development and overall human health. Positive spiritual coping would then involve taking cognitive and behavioural efforts aimed at solving an awkward situation, which–depending on the domain–are manifested in: 1) pursuit of a goal, sense, and meaning, concentration on one's internal life, attempts to overcome one's weaknesses and to acquire more and more self-knowledge, and looking for internal peace and harmony; 2) establishing and maintaining deep and valuable relations with other people, heeding moral values, treating people fair, caring about others, willingness to help, displaying love, empathy and compassion (the social domain); 3) concentration on the sense of attachment and belonging to nature, perceiving harmony and order in it, treating nature as friendly to humans, openness to noticing miracles in nature (the environmental domain); 4) maintaining solid relation with God/the Supreme Power based on the sense of presence, love and trust (the religious domain). Negative spiritual coping makes it impossible for an individual to draw strength from spiritual resources, blocks the pursuit of sense and meaning in life, and hinders its growth 'upward movement'. All areas of development and learning are important. Learning and development follow sequences. Development and learning proceed at varying rates. Development and learning result from an interaction of maturation and experience. Early experiences have profound effects on development and learning.

In a number of situations, spiritualism works for intervention or coping. One of the ways is to enhance the spiritual capacity so that adverse circumstances which are dealt with it. Enhanced cognitive ability and resilience are the main features which directly affect the impact of an adverse event or level of stress.

This is a 'way of being' that involves some capacity for awareness of the sacred qualities of life experiences. Connections in four domains characterise it:

(1) Regards to self,
(2) Others,
(3) Nature and

(4) With a sense of mystery or more significant meaning to life, or whatever one considers being ultimate. Spirituality is not about God but the experience of God.

There have been a reference to many connotations, for example, spirituality, spiritual health, spiritual well-being, spiritual therapy, spiritual intervention, spiritual healing and 'Spiritual-religious' (S-R) intervention. There is significant overlap in the definition and understanding of each one of these. I prefer to use the term 'spiritual-religious intervention (SRI)' as a therapy.

Religious involvement and spirituality are associated with better health outcomes, including greater longevity, coping skills, health-related quality of life (even during terminal illness), less anxiety, depression and suicide. Addressing the spiritual needs of the patient may enhance recovery from illness. Supporting the spiritual needs of a person can be done in a straightforward and non-controversial manner.[431, 432] Spirituality can help patients who are in the process of recovery by facilitating their autonomy and assisting them to live and grow beyond the limitations imposed by their illness.[433]

Spiritual people are less likely

to develop mental illness.

Spirituality determines the outcome status of Treatment.
Spiritual people improve to a treatment than those who are not spiritual

Spiritual people show better quality of outcome.

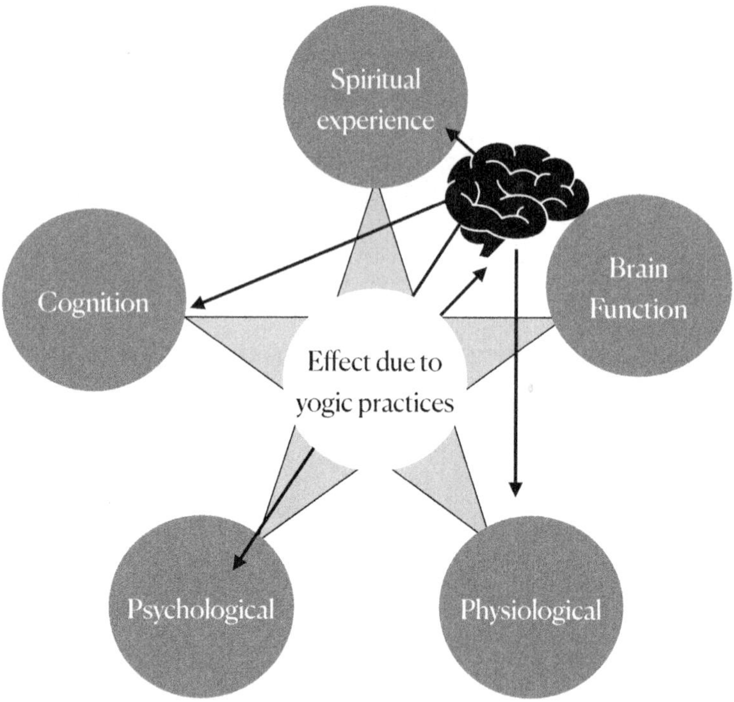
Spiritual experience
Cognition
Brain Function
Effect due to yogic practices
Psychological
Physiological

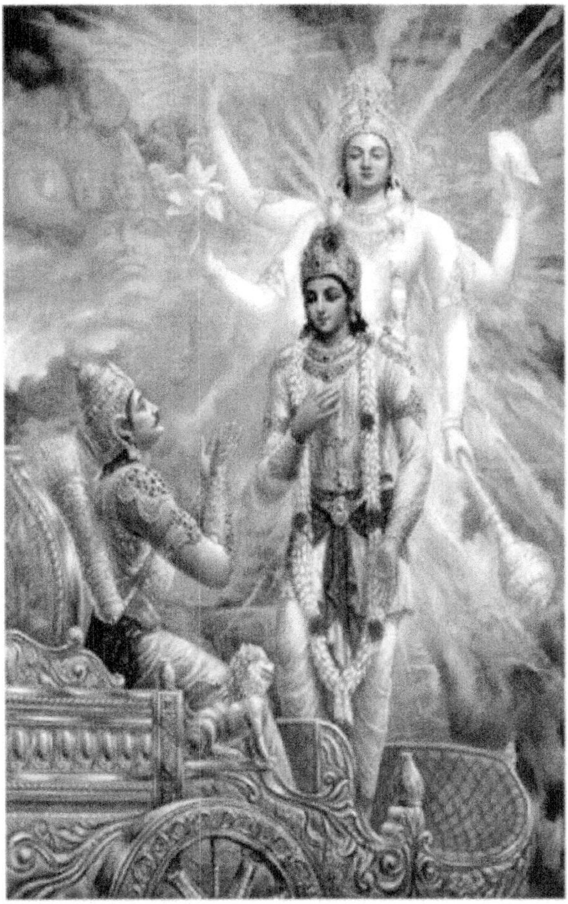

CHAPTER 10
ENHANCING MENTAL GRIT

My objective is to discuss spirituality from the point of view of its relevance for treatment or intervention for psychological problems. I do not mean to give viewpoint but make simple observation about few basic conceptual issues.

As we know spirituality has number of attributes which reflects wisdom and knowledge, resiliency is of particular significance because of its capacity to heal.

I am looking at spirituality as an instrument for behavioural change among people to minimize their problems which they have with (1) them- selves and (2) with others to promote their mental health and prevent a pathology.

Number of scholars have discussed that spirituality can change life; it makes people cope better. No doubt it can, but the larger issue is how? It is an unavoidable question. Modern science has tried to establish the connection however more research is required to answer this question. Another challenge is to find nature and type of intervention using spirituality as a modality to effectively reduce psychological symptoms. Some of the observations are pertinent e.g.:

Why spirituality will help minimize psychological distress?

What type of spiritual practice can be undertaken for different types of problems e.g., for intervention and prevention?

103. YOGIC SCIENCES

Yoga is a spiritual practice which affects our health positively. Yoga was developed in the Indus Saraswati civilisation over 5,000 years ago. The word 'Yog' was first mentioned in the sacred Indian text called The Rigveda. The Vedas are a collection of spiritual text containing songs and mantras. Yoga, is a popular form of treatment or intervention for health-related conditions which are used not only in India, but world over. It is also practised for prevention of mental disorders and for healthy living. Yoga, in fact, is a way of life. People practising yoga attain highest degree of spiritualism. It is said that spirituality arises from yogic practice and experiences. It is a mental activity which is the source of meditation.[434]

Science of yoga gives us the complete essence of way of life. It has been a subject for research in health and behaviour, for the purpose of healthy living. Yoga is adopted in most countries after United Nations declared Yoga day on 21st June. Yoga provides emotional stability and improves learning and concentration. While early text such as *Patanjali's Yoga Sutra* [C. 400AD] described the basic principles of yoga, the technique of this discipline has evolved over last two millennia.

I will discuss here health perspective of yoga, its mechanism and effectiveness in psychiatric disorders here. I will also briefly mention the current research findings.

WHAT IS YOGA?

Yoga is not a form of physical exercise alone.

Yoga is a form of spirituality. The word 'yoga' arises from Sanskrit word *yoga*. It comes from verb root YUJ, which means 'to link' or 'to connect'. By its very meaning it explains that there are two points which are connected with each other, that is, two different entities separated from a third one. The Bhagwad Gita explains these entities as:

1. Individual consciousness
2. Universal or supreme consciousness.

These two have been interpreted and described by different scholars in a different manner. It is likely that individual consciousness is an all-pervading energy and supreme consciousness is God, the all-pervading universal energy, but the very existence of energy implies that there is a processor which controls or regulates this energy 'the energetic who is an intelligent being'. Our individual consciousness or energy is part of manifestation of spirit, or spiritual of the soul inside our body, and the supreme consciousness is outside the body and something connects our inside to outside, that is, a connection between individual consciousness and supreme consciousness. This third energy is yoga.

The core feature of yoga is 'to connect'. The very meaning of connectedness is existence of two points which are connected by a third thing. Our individual consciousness, which is within us, is connected with supreme consciousness, which is an energy outside; what connects these two energies is yoga. The connectedness does not mean that inner consciousness merges with outer or universal consciousness, but it 'connects'. These three forms of energy are described as the individual consciousness, the supreme consciousness and yoga. In Vedic philosophy, yoga is divine, and it is a perfect realisation or experience.

There are several other interpretations of the phenomenon of consciousness concept, however those are outside the scope of this chapter, and readers are encouraged to read about it from standard resources.

1. Visada Yoga - The Path of Dejection. Many times we also seek guidance from a spiritual person when we are utterly frustrated with the sufferings of this material world. That is why this is called the yoga of dejection.
2. Sankhya Yoga – The Path of Analysis. It describes how to understand the Absolute by means of logical analysis and reasoning. Philosophers and intellectuals may prefer this yoga.
3. Karma Yoga – The Path of Action. It decribes actions and reactions. Activity for one's personal sense gratification can cause bondage.
4. Jnana Yoga – The Path of Knowledge. It describes the transcendental knowledge about the form, birth and activities of the Supreme Being. It also stresses that the knowledge about the Supreme has to be obtained in disciple succession, originating from the Supreme Being.
5. Karma-Vairagya Yoga – The Path of Renunciation of Action. Another name of this chapter is Karma-Sanyasa yoga.
6. Abhyasa Yoga – The Path of Practice (Self-Control). Other names of this chapter are dhyana yoga – the path of meditation or Astanga yoga – the path of the eight-fold mystic processes. When we refer to yoga as a system of physical exercises, we actually mean this particular yoga. The purpose of this yoga is to connect one's consciousness to the Supreme Consciousness by controlling one's body, mind and senses.
7. Paramahamsa Vijnana Yoga – The Path of Realisation of the Ultimate Truth.
8. Aksara-Parabrahman Yoga – The Path of Imperishable Brahman. Here, the nature of the living entities, the nature of material activities and the ever-changing material manifestation have been discussed.
9. Raja-Vidya-Guhya Yoga – The Path of the Most Secret of Royal Knowledge. Here, devotion has been stated to be the topmost important means to connect to the Supreme because the Supreme is a person.
10. Vibhuti-Vistara-Yoga – The Path of Manifestation of Opulence (of the Absolute).
11. Visvarupa-Darsana Yoga – The Path of Vision of the Universal Form. It explains how the Supreme Being is pervading the entire cosmic creation and how we can connect to Him by seeing Him in everything.
12. Bhakti Yoga – The Path of Devotion or the Path of Love. It discusses how to link with the Supreme through loving relationship and devotional service. According to the Bhagavad Gita, this is the highest form of yoga and we will come back to this again at the end of our discussion.
13. Ksetra-Ksetrajna Vibhaga Yoga – The Path of Fields and the Knower of the Fields of His energies.
14. Gunatraya-Vibhaga Yoga – The Path of the Three Divisions of Modes.
15. Purusottama Yoga – The Path of the Supreme Enjoyer.
16. Daivasura-Sampad-Vibhaga Yoga – The Path of Divine and Demoniac Qualities. It enlists the qualities of a yogi.
17. Sraddhatraya-Vibhaga Yoga – The Path of the Three Divisions of Faith. It discusses foods, sacrifices, austerity and charity in the three modes (goodness, passion and ignorance) and how they relate to connecting to the Supreme.
18. Moksa-Opadesa Yoga – The Path of Advice for Liberation. Renunciation is a qualification for the perfection of yoga.

Reproduced from: The Ultimate Science of Yoga by Gautam Paul

104. MECHANISM OF YOGA

Yoga is misunderstood as physical exercise, and this is not the whole truth since yoga as a practice of physical exercise was first systematically compiled by sage Patanjali in the Yoga Sutras; the same yoga is also described in Chapter 6 of the Bhagavad Gita.

The original purpose of this *yoga* was to connect one's consciousness to the supreme consciousness by controlling one's body, mind and senses; good health is just a by-product of this endeavour. Because a healthy mind resides in a healthy body, *Abhyasa yoga* is supposed to help focus one's mind upon the Supreme.[435]

The Yoga Sutras of Patanjali are a collection of 196 Sanskrit sutras (aphorisms) on the theory and practice of yoga. The Yoga Sutras were compiled sometime between 500 BCE and 400 CE by the sage Patanjali in India who synthesised and organised knowledge about yoga from much older traditions.

The eight limbs of yoga are yama (abstinences), niyama (observances), asana (yoga postures), pranayama (breath control), pratyahara (withdrawal of the senses), dharana (concentration), dhyana (meditation) and samadhi (absorption).

The classic Sutras (thought-threads), at least 4,000 years old, cover the yogic teachings on ethics, meditation and physical postures, and provide directions for dealing with situations in daily life.

Patanjali's definition considers meditation and its obstacles, i.e., fluctuations of the mind.[436] According to Patanjali, five types of fluctuations of mind should be overcome to attain concentration (meditation): (1) cognition, logical reasoning and verbal communication; (2) illusory imagination; (3) linguistic conceptualisations; (4) sleep and (5) memory.[437, 438]

Mechanism of yoga involves psychological as well as physiological changes. Yoga leads to transcendence effect due to changes in cognition, that is, mental activity involving memory, concentration and reasoning. Yoga is recognised as a form of mind-body medicine which indicates the integration of individual's physical, mental and spiritual dynamics to improve health conditions. It is a form of holistic adaptation for managing trauma and stress. Yoga therapy involves yogic practices and techniques to prevent and alleviate structural, physiological, emotional and spiritual pain.

Yoga has been practiced to treat patients suffering from mental health problems. The scientific evidence is very strong all over the world studies have been conducted to examine if mechanism and effectiveness.

Yoga facilitates progress from disease to a healthy state. The essence is that it preserves this deterioration by restoring any possible biological decay. Yoga is perceived as a form of intelligence, considering it integrates abilities which establish a balance between physiological, emotional, cognitive and motivational processes.[439] Yoga involves different techniques such as physical postures (asanas), controlled breathing (pranayama's), deep relaxation (yogendra) and meditation.[440] Thus yoga allows us to develop and preserve attributes of total well-being, that is, to be a human being with moral and spiritual values in which people can attain a state of peace of mind, remain healthy, do pure deeds, believe in the purity of life and have the ability to relate to others.

It explains the two pathways to 'attainment' or 'reaching the supreme' – (1) Bhakti yoga (devotion) (2) Gyan yoga (knowledge and philosophy). Thus, yoga allows us to develop and preserve attributes of spiritual well-being.

One of the best ways to keep stress at bay is to learn the art of relaxation and cultivate ways which can enhance our sense of well-being. Yoga is a fantastic science which helps us to travel on the road to significant mental and physical health.

Thus, yoga is a way of life that teaches us to live a life based on yogic principles.

105. YOGA AND BRAIN CHANGES

Several studies have been carried out involving normal volunteers, patients who have a mental disorder, cancer, heart disease, diabetes, hormonal problems, chronic pain and many other disorders.

The evolution of the functional brain systems is reflected in changing patterns of local activations and deactivations as revealed by Brain scan called functional Magnetic Resonance Imaging (fMRI). Such studies show changes in neural activity[441] reflecting changes in intentional focus, emotionality, cognitive strategies, processing routines etc. Research into meditation using other sophisticated brains cans like Positron emission tomography PET, SPECT or Functional magnetic Neuro Imaging fMRI.

Modern research in the field of neuroscience is showing us just what's happening in our brains when we engage in yoga.[442]

Neuroimaging brain waves seen in EEG, and neurochemistry had clearly shown how yogic kriya brings about changes in the brain when the changes in emotion, memory, increased awareness and insight take place with yoga.[443,444] It is quite fascinating that we can track that information now, and we can see different parts of the brain lighting up as a result of yogic practice. The intersection of neuroscience, mindfulness, meditation and yoga has been quite profound in terms of understanding exactly what is happening in our mind, brain and body when we meditate, chant or do different breathing practices.[445] Changes are also seen in protein structures similar to those which form a sheath around a brain cell for protection and insulation, as well as various substances which are metabolised molecules involved in the communication of one cell to another. A thick collection of brain cells interconnects all the regions of the brain; these form a track which allows information to travel from one place to another. These are called neuronal circuits.[446]

Experiments have been conducted to measure and compare the changes during, before and after such practices like yoga, TM (transcendental meditation) or relaxation.[447] When such studies are done in various conditions of health and diseases, changes are compared to what is known as standard or 'normal' or what is seen in a person who does not have the same disease. There has always been a problem in defining 'normal' state of rest, in mind and brain function. Such information is available from people who have been doing practice for a long time, and these changes are compared with people who have not been doing yoga or have done only for the experiment. Discussion papers have been written suggesting that when we are thinking positive thoughts, the left prefrontal cortex lights up. We also see what happens in the brain and the body within milliseconds when we are under stress. We see the activation of the middle part of the brain which contains amygdala, hippocampus, adrenal glands and many other areas that are responding to activate the body to respond to the threat.

Beyond doubt, yoga and other methods of mind-body-brain regulation for equilibrium were found effective in reducing severity of psychiatric symptoms, increasing quality of life and reducing general level of stress among patients suffering from mental disorders (particularly in adolescents, elderly people, prison inmates, teachers, military personnel) as well as severe neurological conditions.

106. EXAMPLES OF RESEARCH

Scientific research of yoga has been primarily in the field of Patanjali's Yoga Sutra. It is no doubt a spiritual experience, which maintains physiological and psychological functions, and it helps in ill-health as well.

Psychophysiological research became the focus of attention to study the changes in the brain and body before and after people become ill, during the illness and after they recovered with another type of treatment or by yogic practice. Traditionally these studies had utilised EEG to give the idea of brain functions and giving the information about changes in physiological function.[448]

I have had the privilege of working in the institute where the department for study of Patanjali Yoga Sutra and mental disorder was started somewhere around 1960 at the KEM hospital in Mumbai. It was a team led by Professor N.S. Vahia. He demonstrated rationale for the use of yoga as therapy[449] as well as the results of clinical application of yoga to patients suffering from psychiatric disorders.[450] It is nostalgic to remember some of most commendable studies in those days published in reputed international journals. I had the opportunity of working with him briefly. Many others from that team have also been my teachers (D.R. Doongaji, L.P. Shah and Ashit Seth). One of Dr Vahia's student, Dilip Jeste in USA, has pioneered the theory of 'wisdom' and 'successful aging', which explains why people become more wise as they age and what can be done for a successful aging. Neurobiology of wisdom is a pathbreaking research with promise of unfolding science of intellect, positive psychiatry and spirituality.

Yoga approaches used in several studies include postures (Asanas), breathing techniques (Pranayamas) and chanting (OM). There is evidence that the yoga intervention produced predictable biological changes. These biological changes too were relevant to the therapeutic effects. Yoga also was found beneficial in certain divergent groups, caregivers and children, and acutely ill in-patients. Persons with difficult-to-treat epilepsy attending out-patient care too expressed a need for yoga as an add-on intervention.[451]

1.	For adults with mild-to-major depression, an 8-week hatha yoga intervention resulted in statistically and clinically significant reductions in depression severity.[452]
2.	*During this 12-week intervention of yoga plus coherent breathing, depressive symptoms declined significantly in patients with major mood disorder (MMD).*[453]
3.	His study tentatively supports the hypothesis that one of the mechanisms through which yoga improves mood is by increasing the activity of the GABA system. The observed increase in GABA levels following a YI that was no longer observed 8 days after a YI suggests that the associated increase in GABA after a YI is time limited such that at least one YI a week may be necessary to maintain the elevated GABA levels.[454]
4.	*There is emerging evidence from randomised trials to support popular beliefs about yoga for depression, sleep disorders and as an augmentation therapy. Limitations of literature include inability to do double-blind studies, multiplicity of comparisons within small studies and lack of replication. Biomarker and neuroimaging studies, those comparing yoga with standard pharmcotherapies and psychotherapies, and studies of long-term efficacy are needed to fully translate the promise of yoga for enhancing mental health.*[456]
5.	Yoga can be introduced early in the treatment of psychosis with some benefits. Elevation of oxytocin may be a mechanism of yoga effects in schizophrenia. Certain components of yoga have demonstrated neurobiological effects similar to those of vagal stimulation, indicating this (indirect or autogenous vagal stimulation) as a possible mechanism of its action. It is time psychiatrists exploited the benefits of yoga for a comprehensive care in their patients.[457]
6.	*The literature suggests that yoga can lead to significant symptomatic improvements in psychiatric disorders, along with neurobiological effects which may underlie these changes. This suggests that mental health professionals should be open to the potential benefits of spiritual practices for their patients, either as complementary interventions to modern treatments or as sole treatment in some disorders.*[458]
7.	The study supported the role of add-on yoga therapy in management of schizophrenia and demonstrated an improvement in endogenous plasma oxytocin levels in schizophrenia patients receiving yoga therapy.[459]
8.	*There was a significant improvement in the social cognition composite score after 20 sessions of yoga ($t[13] = -5.37$, $P \leq 0.001$). Clinical symptoms also reduced significantly after twenty sessions of yoga.*[460]
9.	Indian research on remediation in schizophrenia has been eclectic and is reviewed here. Some investigators have focused mainly on symptom control and quality of life, as yoga could be a cost effective and culturally acceptable intervention for remediation and rehabilitation. Although participants were not exhaustively tested for improvement in cognitive function in the majority of such trials, published results are encouraging.[461]
10.	*We found minimal differences between yoga and non-standard care, the latter consisting of another exercise comparator, which could be broadly considered aerobic exercise. Outcomes were largely based on single studies with limited sample sizes and short-term follow-up. Overall, many outcomes were not reported, and evidence presented in this review is of low to moderate quality – too weak to indicate that yoga is superior or inferior to non-standard care control for management of people with schizophrenia.*[462]

11.	The findings of the proposed study are expected to have a major impact on establishing the scientific basis for the effects of yoga in a severe mental disorder such as schizophrenia. The results will have the potential to significantly impact the use of yoga in clinical management of schizophrenia and psychosis in India and the world.[463]
12.	*Though preliminary, our results suggest that memory training induces structural and neurochemical plasticity in seniors with MCI. Further research is needed to determine whether mind-body interventions like yoga yield similar neuroplastic changes.*[464]
13.	In summary, yoga is emerging as a potential therapeutic intervention and has already reached the armamentarium of psychiatrists. There is a need to objectively evaluate yoga therapy further in multicenter trials and integrate yoga into clinical practice. A yoga therapist could become a very useful member of the mental health team in the days to come.[465]
14.	*Biasing toward the local stimuli in the global-local task and negative correlation of previous meditation experience with attentional blink performance is consistent with Isha practices being focused-attention practices. Given the relatively small effect sizes and the absence of a control group, our results do not allow clear support nor rejection of the hypothesis of meditation-driven neuronal plasticity in the attentional system for Isha yoga practice.*[466]
15.	A clear operational definition of yoga-based therapeutic interventions for scientific purposes, as well as a comprehensive theoretical framework from which testable hypotheses can be formulated, is therefore needed. Here we propose such a framework and outline the bottom-up neurophysiological and top-down neurocognitive mechanisms hypothesised to be at play in YBP.[467]

BHAGVAD GITA HAS BEEN WRITTEN BY HUNDREDS OF SCHOLARS. WHAT I AM WRITING HERE IS VERY BASIC MESSAGE WHICH CAN BE HELPFUL TO INITIATE LEARNING ABOUT IT FROM ANY RESOURCE. MY PURPOSE IS TO HIGHLIGHT MERITS OF THIS SPIRITUAL NARRATION TO BRING NECESSARY CHANGES IN DAILY LIFE FROM THE PERSPECTIVE OF SELF-EVOLUTION. THESE MESSAGES FROM BHAGVAD GITA ARE EFFECTIVE BEYOND DOUBT, I BELIEVE. I ALSO QUESTION WHY AM I AM WRITING IT. EVERYBODY KNOWS THAT THE GITA IS A PSYCHCOLOGICAL MASTERPIECE. EVERYONE KNOWS ABOUT ITS SPIRITUAL MERIT. THE REASON FOR MY WRITING IT IN THIS BOOK IS TO INFORM READERS.

107. BHAGAVAD GITA: THE SPIRITUAL NARRATION

INTRODUCTION

Bhagavad Gita is a narration by Lord Krishna to Arjun, the greatest warrior. It was scripted by Maharishi Vyas 5000 years ago, which depicts the conflict between two cousins. Gita was narrated at a time when, in the middle of a battlefield, Arjun becomes hopeless, and puts down his bow and arrow, he had panicked because he had severe doubts about the purpose of such war, in which he had to slay his own relatives. At this point Lord Krishna becomes a spiritual master and explained the essence and principle of life. That the lessons of Gita are useful in elevating the spiritual worth is based upon the insight that people have problems in this world because their connection with the almighty is not adequate.

Bhagavad Gita is an extensive sacred text is 18 chapters with 700 verse. I am mentioning here those essential principles which can be easily understood and practiced in daily life by repeated reading and attending regular discourses and discussion groups.

Bhagavad Gita is supreme text which provides spiritual insight.

It lays down principles of life. It is sacred teaching commonly recited and discussed in family and communities since ancient times; its practice and acceptability as a way of life is a testimony of its effectiveness. It is useful for enhancing coping abilities and resilience. It provides answers to complex questions which confront every one for survival.

One of the important aspects of Bhagavad Gita is that it can be understood, discussed and recited by everyone. Someone may be a common person or a scholar in philosophy or a neuroscientist, everybody has something or the other to take home.

A psychologist will understand it from point of view of mental mechanism and a neuroscientist will be lost in the question of what molecular or cellular changes may be taking place e.g. in mechanism of 'subconscious' and 'conscious' mind, this is why Gita is universal.

My purpose here is to explain in an unequivocal terms that Gita is good for mental health of everybody, those who have learnt and practiced it can deal with problem far more easily and deal with potential problems in life whether it is due to. Longstanding trauma, stress or sudden crisis. It can keep you in ready-state of alert so that you can protect yourself from internal or external factors which may perpetuate in a condition which is detrimental to yourself.

108. WHY DISCUSS BHAGVAD GITA?

Lessons from Bhagavad Gita are one of the best possible methods to learn and practice spirituality and improve spiritual health.

Lessons of Bhagvad Gita provide a unique psychological insight. Much has been written and discussed about Gita and most people have heard about it. At least in India, everyone knows the fundamental lessons and their implications on human life. It is the most respected scripture which has won over everyone's faith. It is a text of 'universality'; applicable to everyone, across all castes, creeds, communities or culture.

'Gita is for everyone'.

In context of the discussion here, the question whether Bhagvad Gita has relevance to mental health or whether it's lessons are effective in improving or treating mental health problems does not arise at all. Several scholars, spiritual leaders, researchers, psychologists and psychiatrists have studied it in depth, and tried to understand the same. They have applied the principles in real life situations, treated patients, guided people for solving their problems and written about their observations. Volumes of literature are available on its relevance to mental health. The principle lessons from Bhagvad Gita are well established

Points for my discussion here are the following:

1. Why is Bhagvad Gita not incorporated d into people's regular reading practices?
2. Why people are not able to utilise these principles in their life to alleviate their sufferings?
3. What necessary steps should be undertaken to facilitate the process for dealing with mental ill-health, pain and sufferings.

Much can be achieved by improving the level of awareness and education.

Bhagvad Gita describes that a good life is one which is lived with 'Righteousness'. Lessons of Bhagvad Gita truly solve complex psychological problems, particularly dealing with conflict resolution.

Bhagavad Gita teaches cognitive training to manage emotions, problem-solving skills, and helps develop a spiritual frame of mind.[468]

THERE IS NO SIGNIFICANT PROBLEM IN LIFE WHICH CANNOT BE REFERRED TO THE BHAGAVAD GITA FOR A PERFECT SOLUTION.[469]

BHAGAVAD GITA IS ENERGY CONSERVING AND MIND PURIFYING FOR IT URGES ONE TO WORK FOR A CAUSE HIGHER THAN ONE'S EGO. UNDERSTANDING OF THE PRINCIPLES OF THE BHAGVAD GITA AND ITS APPLICATION IN DAY-TO-DAY LIFE AS AN EFFECTIVE TOOL FOR MANAGEMENT AND COPING OF STRESS.[470]

IT IS BETTER FOR THE PSYCHIATRIST AND MENTAL HEALTH PRACTITIONERS TO USE SPIRITUALITY AS A PART OF THEIR THERAPEUTIC ARMAMENTARIUM.[471]

THE DIVINE PRINCIPLES IN BHAGVAD GITA IS IN LINE WITH POSITIVE PSYCHOLOGY FOR IT'S APPLICATION.

109. BHAGVAD GITA: THE SPIRITUAL NARRATION

Arjun suddenly develops a sense of despondency in the middle of a battle field.

The theme of Gita is transcendental between the student Arjuna and the master narrator, friend philosopher and guide Lord Krishna in the battlefield of Mahabharat. It is a narration, between a student (the seeker) and the master.

Lord Krishna first listens to Arjuna with apt attention who describes his mental state and the nature of conflict, overtaking him. Arjun had succumbed to the severe pressure the conflict had inflicted on him. He felt a total loss of power and was shaking with uncontrollable emotions. The scene is vividly described and is a great learning experience for any-one who reads or listens.

After listening to the state of Arjun's mind and emotions, Lord Krishna spoke in a manner where he questioned regarding his student's insight, and his understanding of the meaning of life. Krishna wants to make sure if Arjun remembers the most important qualities of righteous-ness and duties. If Arjuna was not aware then why not? What had failed his memory. The conversation is much unique because of his affection towards Arjun but at the same time it is firm and challenging.

One of the first lesson to be learnt is: **'Be a listener'**:

When Arjun drops his Gandiv [the bow], his mind is full of ques-tions, and he presents this state of mind to his charioteer, friend and guide. And how did Lord Krishna respond? He did not speak. He only gave him a good listening. The 'Art of listening' is best demonstrated here. This can apply to all those who are addressing other people's prob-lems, whether it is a psychiatrist, mental health professional, teacher, par-ent or friend, when someone comes to you with their problems, listen to them, hear them out.

DEVOTION

Arjun gets a convincing guidance, motivating him enough to dispel all his fears and misconceptions. He gathers the courage and trust, good enough to pick up the Gandiv (Arjuna's bow) again. How did this hap-pen? Who was the real motivator? Was it because of the narrator, the listener, the content or the setting or situation where this session was conducted? May be, all these could also be the reasons. But the most important one, without which it was not possible was the fact that Arjuna was a devotee of Lord Krishna. Unless the listener has full faith and de-votion, the listener cannot get this grade of benefit. This is explained in

Bhagvad Gita. "So how can a human being understand Lord Krishna without becoming His devotee?" Therefore, Bhagvad Gita should be taken up in a spirit of devotion.[472]

EFFECTIVENESS OF COGNITIVE DISCOURSE

What did Lord Krishna narrate, what was so educative and powerful that Arjuna's mind was transformed. To briefly mention, the entire content was cognitive in nature, it was based upon sound knowledge and logic for 'problem-solving' which was explained with excellent expression of 'How And 'Why'? The content of this nature is called 'cognitive restructuring'. Thus, changing cognition is one of the main principles for mental transformation.

A Man like Arjuna- most virtuous warrior can get confused and develop symptoms, so severe that he lost direction, changed decisions and sank in despair, to such an extent that it could have put the entire war in jeopardy. What if Arjun would have prevailed with his decision not to fight?

But he did not do that.

Think about number of possibilities of consequences of panic an distress which generally people display in such a condition.

What if Arjun would have returned from the battlefield in despair without asking for guidance, (seeking help) or

What if Arjun's thoughts were 'ambivalent' – and not open to suggestibility,

What if he was to have taken a firm decision not to fight (given up)?

These are two main psychological factors which prevailed despite clouding state mind. 1. Hope and 2. Seeking help. In fact one's attempt to seek help is a sign of Hope.

Even under the worst circumstances these two cognitive attributes made it possible to bring Arjuna back to his original state of mind.

Thus Gita begins with the lesson of the 'art of listening' and 'narrating', the form, style and content of thoughts, the spiritualism, devotion and duties. Entire session of spiritual therapy was completed in only one scene on the battle field alone. It methodically addressed the very root of conflict, and demonstrated conflict resolution by cognitive re-structuring in the narration of Lord Krishna.

Likewise, in every verse of Bhagavad-Gita is a discussion which resolves several problems of psychological nature.

This was one such example where a problem-solving was explained.

110. THEORIES/PRINCIPLES

Though there are many principles for life explained, some which have a direct reference to mental health are worth mentioning.

- Theory of consequences
- Defining our identity
- Meditation for mind
- Desires lead to lust
- Change is the law of the universe

(This part of the chapter includes Excerpts from Srimad Bhagavad Gita Chapter 2, Saankhya Yoga: Yoga of Knowledge translated Sanskrit Text)[473]

As explained in Bhagvad Gita:

1. Theory of consequences

Our right is to work only, but never to claim its fruits. Do not become an instrument for making your actions yield fruit, nor let your attachment be to inaction.[474]

Do not become an instrument for making your actions yield fruit, nor let your attachment be to inaction.

This is one of the most quoted verses of the Gita. This famous verse contains the essential principle of disinterestedness in action. When we do our work, we will be side-tracked from disinterestedness if we think of name, fame, income, or any such extraneous consideration. Nothing should matter except the prompt fulfilment of the purpose of God, keeping in mind that success or failure depends upon other forces as well.[475]

The most important and widely applicable principle is about doing or taking actions. We may call it 'theory of consequences.' The lesson means that it is in our control to decide what our deeds are going to be, which means what we want to do. It's for other factors, the supreme, the God to determine the consequences.

We need to keep on doing our deeds and not focus on what will be the consequence. This lesson has a powerful lesson in which you are expected to detach yourself from a positive or negative outcome.

It is a robust motivational lesson, once this concept is understood and accepted it removes the fear and anxiety of failing or facing adverse consequences, allows you to concentrate better on preparing or doing' a task and you are not distracted due to a mental preoccupation with results. It takes away the unnecessary load of responsibility for the consequences and motivates you to do your best We are unable the control or determine the result or the outcome which may make us more anxious, and it will affect our performance. The ability to cope with changes is essential.

2. Defining our identity

It is not that I did not exist before, nor you nor these kings. Nor is it that we shall cease to live in the future.[476]

The lessons that we learn have a strong focus on the existence of man. It describes that man is part of the whole universe; he and she does not exist in isolation. On several occasions, we are engrossed with ideas of 'self-importance or self-identity.' Bhagavad Gita teaches "We did not bring anything to this world; neither are we going to take anything. "that we belong to a larger 'whole' as its parts. And therefore we will integrate into the supreme power.

We came to this world empty-handed. We have made everything over here, be it relations, money, love or respect. Everything would be left over here itself. We should be satisfied with what we have as everything would be left over here in this material world, we won't be able to take anything with us.[477]

There are two things in the world, the soul which is real, and the unreal body. Both of these are not to be grieved for because the soul never ceases to be and the body is ever perishable. Thus Sri Krishna speaks here of the immortality of the Self or the soul. The Self exists in the three periods - past, present and future.

He declares that the embodied soul in every one identifies itself with varied forms temporarily to gain preordained experiences. Neither Krishna himself nor Arjuna nor the other kings who have assembled in the battlefield are mere accidental happenings nor shall they cease to exist in the future. It is not that they came from nowhere nor at their death, they become nothing or non-existent.[478]

3. Meditation for mind

The man whose mind is not under his control has no Self-Knowledge, and to the unsteady no meditation is possible, and to the unmeditative, there can be no peace and to the man who has no order how can there be any happiness?

The necessity for the quietness of mind for practising the technique of Self-perfection is explained here. The unsteady mind cannot practice meditation. The mind which cannot be focused on meditation cannot acquire the Knowledge of the Self.[479]

Bhagavad Gita discusses a lot about meditation and its importance. Meditation is considered extremely helpful for attaining inner peace. Meditation is a way of learning. It is also referred to as a supreme science, which helps complete all desires of life.[480] To achieve our purpose of learning meditation, it needs to be practised sincerely and systematically. The emotional and physical problems can be addressed only after the sustained practice of meditation. This practice also enhances our creative capacities which means that we are better able to contribute to everybody around us, our family, and society.[481]

4. Duties and Desires

He attains peace into whom all desires enter as the waters enter the ocean, which is full to the brim and grounded in stillness, but not the man who is the desire of attractions.

Just as the ocean is not at all affected by the waters flowing into it from all sides, an enlightened person, who rests in his essential nature or Self is not in the least disturbed by desires produced by the objects of enjoyment, which he happens to come across during his sojourn on earth.

Such an individual who maintains true peace in spite of being a target for the stimuli conveyed through his sense organs by many sense objects is called a man of perfection, a true saint.[482]

Every human being must perform. It is an answer to your existence in this world; everyone has a specific role. Once you have completed your role, your body ceases to exist. Duty is the primary obligation of a person. When you ask yourself, why are you here the only answer is that you have to play your dedicated role, there is no question of shying away or feeling regret. Those who do not perform their duties are not on the right path.

There is another message related to desire. One needs to remain a dispassionate witness without getting involved like a spectator merely watching and enjoying the show. Everyone experiences desires, but they should not sway one. They should not bother a person. People often do not follow the right path and become a slave of desires. So, one should not come under the chains of desire.

Desires lead to lust, attachment to material objects, enlarge unnecessary ambitions and expectations. Those who have no control over their desires are at risk of drifting away from the righteous path of life. This drift can be so wide that it may be challenging to return to your original way of achieving your objectives. Gita cautions you and also makes you aware of the consequences. Keeping this caution in mind will help you to remain alert and focused. Too much of anything inevitably leads to the destruction of character and conduct.

111. FEW PSYCHOLOGICAL LESSONS FROM THE BATTLE OF MAHABHARAT

Battle of Mahabharat is a great resource for learning. There are many lessons for self-awareness and improvement, however I think there is one more dimension that will help me promote mental health.

For creating awareness, the knowledge of mental health is translated into a language that people understand. We approach the general public via multiple means like, lectures, workshops, social media etc.

People do not come to seek help because they have very little to very poor knowledge about the illnesses related to mind. Their lack of awareness often becomes the cause of elevated risks responsible for deterioration in health, suicide or violence.

Many challenges of psychological nature can affect the mental health leading to severe mental pain, distress and the resultant dysfunction can affect their capacity to work. They have no idea that these symptoms are reversible when treated in the early phase and therefore they must seek timely help.

The episode of Arjun's suffering, his discussion with Lord Krishna and his recovery to the full extent is a testimony that psychological problems can be treated. These grounds should fairly explain the dire need to know, understand and utilise the most precious resource to maintain good mental health and address the problems related to mental ill health. Bhagavad Gita is 'The most effective' body of knowledge which when translated and imbibed in our lives, will help create awareness and help people handle their life problems with better outcome. Whenever you read Bhagvad Gita or discuss it amongst family members or friends, it is impossible to miss the psychological reference and its implications in everyone's life.

Bhagvad Gita is an unquestionable text. People believe in the events described therein. It is culturally acceptable. It is for everybody and everyone has a take-home message. It is said that what is not in Bhagavad Gita/ Mahabharata, can be nowhere else. There are several messages relevant to people regarding mental health. Some of these can be discussed in a discourse or educational exercise to develop an awareness program.

The following are simple meanings of shlokas related to the episode of psychological distress of Arjun

BG 1.27: Seeing all his relatives present there, Arjun, the son of Kunti, was overwhelmed with compassion, and with deep sorrow, spoke the following words.

BG 1.28: Arjun said: O Krishna, seeing my kinsmen arrayed for battle here and intent on killing each other, my limbs are giving way and my mouth is drying up.

In chapter one of Bhagavad Gita, it is described how Arjuna who suffered an episode of

Anxiety and despondency presented with the belief that he should not fight the war.

BG 1.29-31: My whole-body shudders; my hair is standing on its end. My bow, the Gāṇḍīv, is slipping from my hand, and my skin is burning all over. My mind is in quandary and whirling in confusion; I am unable to hold myself steady any longer. O Krishna, killer of the Keshi demon, I only see omens of misfortune. I do not foresee how any good can come from killing my kinsmen in this battle.

BG 1.32-33: O Krishna, I do not desire the victory, kingdom, or the happiness accruing it. Of what avail will be a kingdom, pleasures, or even life itself, when the very persons for whom we covet them, are standing before us for battle?

BG 1.34-35: Teachers, fathers, sons, grandfathers, maternal uncles, grandsons, fathers-in-law, grand-nephews, brothers-in-law, and other kinsmen are present here, staking their lives and riches. O Madhusudan, I do not wish to slay them, even if they attack me. If we kill the sons of Dhritarashtra, what satisfaction will we derive from the dominion over the three worlds, what to speak of this Earth?

Principles of Gita are being applied in psychotherapy, counselling, healing, behaviour modification techniques etc. Most conditions which are treated with the help of these concepts are stress related conditions, personality difficulties, depression and existential conflicts.

Some of these therapies have been developed based upon the principles of Bhagvad Gita e.g. yoga therapy, meditation, mindfulness, etc. I hope in future there will be further research done so as to examine its application.

Bhagvad Gita is truly a psychological as well as a spiritual text with several concepts which explain human behaviour and symptoms related to mind.

These lessons indeed are a way of life for every breath that we take. It provides understanding about how to deal with the inabilities.[478]

Some characteristics can be named as:

1. Resolving identity crisis
2. Improving learning and cognition, i.e. memory and concentration[483]
3. Personality development (optimizing role, responsibility, and performance[484]

4. Stress management techniques[485]
5. Conflict resolution[486]
6. Teaches art and science of crisis intervention[487]
7. Maintaining a calm state of mind for the long term in cases of a mental health-related problem, e.g., depression or effect of trauma[488]

In Bhagavad Gita, there is the description of a psychological condition from the time Arjun presents his confusion, to the state when he is convinced that he must fight no matter who the enemy is and establish the rule of law, Dharma, to develop a new society.

The mental health implication of lessons we learn from Bhagvad Gita are highly relevant to promote mental health and to help people overcome their problems. In a nutshell for basic understanding, we can derive that psychological conditions may affect any one and the symptoms that create confusion and conflict. Symptoms can be physical or mental. Treatments can be offered, and people can acquire total recovery and at times with the right guidance from teachers, master or counsellors, the improvement may exceed far more than expected. One can be highly motivated, clear-headed and focus and thus accomplish the goals. Those who suffer can recover if treated appropriately, the symptoms do not recur. There are several good factors to help explain his complete recovery, namely: early intervention, therapist in form of a friend and mentor, and above all the complete devotion of Arjun.

1. So what people can gain from Gita regarding mental health: As stated above, people can read and understand the nature of problems one can develop in difficult circumstances. It is important to note that mental conflict can lead to symptoms which can be severe.

2. What people who are suffering, can learn from Gita? a knowledge of how mental symptoms can present themselves, what can be the consequences, and Full Recovery as an effect of intervention and outcome.

3. What the healers, doctors, psychiatrists or psychologists and other mental health professionals can learn; the ethics of therapy, how the therapy is conducted, also the language and style of conversation.

1. Conflicts or source of distress can be social in origin.
2. Anyone can develop the condition.
3. Being strong does not mean one cannot develop psychological symptoms.
4. Presence of a therapist, like a Guru in Indian culture, in a form of psychotherapy or counselling.
5. Treatment is a mental process involving logic, understanding thought process and intellect.

6. Early intervention gives the best results.
7. Psychological symptoms can be reversible.
8. Treatment can be done in any setting.
9. The healer must learn the 'art of listening'.
10. The clients need to have faith and trust.
11. A person who is known, like a friend, philosopher or guide can also be a therapist.

112. SPIRITUAL INSIGHT IS A HEALING

The objective of Gita is to provide learning in which people develop faith in 'the supreme', understand the purpose of life, birth and death, duties, righteousness and the like.

My objective is to discuss spirituality from the point of view of its relevance for treatment or intervention for psychological problems. I do not mean to give a viewpoint but instead make a simple observation about few basic conceptual issues.

As we know, spirituality has a number of attributes which reflect wisdom and knowledge, and resiliency. It is of particular significance because of its capacity to heal.

I am looking at spirituality as an instrument for behavioural change among people to minimise their problems which they have (1) with themselves and (2) with others to promote their mental health and prevent a pathology.

A number of scholars have discussed that spirituality can change life since it makes people cope better. There is no doubt that it can, but a large issue is 'how?'. If we pause and think practically, it is an unavoidable question to elicit the content and style of intervention using spirituality as a modality which will effectively deal with psychological symptoms or causes. Some of these are:

Why will spirituality help minimise psychological distress?

What type of spiritual practice can be undertaken for a different type of problem, for example, for intervention and prevention?

Consider the example of the Bhagavad Gita.

The theme of Gita is transcendental between the student Arjuna and the master, narrator, friend, philosopher and guide Lord Krishan in the battlefield of Mahabharat. It is a narration, in which there is a student (the seeker) and a master.

Lord Krishna first listens to Arjuna with apt attention, who describes his mental state and the nature of the conflict which had taken over him. It was so severe that he succumbed to the pressure. He had started shivering and had become powerless. The scene is vividly described which is a great learning experience for anyone who reads or listens.

After listening to Arjuna, he speaks in a manner in which he questions -the student's insight, understanding the meaning of life. He wants to know if Arjuna remembers righteousness and his duties. If he did not then why not. The conversation is much unique because of his affection towards Arjuna, but it is firm and challenging.

There are certain basic questions raised by the student. The question is very basic: why should he go to war and kill his relative for no gains?

It is about education and learning, and it teaches the lesson of how to understand, analyse, reason and act accordingly.

One of the main themes of Gita is keeping trust and belief in the almighty supreme Lord. He alone can narrate, know and impart its meaning. He alone knows it all and no one else. He alone decides the outcome of every action.

In medical literature, I have not found any definition or context in which spirituality has been defined without reference to God and Almighty, the Supreme. I cannot say if one can be spiritual without believing in God. The dimensions of spirituality is vast, immeasurable and unlimited.

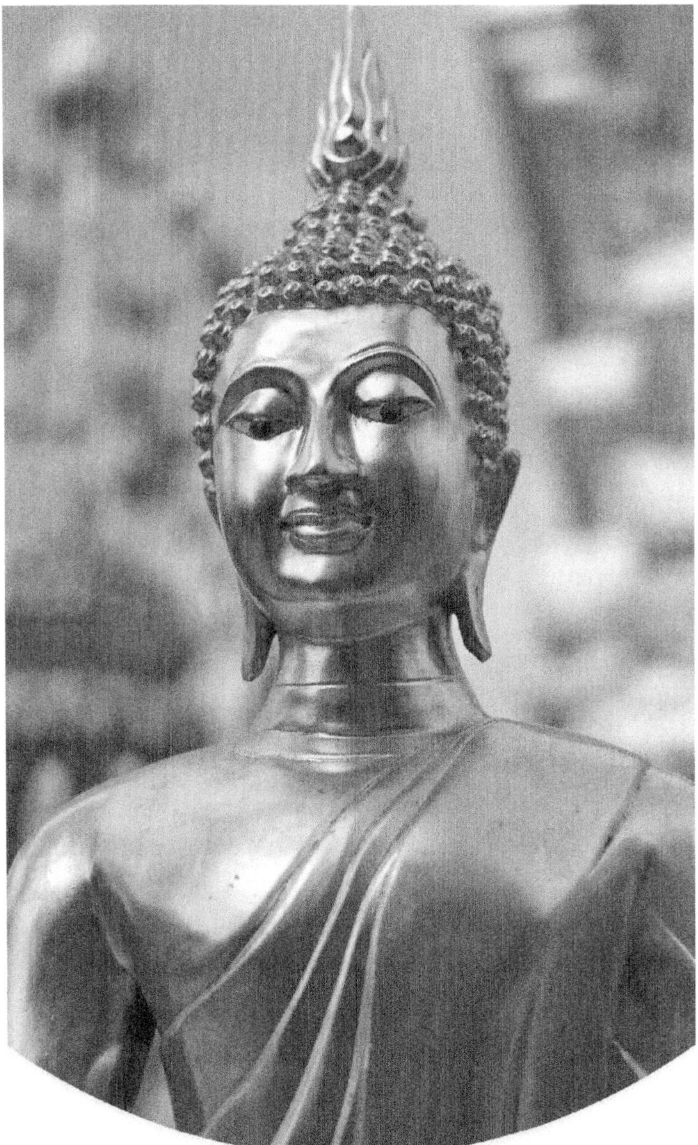

113. TEACHINGS OF GAUTAM BUDDHA (HELP FOR POSITIVE MENTAL HEALTH)

"You will not be punished for your anger; your anger will punish you."

Buddhism is a religion that was founded by Siddhartha Gautama. Or as popularly referred to 'Gautam Buddha'

"Better than a thousand hollow words is one word that brings peace."

One of the ways you can boost your mental health is by following the teachings of the great men in the world. Gautam Buddha was one such man. He not only founded a religion but also taught men how to conquer the ills that plague the mind and attain nirvana.

Buddhism is a religion that was founded by Siddhartha Gautama ("The Buddha") more than 2,500 years ago in India. Buddhism is a major global religion with history and system of beliefs. The following is intended only to introduce Buddhism's history and fundamentals, and by no means covers the religion exhaustively and in totality.

Followers of Buddhism don't acknowledge a supreme God or deity. They instead focus on achieving *enlightenment - a state of inner peace and wisdom.* When followers reach this spiritual state of bliss, they're said to have experienced *nirvana.*

Buddhism encourages its people to avoid self-indulgence but also self-denial. It advocates following a middle path in all walks of life. The path to enlightenment is attained by utilizing morality, meditation and wisdom. If these principles are followed in life, too, your mental health can be robust. Buddhists often meditate because they believe it helps awaken truth. The religion has historically been most prominent in East and Southeast Asia, but its influence is growing in the West. Many Buddhist ideas and philosophies overlap with those of other faiths. The religion's founder, Buddha, is considered an extraordinary man, but not a God. The word Buddha means "enlightened."[306]

When Gautama passed away around 483 B.C., his followers began to organize a religious movement. In the 3rd century B.C. Ashoka the Great, the Mauryan Indian emperor, made Buddhism the state religion of India and helped in its expansion. Buddhist monasteries were built, and missionary work was encouraged. Buddha's teachings became the foundation for what would develop into Buddhism. There are many philosophies and interpretations within Buddhism, making it a tolerant and evolving religion. Some scholars don't recognize Buddhism as an organized religion, but rather, a "way of life" or a "spiritual tradition."[307]

PRINCIPLE FOR MENTAL HEALTH

Following and understanding the teachings of Buddha will undoubtedly bring relief from mental trouble and give peace of mind.

All Buddhists live by five moral precepts, which prohibit:

1. Killing living things
2. Taking what is not given
3. Sexual misconduct
4. Lying
5. Using drugs or alcohol

These noble Truth practiced in Buddhism are a contingency plan for dealing with suffering. It helps improve the quality of life and increases the coping ability.

The **First Truth** identifies the presence of suffering. Every human being who steps on the earth suffers.

The **Second Truth**, on the other hand, seeks to determine the cause of suffering. In Buddhism, desire and ignorance lie at the root of suffering. By desire, Buddhists refer to craving pleasure, material goods, and immortality, all of which are wants that can never be satisfied. As a result, desiring them can only bring suffering.

The **Third Noble Truth,** the truth of the end of suffering, has dual meaning, suggesting either the end of suffering in this life, on earth, or in the spiritual life, through achieving Nirvana. When one has achieved Nirvana, which is a transcendent state free from suffering and our worldly cycle of birth and rebirth, spiritual enlightenment has been reached.

The **Fourth Noble truth** charts the method for attaining the end of suffering, known to Buddhists as the Noble Eightfold Path.

The steps of the Noble Eightfold Path are

1. Right Understanding,
2. Right Thought,
3. Right Speech,
4. Right Action,
5. Right Livelihood,
6. Right Effort,
7. Right Mindfulness and
8. Right Concentration.

Moreover, there are three themes into which the Path is organized:

1. Good moral conduct (Understanding, Thought, Speech);
2. Meditation and mental development (Action, Livelihood, Effort), and
3. Wisdom or insight (Mindfulness and Concentration).

The Buddhist interpretation of karma does not refer to preordained fate. Karma refers to good or bad actions a person does during one's lifetime.

Good actions involve either the absence of bad actions, or actual positive acts, such as generosity, righteousness, and meditation, bring about happiness in the long run. Bad actions, such as lying, stealing or killing, bring about unhappiness in the long run.

Five conditions determine the way as actions carried out:

- Frequent, repetitive action;
- Determined, intentional action;
- Action performed without regret;
- Action against extraordinary persons; and
- Action toward those who have helped one in the past.

To be calm and cool like him, you will have to take in a few of his observations about life which will help bring you mental peace. Like:

1. "Three things cannot be hidden: the sun, the moon and the truth. "No matter how much you try to conceal the truth, it will be known one day or the other. It's foolish to cover up lies because the truth reveals itself most honestly."
2. "You will not be punished for your anger; your anger will punish you. Anger is a lethal weapon. Apart from slaying the enemy, it also slays you. When you're angry, your words deceive you, and they hurt others. Therefore, it's advisable to remain silent and not speak when something annoys you.
3. "You can search throughout the entire universe for someone more deserving of your love and affection than you, but you wont find that person anywhere. You, yourself, as much as anybody in the entire universe, deserves your love and affection." We often expect to receive love and affection from others. In that process, we start neglecting ourselves. We try too hard to get attention. However, we forget that loving oneself comes before loving others. You cannot love selflessly, until and unless you understand yourself.
4. "Our thoughts shape us; we become what we think. When the mind is pure, joy follows like a shadow that never leaves." The message here is to think happy thoughts that will keep you happy throughout the day. Being optimistic is better than having negative thoughts.
5. "You only lose what you cling to." Getting attached to a thing is the biggest mistake we can make in our lives. It is when we get too dependent on it that we start losing it.

6. "Believe nothing, no matter where you read it, or who said it, no matter if I have said it unless it agrees with your reason and your common sense."
7. "Physical charms attract the eyes; goodness attracts the mind." Good looks are an asset - however, a good character is an identity. It's completely wrong to judge someone only by their looks and not by their character.
8. "When you like a flower, you pluck it. But when you love a flower, you water it daily." Buddha teaches us the difference between love and lust. In love, you nurture a relationship. In lust, you only satisfy your physical needs.
9. "A jug fills drop by drop."

5th Jan 2010, The Guardian, Buddhism beats depression: mindfulness meditation goes mainstream in the UK. It's already endorsed as a treatment for depression by the National Institute for Clinical Excellence, and today a major mental health charity is calling for meditation-based courses to be offered much more widely on the NHS… impressive clinical evidence for an approach called mindfulness-based cognitive therapy (MBCT) – the eight-week courses have been shown to reduce relapse rates by half among people who have suffered several episodes of depression have been reported. The report also finds that very few patients who could benefit from mindfulness training are currently being referred for the treatment – just one in 20 GPs prescribes MBCT regularly, even though nearly three-quarters of doctors think it would be helpful for their patients with mental health problems. Changing that could make a massive difference not only to them but to the economy – the cost of depression to the UK has been estimated at £7.5 billion every year.[308]

Mindfulness-based cognitive therapy is indicated for: Maintenance treatment of those who have suffered multiple episodes of unipolar major depression – the evidence suggests that the treatment is effective for patients with a history of at least three episodes; the therapy can be used alone or in conjunction with pharmacotherapy.[309] Regular mindfulness practice is believed to help further psychological insight and emotional healing over time. Mindfulness-based interventions, generally aimed at relieving symptoms of stress, mental health concerns, and physical pain.

ॐ भूर्भुवः स्वः तत्सवितुर्वरेण्यं
भर्गो देवस्य धीमहि
धियो यो नः प्रचोदयात् ॥

oṃ bhūr bhuvaḥ svaḥ
tat savitur vareṇyaṃ
bhargo devasya dhīmahi
dhiyo yo naḥ pracodayāt
– Rigveda 3.62.10[14]

114. GAYATRI MANTRA

EFFECT OF GAYATRI MANTRA ON BRAIN

Sanskrit mantra chanted in the prescribed manner changes brain function. This has been repeatedly demonstrated by scientific studies. A mantra is a word or phrase repeated aloud or silently and used to focus attention. Meditation using mantras is widely practiced in India. However, research on the effects of mantra meditation on the brain is sparse.

Gayatri mantra is taken from the Rig Veda and is a prayer dedicated to the Sun God. It is extremely powerful and effective with widespread use even now. Reciting or listening to the mantra has a positive effect on your mind and wellbeing.[310]

GAYATRI – is a Sanskrit word taken from Vedas.
MANTRA – OM BHUR BHUVAH SWAH
TAT SAVITUR, VARENYAM
BHARGO DEVASYA DHIMAHI
DHIYO YONAH PRACHODYAT

(The light of the sun illumines all the three worlds namely Bahu log, Bhavsar log, and Suva Log. I meditate upon that highly effulgent light. Let that light kindle and illumine my intellect too.)

Given by Saint Vishwamitra, in this mantra, a prayer is offered that God should show us light and take us to the truth. Gayatri Mantra is one of the most influential mantras of Rig Veda.

However, research on the effects of mantra meditation on the brain is sparse. Imaging (FMRI).[311]

The syllables of gayatri mantra are uttered by different parts of the mouth such as throat (larynx), tongue, teeth, lips and the root of the tongue. During speech, the nerve-fibers of the particular parts of the mouth from which sound emits stretch up to various parts of the body and exert pressure on the corresponding glands. There are various large, small, visible and invisible glands in the body. Uttering of different words has its impact on different glands and by such impact the energy of these glands gets stimulated. The twenty-four letters in Gayatri-Mantra which are related to twenty-four such glands located in the body which, on getting stimulated, activate and awaken the powers of mind for righteous wisdom (sattva guna).[312] The landmark study, which was conducted at the All India Institute of Medical Sciences New Delhi demonstrated positive effects of Gayatri Manta on adult males 25-30 years of age, using radiological investigations (MRI). In this research, they have visualized brain centers getting activated listening to the Gayatri mantra. The study duration was for nine months and data were studied for five years. It was concluded that remarkable expansion occurred in certain areas of the brain after listening to Gayatri mantra for a specific duration. It has a calming effect on the mind. Chanting the mantra can help mind and body relax. It helps the free flow of air through your system and reduced the secretion of "cortisol", the stress hormone. It reduces depression. It relaxes the nervous system and strengthens the brain to further regulate the activity of neurotransmitters, which often are deregulated in depression. Improvement in respiration and relaxation help the blood flow to increase in the skin resulting in improvement in the dullness of skin. Chanting Gayatri mantra helps to activate the eyes, brain and pineal glands thus improving the coordination of the body and concentration.[313] This mantra involves deep breathing, therefore it strengthens cardiac muscles and controls blood pressure. It improves breathing as chanting this mantra helps a person breathe deep and clear out the lungs.[314] It relaxes the body and increases spirituality.

REFERENCES

1. Bazargan-Hejazi, S., Bazargan, M., Shaheen, M., Teklehaimanot, S., Ahmadi, A., Cooper, J. S., & Teruya, S. (2016). Depression Symptoms, Acculturation, Needing Care, and Receiving Care: A Study of Adolescents Living in California. *Journal of Health Disparities Research and Practice*, 9(3), 45–66.
2. Adams, R. E., & Boscarino, J. A. (2013). Differences in mental health outcomes by acculturation status following a major urban disaster. *International Journal of Emergency Mental Health*, 15(2), 85–96.
3. Chinmaya Mission www.chinmayamission.com/what-we-do/activities/jnana-yajnas-and-spiritual-camps/
4. Chanen AM1, Kaess M. Developmental pathways to borderline personality disorder. Curr Psychiatry Rep. 2012 Feb;14(1):45–53.
5. Schmidt C. W. (2007). Environmental connections: a deeper look into mental illness. Environmental health perspectives, 115(8), A404–A410. https://doi.org/10.1289/ehp.115-a404
6. Joffe R. T. (2001). Progress in the biology of psychiatry. *Journal of Psychiatry & Neuroscience: JPN*, 26(2), 101–102.
7. Meymandi A. (2009). Eric R. Kandel: my kind of saint. *Psychiatry (Edgmont (Pa. : Township))*, *6*(11), 48–50.
8. Kirsten Weir (2012) The roots of mental illness, American Psychological Association www.apa.org/monitor/2012/06/roots
9. Daré, L.O., Bruand, P., Gérard, D. *et al.* Co-morbidities of mental disorders and chronic physical diseases in developing and emerging countries: a meta-analysis. *BMC Public Health* 19, 304 (2019). https://doi.org/10.1186/s12889-019-6623-6
10. Gururaj G, Varghese M, Benegal V, Rao GN, Pathak K, Singh LK, et al. Bengaluru: National Institute of Mental Health and Neuro Sciences; 2016. National Mental Health Survey of India, 2015-16: Prevalence, Patterns and Outcomes. NIMHANS Publication No. 129; pp. 90–121
11. Singh O. P. (2018). Closing treatment gap of mental disorders in India: Opportunity in new competency-based Medical Council of India curriculum. *Indian Journal of Psychiatry*, *60*(4), 375–376. https://doi.org/10.4103/psychiatry.IndianJPsychiatry_458_18
12. Herrman H (2001). The need for mental health promotion. *The Australian and New Zealand Journal of Psychiatry*, 35:709–715.
13. Marteau TM, Hollands GJ, Kelly MP. (2015). Changing population behaviour and reducing health disparities: Exploring the potential of 'choice architecture' interventions. In: Kaplan R, Spittel M, David D (Eds). Population Health: Behavioral and Social Science Insights. AHRQ Publication No. 15-0002. Rockville, MD: Agency for Healthcare Research and Quality and Office of Behavioral and Social Sciences Research, National Institutes of Health
14. Chen L, Magliano DJ, Zimmet PZ. The worldwide epidemiology of type 2 diabetes mellitus-present and future perspectives. *Nat Rev Endocrinol.* 2011 Nov 8; 8(4):228–236
15. Laslett LJ, Alagona P Jr, Clark BA 3rd, Drozda JP Jr, Saldivar F, Wilson SR, Poe C, & Hart M (2012). The worldwide environment of cardiovascular disease: prevalence, diagnosis, therapy, and policy issues: a report from the American College of Cardiology. *J Am Coll Cardiol.* 60(25 Suppl): S1-49.
16. Jang, H. W. & Park, S. W. (2016). Effects of personality traits on collaborative performance in problem-based learning tutorials. *Saudi Medical Journal, 37*(12), 1365–1371.
17. Duckworth, A. L., Quirk, A., Gallop, R., Hoyle, R. H., Kelly, D. R., & Matthews, M. D. (2019). Cognitive and noncognitive predictors of success. *Proceedings of the National Academy of Sciences of the United States of America, 116*(47), 23499–23504.
18. Briley, D. A., Domiteaux, M., & Tucker-Drob, E. M. (2014). Achievement-Relevant Personality: Relations with the Big Five and Validation of an Efficient Instrument. *Learning and Individual Differences, 32*, 26–39.

19. Bergold, S. & Steinmayr, R. (2018). Personality and Intelligence Interact in the Prediction of Academic Achievement. Journal of Intelligence, *6*(2), 27.
20. Rammstedt, B., Lechner, C. M., & Danner, D. (2018). Relationships between Personality and Cognitive Ability: A Facet-Level Analysis. Journal of Intelligence, *6*(2), 28.
21. Committee on the Science of Children Birth to Age 8: Deepening and Broadening the Foundation for Success; Board on Children, Youth, and Families; Institute of Medicine; National Research Council; Allen LR, Kelly BB, editors. Transforming the Workforce for Children Birth Through Age 8: A Unifying Foundation. Washington (DC): National Academies Press (US); 2015 Jul 23. 6, Educational Practices. Available from: www.ncbi.nlm.nih.gov/books/NBK310528/
22. Chang LJ, Sanfey AG. Emotion, decision-making and the brain. Adv Health Econ Health Serv Res. 2008;20:31-53. PMID: 19552303.
23. Lee, V. K. & Harris, L. T. (2013). How social cognition can inform social decision making. Frontiers in Neuroscience, 7, 259. doi:10.3389/fnins.2013.00259
24. Fraser, L., Burnell, M., Salter, L. C., Fourkala, E. O., Kalsi, J., Ryan, A., ... Menon, U. (2014). Identifying hopelessness in population research: a validation study of two brief measures of hopelessness. BMJ Open, 4(5), e005093.
25. Everson SA, Kaplan GA, Goldberg DE, et al. (2000). Hypertension incidence is predicted by high levels of hopelessness in Finnish men. Hypertension; 35:561–7
26. David Klonsky, E., Kotov, R., Bakst, S., Rabinowitz, J., & Bromet, E. J. (2012). Hopelessness as a predictor of attempted suicide among first admission patients with psychosis: a 10-year cohort study. Suicide & life-threatening behavior, 42(1), 1–10. https://doi.org/10.1111/j.1943-278X.2011.00066.x
27. Keenan, K., Hipwell, A., Feng, X., Babinski, D., Hinze, A., Rischall, M., & Henneberger, A. (2008). Subthreshold symptoms of depression in preadolescent girls are stable and predictive of depressive disorders. *Journal of the American Academy of Child and Adolescent Psychiatry, 47*(12), 1433–1442. doi:10.1097/CHI.0b013e3181886eab
28. Burcusa, S. L., & Iacono, W. G. (2007). Risk for recurrence in depression. Clinical Psychology *Review, 27*(8), 959–985. doi:10.1016/j.cpr.2007.02.005
29. Krakowski, M. I., & Czobor, P. (2014). Depression and impulsivity as pathways to violence: implications for antiaggressive treatment. Schizophrenia Bulletin, *40*(4), 886–889. https://doi.org/10.1093/schbul/sbt117
30. Mestre, T. A., Strafella, A. P., Thomsen, T., Voon, V., & Miyasaki, J. (2013). Diagnosis and treatment of impulse control disorders in patients with movement disorders. Therapeutic Advances in Neurological Disorders, 6(3), 175–188.
31. Hamzaoglu O, Ozkan O, Ulusoy M, Gokdogan F. The prevalence of hopelessness among adults: disability and other related factors. Int J Psychiatry Med. 2010;40(1):77-91. doi:10.2190/PM.40.1.f
32. Haatainen K, Tanskanen A, Kylmä J, et al. Factors associated with hopelessness: a population study. Int J Soc Psychiatry. 2004;50(2):142-152.
33. Miller, A. B., Esposito-Smythers, C., Weismoore, J. T., & Renshaw, K. D. (2013). The relation between child maltreatment and adolescent suicidal behavior: a systematic review and critical examination of the literature. Clinical Child and Family Psychology Review, 16(2), 146–172. doi:10.1007/s10567-013-0131-5
34. Gottschalk, L. A., Fronczek, J., & Buchsbaum, M. S. (1993). The cerebral neurobiology of hope and hopelessness. Psychiatry: Interpersonal and Biological Processes, *56*(3), 270–281.
35. Burcusa, S. L., & Iacono, W. G. (2007). Risk for recurrence in depression. Clinical Psychology Review, 27(8), 959–985. doi:10.1016/j. cpr.2007.02.005
36. Keenan, K., Hipwell, A., Feng, X., Babinski, D., Hinze, A., Rischall, M., & Henneberger, A. (2008). Subthreshold symptoms of depression in preadolescent girls are stable and predictive of depressive disorders. Journal of the American Academy of Child and Adolescent Psychiatry, 47(12), 1433–1442. doi:10.1097/CHI.0b013e3181886eab
37. Lépine, J. P., & Briley, M. (2011). The increasing burden of depression. Neuropsychiatric Disease and Treatment, 7(Suppl 1), 3–7. doi:10.2147/NDT. S19617
38. Burcusa, S. L., & Iacono, W. G. (2007). Risk for recurrence in depression. Clinical Psychology Review, 27(8), 959–985. doi:10.1016/j. cpr.2007.02.005
39. Lépine, J. P., & Briley, M. (2011). The increasing burden of depression. Neuropsychiatric Disease and Treatment, 7(Suppl 1), 3–7. doi:10.2147/NDT. S19617

40. American Psychiatric Association, www.psychiatry.org/patients-families/warning-signs-of-mental-illness
41. Tan, S. Y., & Yip, A. (2018). Hans Selye (1907-1982): Founder of the stress theory. Singapore Medical Journal, 59(4), 170–171
42. Rajesh, S. K., Ilavarasu, J. V., Srinivasan, T. M., & Nagendra, H. R. (2014). Stress and its Expression According to Contemporary Science and Ancient Indian Wisdom: Perseverative Cognition and the Pañca. Mens sana monographs, 12(1), 139–152.
43. Tiwari, S. C., & Pandey, N. M. (2013). The Indian concepts of lifestyle and mental health in old age. Indian Journal of Psychiatry, 55(Suppl 2), S288–S292. https://doi.org/10.4103/0019-5545.105553
44. Rastogi S. (2010). Building bridges between Ayurveda and Modern Science. International Journal of Ayurveda Research, 1(1), 41–46.
45. Bhui, K., Dinos, S., Galant-Miecznikowska, M., de Jongh, B., & Stansfeld, S. (2016). Perceptions of work stress causes and effective interventions in employees working in public, private and non-governmental organisations: a qualitative study. BJPsych Bulletin, 40(6), 318–325.
46. National Collaborating Centre for Mental Health (UK). Post-Traumatic Stress Disorder: The Management of PTSD in Adults and Children in Primary and Secondary Care. Leicester (UK): Gaskell; 2005. (NICE Clinical Guidelines, No. 26.) 2, Post-traumatic Stress Disorder. Available
47. Montero-Marín, J., García-Campayo, J., Mosquera Mera, D., & López del Hoyo, Y. (2009). A new definition of burnout syndrome based on Farber's proposal. Journal of Occupational Medicine and Toxicology (London, England), 4, 31.
48. McEwen B. S. (2006). Protective and damaging effects of stress mediators: central role of the brain. Dialogues in Clinical Neuroscience, 8(4), 367–381.
49. Pulliam JV, Dawaghreh AM, Alema-Mensah E, $ Plotsky PM. (2010). Social defeat stress produces prolonged alterations in acoustic startle and body weight gain in male Long Evans rats. J Psychiatr Res. 44(2):106-111. doi:10.1016/j.jpsychires.2009.05.005
50. McEwen B. S. (2006). Protective and damaging effects of stress mediators: central role of the brain. Dialogues in Clinical Neuroscience, 8(4), 367–381.
51. Koinis, A., Giannou, V., Drantaki, V., Angelaina, S., Stratou, E., & Saridi, M. (2015). The Impact of Healthcare Workers Job Environment on Their Mental-emotional Health. Coping Strategies: The Case of a Local General Hospital. Health Psychology Research, 3(1),
52. Desbordes, G., Gard, T., Hoge, E. A., Hölzel, B. K., Kerr, C., Lazar, S. W., Olendzki, A., & Vago, D. R. (2014). Moving beyond Mindfulness: Defining Equanimity as an Outcome Measure in Meditation and Contemplative Research. Mindfulness, 2014(January), 356–372. https://doi.org/10.1007/s12671-013-0269-
53. Bhui, K., Dinos, S., Galant-Miecznikowska, M., de Jongh, B., & Stansfeld, S. (2016). Perceptions of work stress causes and effective interventions in employees working in public, private and non-governmental organisations: a qualitative study. BJPsych Bulletin, 40(6), 318–325. https://doi.org/10.1192/pb.bp.115.050823
54. Richardson, G. E. (2002). The metatheory of resilience and resiliency. Journal of Clinical Psychology, 58, 307-321.
55. Shrivastava, A., & Desousa, A. (2016). Resilience: A psychobiological construct for psychiatric disorders. Indian Journal of Psychiatry, 58(1), 38–43.
56. Norris FH, Tracy M, & Galea S. (2009). Looking for resilience: Understanding the longitudinal trajectories of responses to stress. Soc Sci Med. 68:2190–2198.
57. Bonanno GA. (2004). Loss, trauma, and human resilience: Have we underestimated the human capacity to thrive after extremely aversive events? Am Psychol. 59:20–28
58. Rutter M. (2012). Resilience as a dynamic concept. Dev Psychopathol. May; 24(2): 335-344.
59. Montgomery, S. A. (2006). Major Depressive Disorders: Clinical Efficacy And Tolerability Of Agomelatine, A New Melatonergic Agonist. European Neuropsychopharmacology. 16 (5), 633-638.
60. Bowes L, Jaffee Sr. (2013). Biology, Genes, and Resilience: Toward a Multidisciplinary Approach Trauma Violence Abuse. Jul;14(3):195-208.
61. United Nations Drug Control Program. Twentieth general assembly special session; World Drug Problem; June 1998; New York.

62. Snoek, A., Levy, N., & Kennett, J. (2016). Strong-willed but not successful: The importance of strategies in recovery from addiction. Addictive Behaviours Reports, 4, 102–107. DOI:10.1016/j.abrep.2016.09.002
63. Drake, R. E., Mueser, K. T., & Brunette, M. F. (2007). Management of persons with co-occurring severe mental illness and substance use disorder: program implications. World psychiatry: official journal of the World Psychiatric Association (WPA), 6(3), 131–136.
64. www.camh.ca/en/health-info/mental-illness-and-addiction-index/addiction
65. Gordon R. An operational classification of disease prevention. In: Steinberg JA, editor; Silverman MM, editor. Preventing mental disorders: a research perspective. Rockville: US Department of Health and Human Services; 1987. pp. 20–26.
66. World Health Organization. Prevention of mental disorders. Effective interventions and policy options. Summary report. Geneva: World Health Organization; 2004.
67. Villatoro JA, Medina-Mora ME, Juárez F, Rojas E, Carreño S, & Berenzon S. (1998). Drug use pathways among high school students of Mexico. Addiction. Oct; 93(10):1577-1588.
68. Villatoro JA, Medina-Mora ME, Juárez F, Rojas E, Carreño S, Berenzon S,(1998) Drug use pathways among high school students of Mexico. Addiction. Oct; 93(10):1577-1588.
69. National Institute on Drug Abuse. Preventing drug use among children and adolescents. A research-based guide. Rockville: 1997. NIH Publication No. 97-4212.
70. Phillipson S. When the going gets tough … the Perfectionist takes control. OCD Online, 2016. Available at: www.ocdonline.com/going-gets-tough
71. Rowland, T. A., Jainer, A. K., & Panchal, R. (2017). Living with obsessional personality. BJPsych Bulletin, *41*(6), 366–367. https://doi.org/10.1192/pb.41.6.366a
72. Healthline www.healthline.com/health/obsessive-compulsive-personality-disorder
73. Stuyt E. (2018). The Problem with the Current High Potency THC Marijuana from the Perspective of an Addiction Psychiatrist. Missouri Medicine, 115(6), 482–486.
74. Shrivastava A, Johnston M, Terpstra K, & Bureau Y. (2015). Pathways to psychosis in cannabis abuse. Clin Schizophr Relat Psychoses. 9(1):30-35. doi:10.3371/CSRP.SHJO.030813
75. Shrivastava A, Johnston M, & Tsuang M. (2011). Cannabis use and cognitive dysfunction. Indian J Psychiatry; 53:187-191
76. World Healh Organisation.(2016) Health and social effet of nonmedical cananbis. www.who.int/substance_abuse/publications/msbcannabis.pdf?ua=1
77. Welch, K. A., McIntosh, A. M., Job, D. E., Whalley, H. C., Moorhead, T. W., Hall, J., Owens, D. G., Lawrie, S. M., & Johnstone, E. C. (2011). The impact of substance use on brain structure in people at high risk of developing schizophrenia. Schizophrenia Bulletin, 37(5), 1066–1076. https://doi.org/10.1093/schbul/sbq013
78. Practical Stress Management: A Comprehensive Workbook Academic Press. (Ed. John A. Romas, Manoj Sharma (2017) UK
79. Compas, B. E., Jaser, S. S., Dunbar, J. P., Watson, K. H., Bettis, A. H., Gruhn, M. A., & Williams, E. K. (2014). Coping and Emotion Regulation from Childhood to Early Adulthood: Points of Convergence and Divergence. Australian Journal of Psychology, 66(2), 71–81. https://doi.org/10.1111/ajpy.12043
80. A.F. Alves, C.M.A. Gomes, A. & Martins, L.S. (2016). AlmeidaSocial and cultural contexts change but intelligence persists as incisive to explain children's academic achievement Ponte International Scientific Researches Journal, 72, 70-89,
81. Donnelly, J. E., Hillman, C. H., Castelli, D., Etnier, J. L., Lee, S., Tomporowski, P., … Szabo-Reed, A. N. (2016). Physical Activity, Fitness, Cognitive Function, and Academic Achievement in Children: A Systematic Review. Medicine and Science in Sports and Exercise, 48(6), 1197–1222.
82. Krapohl, E., Rumsfeld, K., Shakeshaft, N. G., Trzaskowski, M., McMillan, A., Pingault, J. B., … Plomin, R. (2014). The high heritability of educational achievement reflects many genetically influenced traits, not just intelligence. Proceedings of the National Academy of Sciences of the United States of America, 111(42), 15273–15278.
83. Committee on the Science of Children Birth to Age 8: Deepening and Broadening the Foundation for Success; Board on Children, Youth, and Families; Institute of Medicine; National Research Council; Allen LR, Kelly BB, editors. A Unifying Foundation. Washington (DC): National Academies Press (US); 2015 Jul 23. 4, Child Development and Early Learning. Available from: www.ncbi.nlm.nih.gov/ books/ NBK310550/
84. Jotterand F. (2018). Childhood Brain Development, the Educational Achievement Gap, and Cognitive Enhancement. Frontiers in Pharmacology, 9, 1142.
85. Mayer, J. (2018). Intelligence about Things and Intelligence about People. In R. Sternberg (Ed.), The Nature of Human Intelligence (pp. 270286). Cambridge: Cambridge University Press.

86. Demetriou, A., & Spanoudis, G. (2017). From Cognitive Development to Intelligence: Translating Developmental Mental Milestones into Intellect. Journal of Intelligence, 5(3), 30.
87. Institute of Medicine (US) Committee on the Health Professions Education Summit; Greiner AC, Knebel E, editors. Health Professions Education: A Bridge to Quality. Washington (DC): National Academies Press (US); 2003. Chapter 4, Current Educational Activities in the Core Competencies. Available from: www.ncbi.nlm.nih.gov/ books/ NBK221517
88. Kuo, M., Barnes, M., & Jordan, C. (2019). Do Experiences With Nature Promote Learning? Converging Evidence of a Cause-and-Effect Relationship. Frontiers in psychology, 10, 305.
89. Bijwaard, G. E., van Kippersluis, H., & Veenman, J. (2015). Education and health: The role of cognitive ability. Journal of Health Economics, 42, 29–43.
90. Szumowska, E., Kossowska, M., & Roets, A. (2018). Motivation to comply with task rules and multitasking performance: The role of need for cognitive closure and goal importance. Motivation and Emotion, 42(3), 360–376.
91. Kern, M. L., & Friedman, H. S. (2008). Early educational milestones as predictors of lifelong academic achievement, midlife adjustment, and longevity. Journal of Applied Developmental Psychology, 30(4), 419–430.
92. Park, D. C., & Bischof, G. N. (2013). The aging mind: neuroplasticity in response to cognitive training. Dialogues in Clinical Neuroscience, 15(1), 109–119.
93. www.youtube.com/watch?v=KPn3ZUcaBOY
94. Tyng, C. M., Amin, H. U., Saad, M., & Malik, A. S. (2017). The Influences of Emotion on Learning and Memory. Frontiers in Psychology, 8, 1454.
95. Ackerman S. Discovering the Brain. Washington (DC): National Academies Press (US); 1992. 2, Major Structures and Functions of the Brain. Available from: www.ncbi.nlm.nih.gov/books/ NBK234157/
96. Luo, Y., Chen, X., Qi, S., You, X., & Huang, X. (2018). Well-being and Anticipation for Future Positive Events: Evidences from an fMRI Study. Frontiers in Psychology, 8, 2199.
97. Salzman, C. D., & Fusi, S. (2010). Emotion, cognition, and mental state representation in amygdala and prefrontal cortex. Annual Review of Neuroscience, 33, 173–202.
98. Kim, S., & Lee, D. (2011). Prefrontal cortex and impulsive decision making. Biological Psychiatry, 69(12), 1140–1146
99. Glimcher PW. (2003). The neurobiology of visual-saccadic decision making. Annu Rev Neurosci.; 26(1):133-179.
100. Wahlstrom, D., Collins, P., White, T., & Luciana, M. (2010). Developmental changes in dopamine neurotransmission in adolescence: behavioral implications and issues in assessment. Brain and Cognition, 72(1), 146–159.
101. Dfarhud, D., Malmir, M., & Khanahmadi, M. (2014). Happiness & Health: The Biological Factors- Systematic Review Article. Iranian Journal of Public Health, 43(11), 1468–1477.
102. Office of the Surgeon General (US) (2001) : A Report of the Surgeon General. Rockville (MD): Substance Abuse and Mental Health Services Administration (US)
103. National Academies of Sciences, Engineering, and Medicine; Division of Behavioral and Social Sciences and Education; Board on Children, Youth, and Families; Committee on Supporting the Parents of Young Children; Briner H, Ford M, Gadsden VL, editors. Parenting Matters: Supporting Parents of Children Ages 0-8. Washington (DC): National Academies Press (US); 2016 Nov 21. 2,
104. Luthar S. S. (2003). The culture of affluence: psychological costs of material wealth. Child Development, 74(6), 1581–1593.
105. Bandura A, Barbaranelli C, Caprara GV, & Pastorelli C. (2001). Self-efficacy beliefs as shapers of children's aspirations and career trajectories. Child Development.;72:187–206
106. Cherian VI. (1991). Parental aspirations and academic achievement of Xhosa children. Psychological Reports.;68:547–555
107. Jang, H. W., & Park, S. W. (2016). Effects of personality traits on collaborative performance in problem-based learning tutorials. Saudi Medical Journal, 37(12), 1365–1371.
108. Levy JJ, & Lounsbury JW. (2011). Big Five personality traits and performance anxiety in relation to marching arts satisfaction. *Work*.;40(3):297-302. doi:10.3233/WOR-2011-1233
109. Duckworth, A. L., Quirk, A., Gallop, R., Hoyle, R. H., Kelly, D. R., & Matthews, M. D. (2019). Cognitive and noncognitive predictors of success. Proceedings of the National Academy of Sciences of the United States of America, 116(47), 23499–23504.
110. Committee on the Science of Children Birth to Age 8: Deepening and Broadening the Foundation for Success; Board on Children, Youth, and Families; Institute of Medicine; National Research Council; Allen LR, Kelly BB, editors. Transforming the Workforce

for Children Birth Through Age 8: A Unifying Foundation. Washington (DC): National Academies Press (US); 2015 Jul 23. 6,

111. Kessler RC, Foster CL, Saunders WB, Stang PE: Social consequences of psychiatric disorders. I am educational attainment. Am J Psychiatry. 1995, 152 (7): 1026-1032
112. Pascale Esch, Valéry Bocquet, Charles Pull, Sophie Couffignal, Torsten Lehnert, Marc Graas, Laurence Fond-Harman, Marc Ansseau (2014) The downward spiral of mental disorders and educational attainment: a systematic review on early school leaving BMC Psychiatry volume 14, 237
113. Adams T, & Moore M. (2007). High-risk health and credit behaviour among 18- to 25-year-old students. J Am Coll Health.; 56:101–108
114. Blanco C, Okuda M, Wright C, Hasin DS, Grant BF, Liu SM, et al. (2008). Mental health of college students and their non-college-attending peers: results from the National Epidemiologic Study on Alcohol and Related Conditions. Arch Gen Psychiat.; 65:1429–1437.
115. Auerbach RP, Alonso J, Axinn WG, Cuijpers P, Ebert DD, Green JG, Hwang I, et al. (2016). Mental disorders among college students in the World Health Organization World Mental Health Surveys. Psychol Med Aug.; 3:1–16.
116. Scott KM, Lim C, Al-Hamzawi A, Alonso J, Bruffaerts R, & Caldasde- Almeida JM. (2016). Association of Mental Disorders With Subsequent Chronic Physical Conditions: World Mental Health Surveys From 17 Countries. JAMA Psychiatr.; 73:150–158.
117. Kerr DC, & Capaldi DM. (2011). Young men's intimate partner violence and relationship functioning: long-term outcomes associated with suicide attempt and aggression in adolescence. Psychol Med.; 41:759–769
118. Ibrahim AK, Kelly SJ, Adams CE, Glazebrook C. (2013). A systematic review of studies of depression prevalence in university students. J Psych Res.; 47:391–400.
119. 172 www.supportive relation ships.org/home/ relationship-problems-are-a-leading cause-for-suicide/
120. Slade M. (2010). Mental illness and well-being: the central importance of positive psychology and recovery approaches. BMC Health Services Research, 10, 26.
121. DeSocio, J. and Hootman, J. (2004). Children's mental health and school success. The Journal of School Nursing 20(4):189-196.
122. Kirmayer LJ, Gomez-Carrillo A, & Veissière S. (2017). Culture and depression in global mental health: An ecosocial approach to the phenomenology of psychiatric disorders. *Soc Sci Med.*;183:163-168. doi:10.1016/j.socscimed.2017.04.034
123. Kovacs, M. (1996). Presentation and course of major depressive disorder during childhood and later years of the life span. Journal of the American Academy of Child and Adolescent Psychiatry 35(6):705-715
124. Kessler, R.C. (2003). The impairments caused by social phobia in the general population: Implications for intervention. Acta Psychiatrica Scandinavica 417(Suppl.):19-27.
125. Stein, M. and Kean, Y.M. (2000). Disability and quality of life in social phobia: Epidemiologic findings. American Journal of Psychiatry 157: 1606-1613.
126. Kieling C, Baker-Henningham H, Belfer M, et al. (2011). Child and adolescent mental health worldwide: evidence for action. Lancet.;378:1515 –1525.
127. Hjorth, C. F., Bilgrav, L., Frandsen, L. S., Overgaard, C., Torp- Pedersen, C., Nielsen, B., & Bøggild, H. (2016). Mental health and school dropout across educational levels and genders: a 4.8-year fol- low-up study. BMC Public Health, 16, 976.
128. Auerbach, R. P., Mortier, P., Bruffaerts, R., Alonso, J., Benjet, C., Cuijpers, P., WHO WMH-ICS Collaborators (2018). WHO World Mental Health Surveys International College Student Project: Prevalence and distribution of mental disorders. Journal of Abnormal Psychology, 127(7), 623–638.
129. Ibrahim AK, Kelly SJ, Adams CE, Glazebrook C. A systematic review of studies of depression prevalence in university students. J Psych Res. 2013; 47:391–400.
130. Freudenberg N, Ruglis J. Reframing school dropout as a public health issue. Prev Chronic Dis, 2007;4:A107.
131. Cutler, D.; Lleras-Muney, (2006) A. Education and Health: Evaluating Theories and Evidence. National Poverty Center Working Paper Series. National Poverty Center; Washington, DC.
132. Fronstin P, Greenberg DH, & Robins PK. The Labor Market Consequences of Childhood Maladjustment. Social Science Quarterly 2005;86s:1170–1195.

133. Huurre T, Aro H, Rahkonen O, & Komulainen E. (2006). Health, lifestyle, family and school factors in adolescence: predicting adult educational level. Educational Research;48:41–53.
134. Joshua Breslau, PhD, ScD, Michael Lane, MS, Nancy Sampson, BA, and Ronald C. Kessler, Mental Disorders and Subsequent Educational Attainment in a US National Sample J Psychiatr Res. 2008 July; 42(9): 708–716.
135. Tungpunkom P, Maayan N, Soares-Weiser K. Life skills programmes for chronic mental illnesses. Cochrane Database Syst Rev. 2012;1:CD000381. Published 2012 Jan 18. doi:10.1002/14651858.CD000381.pub3
136. Pujar, L.L., Hunshal, S.C., Bailur, K.B., 2004. Impact of intervention on life skill development among adolescent girls. Karnataka J. Agric. Sci. 27 (1).
137. Promoting Mental Health World Health Organization Geneva, 2004, www.who.int/mental_health/evidence/en/promoting_mhh. pdf
138. Simran www.youthkiawaaz.com/2018/05/ mental-health-| situation-in-indian-colleges/
139. Demographic indicators. National Health Profile 2011. New Delhi: Prabhat Publicity; 2011. Central Bureau of Health Intelligence. Available from: www.cbhidghs.nic.in/writeread-data/mainlink- File/01%20Cover%20page%202011.pdf.
140. Rao VG, Aggrawal MC, Yadav R, Das SK, Sahara LK, Bondley MK, et al. Intestinal parasitic infections, anaemia and undernutrition among tribal adolescents of Madhya Pradesh. Indian J Community Med. 2003;28:26–29.
141. World Health Survey, 2003, India. International Institute for Population Sciences (IIPS), Mumbai. World Health Organization (WHO), Geneva and WHO - India-WR Office. Available from: www.who.int/healthinfo/survey/whs_hspa_book.pdf.
142. Parasuraman S, Kishor S, Singh SK, Vaidehi Y. National Family Health Survey (NFHS-3), India, 2005-06. Mumbai: International Institute for Population Sciences. Calverton, Maryland, USA: ICF Macro; 2009 A profile of youth in India. Available from: www.rchiips.org/ NFHS/youth_report_for_website_18sep09.pdf.
143. Veena N, Shailaja Shastri 2016. Stress and Academic Performance, The International Journal of Indian Psychology, Volume 3, Issue 3, No. 4,
144. Sahoo SI, & Khess CR. (2010). Prevalence of depression, anxiety, and stress among young male adults in India: a dimensional and categorical diagnoses-based study. J Nerv Ment Dis. Dec;198(12):901-904.
145. Mohan S, Sathya Devi, R, A study on stress and its effects on college students, International Journal of Scientific Engineering and Applied Science (IJSEAS) - Volume-1, Issue-7, October 2015
146. Schneiderman, N., Ironson, G., & Siegel, S. D. (2005). Stress and health: psychological, behavioral, and biological determinants. Annual review of clinical psychology, 1, 607–628.
147. Michaela C. Pascoe, Sarah E. Hetrick & Alexandra G. Parker (2020) The impact of stress on students in secondary school and higher education, International Journal of Adolescence and Youth, 25:1, 104-112,
148. Gregg Henriques, Psychology Today, www.psychologytoday. com/ca/experts/gregg-henriques-phd
149. Students and College, A Stressful Time of Life: Parents and Students Beware, MentalHelp.net www.mentalhelp.net/stress/ students-and-college-a-stressful-time-of-life/
150. Merlin, A., Bonis, A., Damgaard, C. F., & Mesléard, F. (2015). Competition Is a Strong Driving Factor in Wetlands, Peaking during Drying Out Periods. PloS one, 10(6), e0130152.
151. Kim S. I. (2013). Neuroscientific model of motivational process. Frontiers in psychology, 4, 98.
152. Leibbrandt, A., Gneezy, U., & List, J. A. (2013). Rise and fall of competitiveness is the nature of individualistic and collectivistic societies. Proceedings of the National Academy of Sciences of the United States of America, 110(23), 9305–9308.
153. Carter TM. The effects of spiritual practices on recovery from substance abuse. J Psychiatr Ment Health Nurs. 1998 Oct;5(5):409-13. doi: 10.1046/j.1365-2850.1998.00153.x. PMID: 10067489.
154. Manning L. K. (2012). Spirituality is a lived experience: exploring the essence of spirituality for women in late life. International Journal of Ageing & Human Development, 75(2), 95–113.
155. Rudolfsson, G., Berggren, I., & da Silva, A. B. (2014). Experiences of spirituality and spiritual values in the context of nursing - an integrative review. The Open Nursing Journal, 8, 64–70.

156. 6 Signs You Feel Stuck and Need To Make a Change In Your Life, https://themindsjournal.com/signs-time-to-move-on/
157. Li X, Weissman M, Talati A, Svob C, Wickramaratne P, Posner J, Xu D. A diffusion tensor imaging study of brain microstructural changes related to religion and spirituality in families at high risk for depression. Brain Behav. 2019 Feb;9(2):e01209.
158. Malhi, G. S., Das, P., Bell, E., Mattingly, G., & Mannie, Z. (2019). Modelling resilience in adolescence and adversity: a novel framework to inform research and practice. Translational psychiatry, 9(1), 316.
159. Banquet Spectral analysis of the EEG in meditation. Electroencephalogr Clin Neurophysiol. 1973 Aug; 35(2):143-51
160. Newberg A. B. (2014). The neuroscientific study of spiritual practices. Frontiers in Psychology, 5, 215.
161. Corby JC, Roth WT, Zarcone VP Jr, Kopell BS Psychophysiological correlates of the practice of Tantric Yoga meditation. Arch Gen Psychiatry. 1978 May; 35(5):571-577
162. Sudsuang R, Chentanez V, Veluvan K, Effect of Buddhist meditation on serum cortisol and total protein levels, blood pressure, pulse rate, lung volume and reaction time. Physiol Behav. 1991 Sep; 50(3):543-548.
163. O'Halloran JP, Jevning R, Wilson AF, Skowsky R, Walsh RN, Alexander C, Hormonal control in a state of decreased activation: potentiation of arginine vasopressin secretionPhysiol Behav. 1985 Oct; 35(4):591-5
164. Ackerman S. Discovering the Brain. Washington (DC): National Academies Press (US); 1992. 2, Major Structures and Functions of the Brain. Available from: https://www.ncbi.nlm.nih.gov/books/ NBK23415
165. Lanciego JL, Luquin N, Obeso JA. Functional neuroanatomy of the basal ganglia. Cold Spring Harb Perspect Med. 2012;2(12):a009621.
166. Jawabri KH, Sharma S. Physiology, Cerebral Cortex Functions. [Updated 2019 Jun 29]. In: StatPearls [Internet]. Treasure Island (FL): StatPearls Publishing; 2019 Jan.
167. Park, J E. (2012) Park's textbook of Preventive and Social Medicine Chapter-2., 22nd Vol.
168. Hogeveen, J., Salvi, C., & Grafman, J. (2016). 'Emotional Intelligence': Lessons from Lesions. Trends in neurosciences, 39(10), 694–705.
169. Ackerman S. Discovering the Brain. Washington (DC): National Academies Press (US); 1992. 4. The Role of the Brain in Mental Illness. Available from: https://www.ncbi.nlm.nih.gov/books/NBK234144
170. Colver, A., & Longwell, S. (2013). New understanding of adolescent brain development: relevance to transitional healthcare for young people with long term conditions. Archives of disease in childhood, 98(11), 902–907.
171. Biran J, Tahor M, Wircer E, Levkowitz G. (2015) Role of developmental factors in hypothalamic function. Front Neuroanat. 20er15;9:47.
172. Fama R, Sullivan EV.(2015) Thalamic structures and associated cognitive functions: Relations with age and ageing. Neurosci Biobehav Rev. 2015;54:29-37.
173. Anand KS, Dhikav V. (2012) Hippocampus in health and disease: An over-view. Ann Indian Acad Neurol;15(4):239-46.
174. Krabbendam, L., Hooker, C. I., & Aleman, A. (2014). Neural effects of the social environment. Schizophrenia bulletin, 40(2), 248–251.
175. Rees, C. L., White, C. M., & Ascoli, G. A. (2017). Neurochemical Markers in the Mammalian Brain: Structure, Roles in Synaptic Communication, and Pharmacological Relevance. Current medicinal chemistry, 24(28), 3077–3103.
176. National Research Council (US) and Institute of Medicine (US) Committee on Integrating the Science of Early Childhood Development; Shonkoff JP, Phillips DA, editors. From Neurons to Neighborhoods: The Science of Early Childhood Development. Washington (DC): National Academies Press (US); 2000. 8, The Developing Brain. Available from: https://www.ncbi.nlm.nih.gov/ books/NBK225562/
177. Boly M, Massimini M, Tsuchiya N, Postle BR, Koch C, Tononi G. Are the Neural Correlates of Consciousness in the Front or the Back of the Cerebral Cortex? Clinical and Neuroimaging Evidence. J Neurosci. 2017;37(40):9603-9613.
178. Johnson, S. B., Blum, R. W., & Giedd, J. N. (2009). Adolescent matu-rity and the brain: the promise and pitfalls of neuroscience research in adolescent health policy. The Journal of adolescent health: official publication of the Society for Adolescent Medicine, 45(3), 216–221.
179. Mittal, R., Debs, L. H., Patel, A. P., Nguyen, D., Patel, K., O'Connor, G., Grati, M., Mittal, J., Yan, D., Eshraghi, A. A., Deo, S. K., Daunert, S., ... Liu, X. Z. (2017). Neurotransmitters:

The Critical Modulators Regulating Gut-Brain Axis. Journal of cellular physiology, 232(9), 2359-2372.

180. Bernstein, K. E., Ong, F. S., Blackwell, W. L., Shah, K. H., Giani, J. F., Gonzalez-Villalobos, R. A., ... Touyz, R. M. (2012). A modern understanding of the traditional and nontraditional biological func-tions of angiotensin-converting enzyme. Pharmacological reviews, 65(1), 1–46.
181. De Sousa A. (2013). Towards an integrative theory of consciousness: part 2 (an anthology of various other models). Mens sana monographs, 11(1), 151–209. https://doi.org/10.4103/0973-1229.109341
182. Sowell ER, Toga AW, (2000)A sarnow R. Brain abnormalities observed in childhood-onset schizophrenia: A review of the structural magnetic resonance imaging literature. Mental Retardation and Developmental Disabilities Research Review. ;6:180–185
183. Marvel, C. L., & Paradiso, S. (2004). Cognitive and neurological impairment in mood disorders. The Psychiatric clinics of North America, 27(1), 19–viii. https://doi.org/10.1016/S0193-953X(03)00106-0
184. Ackerman S. Discovering the Brain. Washington (DC): National Academies Press (US); 1992. 6, The Development and Shaping of the Brain. Available from: https://www.ncbi.nlm.nih.gov/books/NBK234146/
185. Trivedi J. K. (2006). Cognitive deficits in psychiatric disorders: Current status. Indian journal of psychiatry, 48(1), 10–20. https://doi.org/10.4103/0019-5545.31613
186. U.S. Department of Health and Human Services (HHS), Office of the Surgeon General, Facing Addiction in America: The Surgeon General's Report on Alcohol, Drugs, and Health. Washington, DC: HHS, November 2016.
187. Sullivan, E. V., Harris, R. A., & Pfefferbaum, A. (2010). Alcohol's effects on brain and behavior. Alcohol research & health : the journal of the National Institute on Alcohol Abuse and Alcoholism, 33(1-2), 127–143.
188. Berridge, K. C., & Kringelbach, M. L. (2015). Pleasure systems in the brain. Neuron, 86(3), 646–664.
189. Kendra Cherry,How experiences change brain plasticity,Septermber 26,2019, https://www.verywellmind.com/what-is-brain-plasticity- .(last accessed on 21.07.2020)
190. Keng, S. L., Smoski, M. J., & Robins, C. J. (2011). Effects of mind- fulness on psychological health: a review of empirical studies. Clinical psycholog y review, 31(6), 1041–1056.
191. Lenroot, R. K., & Giedd, J. N. (2008). The changing impact of genes and environment on brain development during childhood and adolescence: initial findings from a neuroimaging study of pediatric twins. Development and psychopathology, 20(4), 1161–1175. https://doi.org/10.1017/S0954579408000552
192. Wang MT, Eccles JS, Kenny S. Not lack of ability but more choice: individual and gender differences in choice of careers in science, technology, engineering, and mathematics. Psychol Sci. 2013;24(5):770-775. doi:10.1177/0956797612458937
193. Shaffer J. (2016). Neuroplasticity and Clinical Practice: Building Brain Power for Health. Frontiers in psychology, 7, 1118. https://doi.org/10.3389/fpsyg.2016.01118
194. American Psychological Association, https://www.apa.org/news/ press/releases/2018/01/perfectionism-young-people
195. Milestones and millennials, Mayo Clinic Proceedings, https:// www.mayoclinicproceedings.org/article/s0025-6196(16)30690-5/ fulltext?linkid=34479498
196. Gong D, He H, Liu D, et al. Enhanced functional connectivity and increased gray matter volume of insula related to action video game playing. Sci Rep. 2015;5:9763. Published 2015 Apr 16. doi:10.1038/srep0976
197. Bavelier, D., Green, C. S., Han, D. H., Renshaw, P. F., Merzenich, M. M., & Gentile, D. A. (2011). Brains on video games. Nature reviews. Neuroscience, 12(12), 763–768. https://doi.org/10.1038/nrn3135
198. Park, D. C., & Bischof, G. N. (2013). The aging mind: neuroplasticity in responsetocognitivetraining.Dialoguesin clinical neuroscience, 15(1),109–119.
199. Shaffer J. (2016). Neuroplasticity and Clinical Practice: Building Brain Power for Health. Frontiers in psychology, 7, 1118. doi:10.3389/ fpsyg.2016.01118
200. Froeliger, B., Garland, E. L., & McClernon, F. J. (2012). Yoga meditation practitioners exhibit greater gray matter volume and fewer reported cognitive failures: results of a preliminary voxel-based morphometric analysis. Evidence-based complementary and alternative medicine : eCAM, 2012, 821307. https://doi.org/10.1155/2012/821307
201. Cicchetti D, Curtis J. (2006)The Developing Brain and Neural Plasticity: Implications for Normality, Psychopatholgy, and Resilience. ; 2:1–64

202. Leuner B, Gould E: (2010)Structural plasticity and hippocampal function. Annu Rev Psychol 61:111–140, C1–C3
203. Agarwal N, Port JD, Bazzocchi M, et al: (2010); Update on the use of MR for assessment and diagnosis of psychiatric diseases. Radiology 255:23–41
204. Jill L. Kays, Psy.D., Robin A. Hurley, M.D., Katherine H. Taber, Ph.D. The Dynamic Brain: Neuroplasticity and Mental Health, WINDOWS TO THE BRAIN https://neuro.psychiatry-online.org/doi/pdf/10.1176/appi.neuropsych.12050109(last accessed on 21.7.2020)
205. Palmer, S. (1989). Occupational Stress. The Health and Safety Practitioner, 7, (8), 16-18.
206. Tyrka AR, Burgers DE, Philip NS, Price LH, Carpenter LL. The neu-robiological correlates of childhood adversity and implications for treatment. Acta Psychiatr Scand. 2013;128:434–447
207. Nicolaides NC, Pavlaki AN, Maria Alexandra MA, et al. Glucocorticoid Therapy and Adrenal Suppression. [Updated 2018 Oct 19]. In: Feingold KR, Anawalt B, Boyce A, et al., editors. Endotext [Internet]. South Dartmouth (MA): MDText.com, Inc.; 2000-. Available from: https://www.ncbi.nlm.nih.gov/books/NBK279156/
208. Kowianski P, Lietzau G, Czuba E, Waskow M, Steliga A, Morys J. BDNF: a key factor with multipotent impact on brain signaling and synaptic plasticity. Cell Mol Neurobiol (2018) 38(3):579–93. doi: 10.1007/ s10571-017-0510-4
209. Thoma, M. V., La Marca, R., Brönnimann, R., Finkel, L., Ehlert, U., & Nater, U. M. (2013). The effect of music on the human stress response. PloS one, 8(8), e70156. https://doi.org/10.1371/journal.pone.0070156
210. Borson S. (2010). Cognition, aging, and disabilities: conceptual issues. Physical medicine and rehabilitation clinics of North America, 21(2), 375–382. https://doi.org/10.1016/j.pmr.2010.01.001
211. Campbell RJ. Campbell's psychiatric dictionary. 8th ed. Oxford: Oxford University Press; 2004. p. 131.
212. Chan RCK, Chen EYH. Assessment of executive functions for schizophrenia in Hong Kong. Hong Kong J Psychiatry. 2005;15:23–8.
213. Goldman-Rakic PS. Working memory dysfunction in schizophrenia. J Neuropsychiatry Clin Neurosci. 1994;6:348–57.
214. Cummings JL. Frontal-subcortical circuits and human behavior. Arch Neurol. 1993;50:873–80
215. National Research Council (US) Panel to Review the Status of Basic Research on School-Age Children; Collins WA, editor. Development During Middle Childhood: The Years From Six to Twelve. Washington (DC): National Academies Press (US); 1984. Chapter 3, Cognitive Development In School-Age Children: Conclusions And New Directions. Available from: https://www.ncbi.nlm.nih.gov/books/NBK216774/
216. Cowan, N. (2008). What are the differences between long-term, short-term, and working memory?. Progress in brain research, 169, 323–338.
217. Aben, B., Stapert, S., & Blokland, A. (2012). About the Distinction between Working Memory and Short-Term Memory. *Frontiers in psychology*, *3*, 301. https://doi.org/10.3389/fpsyg.2012.00301
218. Campbell, J. M., Brown, R. T., Cavanagh, S. E., Vess, S. F., & Segall, M. J. (2008). Evidence-based assessment of cognitive functioning in pediatric psychology. Journal of pediatric psycholog y, 33(9), 999–1020.
219. Baddeley, Alan (2007) Working Memory, Thought, and Action. Oxford University Press. UK
220. Cowan, N. (2008). What are the differences between long-term, short-term, and working memory?. Progress in brain research, 169, 323–338.
221. Camina, E., & Güell, F. (2017). The Neuroanatomical, Neurophysiological and Psychological Basis of Memory: Current Models and Their Origins. Frontiers in pharmacology, 8, 438. https://doi.org/10.3389/fphar.2017.00438
222. Norris D. (2017). Short-term memory and long-term memory are still different. Psychological bulletin, 143(9), 992–1009. https://doi.org/10.1037/bul0000108
223. Rolls ET. Memory systems in the brain. Annu Rev Psychol. 2000;51:599-630. doi:10.1146/annurev.psych.51.1.599
224. National Research Council (US) and Institute of Medicine (US) Committee on Depression, Parenting Practices, and the Healthy Development of Children; England MJ, Sim LJ, editors. Depression in Parents, Parenting, and Children: Opportunities to Improve Identification, Treatment, and Prevention. Washington (DC): National Academies Press

(US); 2009. 4, Associations Between Depression in Parents and Parenting, Child Health, and Child Psychological Functioning.
225. Committee on Psychological Testing, Including Validity Testing, for Social Security Administration Disability Determinations; Board on the Health of Select Populations; Institute of Medicine. Psychological Testing in the Service of Disability Determination. Washington (DC): National Academies Press (US); 2015 Jun 29. 5, Cognitive Tests and Performance Validity Tests.
226. Lauralee Sherwood 2015). Human Physiology: From Cells to Systems. Cengage Learning. pp. 157–162.
227. Cowan, N. (2008). What are the differences between long-term, short- term, and working memory?. Progress in brain research, 169, 323–338.
228. Buchanan T. W. (2007). Retrieval of emotional memories. Psychological Bulletin, 133(5), 761–779.
229. Pino, M., & Mortari, L. (2014). The inclusion of students with dyslexia in higher education: a systematic review using narrative synthesis. Dyslexia (Chichester, England), 20(4), 346–369.
230. Borghans, Lex, Angela L. Duckworth, James J. Heckman, and Bas ter Weel. 2008. "The Economics and Psychology of Personality Traits." Journal of Human Resources, vol. 43, no. 4, 972–1059.
231. Campbell, J. M., Brown, R. T., Cavanagh, S. E., Vess, S. F., & Segall, M. J. (2008). Evidence-based assessment of cognitive functioning in pe- diatric psychology. Journal of pediatric psychology, 33(9), 999–1020.
232. World Health Organization, South east Asian Countries, Depression in India, http://www.searo.who.int/india/depression_in_india.pdf
233. Paris J. (2007). Why Psychiatrists are Reluctant to Diagnose: Borderline Personality Disorder. Psychiatry (Edgmont (Pa. : Township)), 4(1), 35–39.
234. Negele, A., Kaufhold, J., Kallenbach, L., & Leuzinger-Bohleber, M. (2015). Childhood Trauma and Its Relation to Chronic Depression in Adulthood. Depression research and treatment, 2015, 650804.
235. Jha KK1, Singh SK2, Nirala SK2, Kumar C2, Kumar P2, Aggrawal N2. Prevalence of Depression among School-going Adolescents in an Urban Area of Bihar, India. Indian J Psychol Med. 2017 May-Jun; 39(3):287-292.
236. Deb sl, Banu PR, Thomas S, Vardhan RV3, Rao PT3, Khawaja N, Depression among indian university students and its association with perceived university academic environment, living arrangements and personal issues. Asian j psychiatr. 2016 oct;23:108-117
237. American Association, http://www.workplacementalhealth.org/ Mental-Health-Topics/Depression/Quantifying-the-Cost-of- Depression
238. Bandelow, B., & Michaelis, S. (2015). Epidemiology of anxiety disor- ders in the 21st century. Dialogues in clinical neuroscience, 17(3), 327–335.
239. Grover, S., Raju, V. V., Sharma, A., & Shah, R. (2019). Depression in Children and Adolescents: A Review of Indian studies. Indian journal of psychological medicine, 41(3), 216–227.
240. Deb sl, Banu PR, Thomas S, Vardhan RV3, Rao PT3, Khawaja N, Depression among indian university students and its association with perceived university academic environment, living arrangements and personal issues. Asian j psychiatr. 2016 oct;23:108-117
241. Patel V, Rodrigues M, DeSouza N. Gender, poverty, and postna- tal depression: a study of mothers in Goa, India. Am J Psychiatry. 2002;159:43–7.
242. Ram D, Darshan MS, Rao TS, Honagodu AR. Suicide prevention is possible: A perception after a suicide attempt. Indian Journal of Psychiatry. 2012 Apr;54(2):172-176. DOI: 10.4103/0019-5545.99535.
243. The World health report: 2001: Mental health: new understanding, new hope, World Health Organization, Geneva
244. Leff J, Gamble C (1995). Training of community psychiatric nurses in family work for schizophrenia. International Journal of Mental Health, 24: 76–88.
245. Dixon LB, Lehman AF, Levine J (1995). Conventional antipsychotic medications for schizophrenia. Schizophrenia Bulletin, 21(4): 567–577
246. Pharaoh FM, Marij J, Streiner D (2000). Family intervention for schizophrenia. Cochrane Collaboration database of systematic reviews, 1: 1–36.
247. Center for Substance Abuse Treatment. Substance Abuse Treatment and Family Therapy. Rockville (MD): Substance Abuse and Mental Health Services Administration (US); 2004.

(Treatment Improvement Protocol (TIP) Series, No. 39.) Chapter 1 Substance Abuse Treatment and Family Therapy. Available from: https://www.ncbi.nlm.nih.gov/books/NBK64269/
248. Nasser EH, Overholser JC. Recovery from major depression: the role of support from family, friends, and spiritual beliefs. *Acta Psychiatr Scand.* 2005;111(2):125-132.
249. Sander, J. B., & McCarty, C. A. (2005). Youth depression in the family context: familial risk factors and models of treatment. *Clinical child and family psychology review, 8*(3), 203–219.
250. Hemovich, V., & Crano, W. D. (2009). Family structure and adolescent drug use: an exploration of single-parent families. *Substance use & misuse, 44*(14), 2099–2113. https://doi.org/10.3109/10826080902858375
251. Chadda R. K. (2018). Youth & mental health: Challenges ahead. The Indian journal of medical research, 148(4), 359–361.
252. Amresh Srivastava Rahel Eynan Ravi Shah Lakshaman Dutt, Shubhangi Parkar TSS Rao Giridhar , Rakesh Bhandari MD & Paul Links Mental Health of University Students: Perspectives for Intervention and Prevention: An Indo-Canadian Collaborative Project , Research Insights of the Regional Mental Health Care London and St. Thomas; Vol. 11, No.1, 2014
253. Boak et al. (2016). The mental health and well-being of Ontario stu- dents, 1991-2015: Document Series . Detailed OSDUHS findings. CAMH Research
254. Canadian Mental health Association https://www.camh.ca/en/driving-change/the-crisis-is-real/ mental-health-statistics
255. The Guardian https://www.theguardian.com/education/2019/mar/05/ levels-of-distress-and-illness-among-students-in-uk-alarmingly-high
256. Odgers CL, Jensen MR. Annual Research Review: Adolescent mental health in the digital age: facts, fears, and future directions. J Child Psychol Psychiatry. 2020 Mar;61(3):336-348. doi: 10.1111/jcpp.13190. Epub 2020 Jan 17. PMID: 31951670; PMCID: PMC8221420.
257. Seligman MEP, Csikszentmihalyi M. Positive psychology: an introduction. Am Psychol. 2000;55:5-14.
258. Peterson C., Seligman M.E.P. Character Strengths and Virtues: A Classification and Handbook. American Psychological Association; Washington, DC, USA: 2004
259. Peterson C, Park N. Positive psychology as the evenhanded positive psychologist views it. Psychol Inq. 2003;14:141-146.
260. Park, N., Peterson, C., Szvarca, D., Vander Molen, R. J., Kim, E. S., & Collon, K. (2014). Positive Psychology and Physical Health: Research and Applications. *American journal of lifestyle medicine, 10*(3), 200–206. https://doi.org/10.1177/1559827614550277
261. Cuijpers P, van Straten A, Warmerdam L. Problem solving therapies for depression: a meta-analysis. Eur Psychiatry. 2007;22:9–15
262. CuijpersP,GeraedtsAS,vanOppenP,AnderssonG,MarkowitzJC,vanStratenA.Interpersonal psychotherapy for depression: a meta-analysis. Am J Psychiatry. 2011;168:581–592
263. Rupke SJ, Black D, Renfrow M. Cognitive Therapy for Depression. Am Fam Physician. 2006;73:83–86.
264. World Health Organization,Preventing suicide(2000) https://www.who.int/mental_health/media/en/56.pdf
265. Shrivastava A, Johnston M, Shah N, Bureau Y. Redefining outcome measures in schizophrenia: integrating social and clinical parameters. Curr Opin Psychiatry. 2010;23(2):120-126. doi:10.1097/YCO.0b013e328336662e
266. Chanen AM1, Kaess M.Developmental pathways to borderline per-sonality disorder. Curr Psychiatry Rep. 2012 Feb;14(1):45-53.
267. National Institute of Health, https://www. n i h . g o v/n e w s - e v e n t s /n i h - r e s e a r c h - m a t t e r s / common-genetic-factors-found-5-mental-disorders
268. Shrivastava, A., McGorry, P. D., Tsuang, M., Woods, S. W., Cornblatt, B. A., Corcoran, C., & Carpenter, W. (2011). "Attenuated psychotic symptoms syndrome" as a risk syndrome of psychosis, diagnosis in DSM-V: The debate. Indian journal of psychiatry, 53(1), 57–65. https://doi.org/10.4103/0019-5545.75560
269. Larson, M. K., Walker, E. F., & Compton, M. T. (2010). Early signs, diagnosis and therapeutics of the prodromal phase of schizophrenia and related psychotic disorders. Expert review of neurotherapeutics, 10(8), 1347–1359. https://doi.org/10.1586/ern.10.93
270. National Institute of Health, https://www. n i h . g o v/n e w s - e v e n t s /n i h - r e s e a r c h - m a t t e r s / common-genetic-factors-found-5-mental-disorders

271. Cash, H., Rae, C. D., Steel, A. H., & Winkler, A. (2012). Internet Addiction: A Brief Summary of Research and Practice. Current psychiatry reviews, 8(4), 292–298. https://doi.org/10.2174/157340012803520513
272. Rikkers, W., Lawrence, D., Hafekost, J., & Zubrick, S. R. (2016). Internet use and electronic gaming by children and adolescents with emotional and behavioural problems in Australia - results from the second Child and Adolescent Survey of Mental Health and Wellbeing. *BMC public health, 16,* 399. doi:10.1186/s12889-016-3058-1
273. Love, T., Laier, C., Brand, M., Hatch, L., & Hajela, R. (2015). Neuroscience of Internet Pornography Addiction: A Review and Update. *Behavioral sciences (Basel, Switzerland), 5*(3), 388–433. doi:10.3390/bs5030388
274. Anand, N., Jain, P. A., Prabhu, S., Thomas, C., Bhat, A., Prathyusha, P. V., ... Cherian, A. V. (2018). Internet Use Patterns, Internet Addiction, and Psychological Distress Among Engineering University Students: A Study from India. *Indian journal of psychological medicine, 40*(5), 458–467. doi:10.4103/IJPSYM.IJPSYM_135_18
275. Kumar, S., Kumar, A., Badiyani, B., Singh, S. K., Gupta, A., & Ismail, M. B. (2018). Relationship of internet addiction with depression and academic performance in Indian dental students. *Clujul medical (1957), 91*(3), 300–306. doi:10.15386/cjmed-796
276. National Institute of Mental Health, https://www.nimh.nih.gov/health/topics/depression/index.shtmlMany chronic mood and anxiety disorders in adults begin as high levels of anxiety in children. At its worst, depression can lead to suicide.
277. World Health Organization, South east Asian Countries, Depression in India, http://www.searo.who.int/india/depression_in_india.pdf
278. Paris J. (2007). Why Psychiatrists are Reluctant to Diagnose: Borderline Personality Disorder. Psychiatry (Edgmont (Pa. : Township)), 4(1), 35–39.
279. Jha KK, Singh SK, Nirala SK, Kumar C, Kumar P, Aggrawal N.,Prevalence of Depression among School-going Adolescents in an Urban Area of Bihar, India. Indian J Psychol Med. 2017 May-Jun;39(3):287-292.
280. Negele, A., Kaufhold, J., Kallenbach, L., & Leuzinger-Bohleber, M. (2015). Childhood Trauma and Its Relation to Chronic Depression in Adulthood. Depression research and treatment, 2015, 650804. doi:10.1155/2015/650804
281. American Psychiatric Association, http://www.workplacementalhealth.org/Mental-Health-Topics/Depression/Quantifying-the-Cost-of-Depression
282. What causes depression HTTPs, Harvard Health Publishing , Harvard Medical School. ://www.health.harvard.edu/mind-and-mood/what-causes-depression.
283. Thapar, A., Collishaw, C., Pine, D. S., Thapar, A. K., (2012). "Dépressions in adolescence". Lancet, 379(9820): 1056-1067.
284. World Health Organization https://www.who.int/campaigns/world-health-day/2017/handouts-depression/yourself/en/
285. Gram glia Carla, Zapping Patrizi, Medical Students and Suicide Prevention: Training, Education, and Personal Risks JOURNAL=Frontiers in Psychology vol 9, 2018 -p 452
286. (https://www.betterhealth.vic.gov.au/health/ConditionsAndTreatments/suicide-family-and-friends)
287. Keller, S., McNeill, V., Honea, J., & Paulson Miller, L. (2019). A Look at Culture and Stigma of Suicide: Textual Analysis of Community Theatre Performances. International journal of environmental research and public health, 16(3), 352. doi:10.3390/ijerph16030352
288. Thorndike, E.L. (1920). Intelligence and its use. Harper's Magazine, 140, 227–235.,
289. Bloom, Benjamin S. 1964. Stability and Change in Human Characteristics: New York: Wiley
290. Anju Sharma, Speeckingtree.IN https://www.speakingtree.in/ a l l s l i d e s /s e v e n t e e n - q u a l i t i e s - o f - s p i r i t u a l l y - i n t e l l i g e n t - p e o p l e - a c c o r d i n g - t o - b h a g w a d g i t a / cleanliness
291. Dipak Shukla1, Kaustubh Shukla, Healthcare Transition and Spiritual Health, Journal of The Association of Physicians India Vol. 64 June 2016
292. Huppert FA, Whittington JE (2003) Evidence for the independence of positive and negative well-being: implications for quality of life assessment. Br J Health Psychol. Feb; 8(Pt 1):107-22
293. Danitz SB, Orsillo SM, Beard C, Björgvinsson T. The relationship between personal growth and psychological functioning in individuals treated in a partial hospital setting. J Clin Psychol. 2018 Oct;74(10):1759-1774. doi: 10.1002/jclp.22627. Epub 2018 Apr 26. PMID: 29696645.
294. Wellness and personal development, Gulf Bend Centre, https://www.gulfbend.org/poc/center_index.php?cn=110 (last accessed on 31.8.2020)

295. Cloninger CR. Cloninger CR. (2004.)Feeling good: the science of well-being. New York: Oxford University Press;
296. Personal Development, https://www.workplacestrategiesformentalhealth.com/employee-resources/personal-development (last accessed on 1.8.2020)
297. Health and Counselling,https://www.rwu.edu/undergraduate/student-life/health-and-counseling/health-education-program/dimensions-wellness (last accessed on 1.8.2020)
298. McLaughlin KJ, Gomez JL, Baran SE, Conrad CD. The effects of chronic stress on hippocampal morphology and function: an evaluation of chronic restraint paradigms. Brain Res. 2007;1161:56-64. doi:10.1016/j.brainres.2007.05.042
299. Personal development and mental health , Career in Government, https://www.careers-ingovernment.com/tools/gov-talk/covid-19/personal-development-and-mental-health-issues-during-this-crisis/#:~:text=The%20state%20of%20your%20mental,express%20positive%20and%20negative%20emotions. (Last accessed on1.8.2020)
300. Petrides J, Collins P, Kowalski A, Sepede J, Vermeulen M. Lifestyle Changes for Disease Prevention. Prim Care. 2019;46(1):1-12. doi:10.1016/j.pop.2018.10.003
301. Bauer, I. E., Gálvez, J. F., Hamilton, J. E., Balanzá-Martínez, V., Zunta-Soares, G. B., Soares, J. C., & Meyer, T. D. (2016). Lifestyle interventions targeting dietary habits and exercise in bipolar disorder: A systematic review. Journal of psychiatric research, 74, 1–7. https://doi.org/10.1016/j.jpsychires.2015.12.006
302. Tessier JM, Erickson ZD, Meyer HB, et al. Therapeutic Lifestyle Changes: Impact on Weight, Quality of Life, and Psychiatric Symptoms in Veterans With Mental Illness. Mil Med. 2017;182(9):e1738-e1744. doi:10.7205/MILMED-D-16-00405
303. Foreyt JP. Need for lifestyle intervention: how to begin. Am J Cardiol. 2005;96(4A):11E-14E. doi:10.1016/j.amjcard.2005.05.009
304. **Kristalyn Salters- Pedneault,What Are DSM Personality Disorders?** https://www.verywellmind.com/personality-disorders-a2-425427
305. Hopwood, C. J., Thomas, K. M., Markon, K. E., Wright, A. G., & Krueger, R. F. (2012). DSM-5 personality traits and DSM-IV personality disorders. Journal of abnormal psychology, 121(2), 424–432. https://doi.org/10.1037/a0026656
306. https://addicted2success.com/life/how-spiritual-beliefs-can-help-you-reach-success/
307. Kimberly A Greenway (2006) The Role of Spirituality in Purpose in Life and Academic Engagement, Journal of College and Character, 7: 6, DOI: 10.2202/1940-1639.1212
308. Emily Chandler (2012) Religious and Spiritual Issues in DSM-5: Matters of the Mind and Searching of the Soul, Issues in Mental Health Nursing, 33:9, 577-582, DO
309. van Ments, L., Roelofsma, P., & Treur, J. (2018). Modelling the effect of religion on human empathy based on an adaptive temporal-causal network model. Computational social networks, 5(1), 1. doi:10.1186/s40649-017-0049-z
310. Helen Harris, James W. Ellor & Gaynor Yancey (2017) DSM-5: The intersectionality of spirituality, culture, and aging, Journal of Religion, Spirituality & Aging, 29:1, 3-17, DOI:
311. Center for Substance Abuse Treatment (US). Improving Cultural Competence. Rockville (MD): Substance Abuse and Mental Health Services Administration (US); 2014. (Treatment Improvement Protocol (TIP) Series, No. 59.) Appendix E, Cultural Formulation in Diagnosis and Cultural Concepts of Distress. Available from: https://www.ncbi.nlm.nih.gov/books/NBK248426/
312. Jacek Prusak, Differential diagnosis of "Religious or Spiritual Problem" – possibilities and limitations implied by the V-code 62.89 in DSM-5 Psychiatr. Pol. 2016; 50(1): 175–186
313. Michaelson, V., Brooks, F., Jirásek, I., Inchley, J., Whitehead, R., King, N., … HBSC Child Spiritual Health Writing Group (2016). Developmental patterns of adolescent spiritual health in six countries. SSM - population health, 2, 294–303.
314. Shek D. T. (2012). Spirituality as a positive youth development construct: a conceptual review. The Scientific World Journal, 2012, 458953. doi:10.1100/2012/458953
315. https://www.spiritualcareassociation.org/docs/resources/hccn_whitepaper_spirituality_and_physicians.pdf
316. Pew Research Center. "America's Changing Religious Landscape". 2015.
317. Pew Research Center. "Nones" on the Rise: One-in-Five Adults Have No Religious Affiliation. 2012.
318. Bansal R, Maroof KA, Parashar P, Pant B. Spirituality and health: a knowledge, attitude and practice study among doctors of North India. Spiritual Health Int. 2008 9:263–9. In Wiley Inter Science. Available from: http://www.interscience.wiley.com. [Google Scholar]
319. Dhar, N., Chaturvedi, S., & Nandan, D. (2011). Spiritual health scale 2011: defining and measuring four dimensions of health. Indian journal of community medicine:

official publication of Indian Association of Preventive & Social Medicine, 36(4), 275–282. doi:10.4103/0970-0218.91329

320. Spirituality and well-being,Royal College of psychiatrist https:// www.rcpsych.ac.uk/mental-health/treatments-and-wellbeing/ spirituality-and-mental-health
321. Dhar, N., Chaturvedi, S., & Nandan, D. (2011). Spiritual health scale 2011: defining and measuring 4 dimension of health. Indian journal of community medicine : official publication of Indian Association of Preventive & Social Medicine, 36(4), 275–282. https://doi.org/10.4103/0970-0218.91329
322. Megari K. (2013). Quality of Life in Chronic Disease Patients. Health psychology research, 1(3), e27. https://doi.org/10.4081/hpr.2013.e27
323. Marilyn Baetz,,Ron Griffin, Rudy Bowen, Gene Marcoux, Spirituality and Psychiatry in Canada: Psychiatric Practice Compared With Patient Expectations, (Can J Psychiatry 2004;49:265–271)
324. Varghese A. (2008). Spirituality and mental health. Indian journal of psychiatry, 50(4), 233–237. doi:10.4103/0019-5545.44742
325. Humphreys, J., 2000, Spirituality and distress in sheltered battered women: J.Nurs. Scholarsh., v. 32, no. 3, p. 273-278
326. McSherry, W., 2000, Education issues surrounding the teaching of spirituality: Nurs. Stand., v. 14, no. 42, p. 40-43.
327. Thomas, S., Jenkins, R., Burch, T., Calamos Nasir, L., Fisher, B., Giotaki, G., ... Wright, F. (2016). Promoting Mental Health and Preventing Mental Illness in General Practice. London journal of primary care, 8(1), 3–9.
328. World Healtyh Assembly, Sixty sevent , WHA67.19. Agenda item 15.5. Strengthening of pal- liative care as a component of comprehensive care throughout the life course 2014; http:// apps.who.int/medicinedocs/documents/s21454en/s21454en.pdf. Accessed May 23, 2017.
329. Marin DB, Sharma V, Sosunov E, Egorova N, Goldstein R, Handzo GF. Relationship between chaplain visits and patient satisfaction. J Health Care Chaplain. 2015;21(1):14-24.
330. Balboni T, Balboni M, Paulk ME, et al. Support of cancer patients' spiritual needs and associations with medical care costs at the end of life. Cancer. 2011;117(23):5383-5391.
331. Balboni TA, Paulk ME, Balboni MJ, et al. Provision of Spiritual Care to Patients With Advanced Cancer: Associations With Medical Care and Quality of Life Near Death. J Clin Oncol. 2010;28(3):445-452.
332. Balboni TA, Balboni M, Enzinger AC, et al. Provision of spiritual support to patients with advanced cancer by religious communities and associations with medical care at the end of life. JAMA Intern Med. 2013;173(12):1109-1117.
333. Astrow AB, Wexler A, Texeira K, He MK, Sulmasy DP. Is Failure to Meet Spiritual Needs Associated With Cancer Patients' Perceptions of Quality of Care and Their Satisfaction With Care? J Clin Oncol. 2007;25(36):5753-5757.
334. Dhar, N., Chaturvedi, S., & Nandan, D. (2011). Spiritual health scale 2011: defining and measuring 4 dimension of health. Indian journal of community medicine : official publication of Indian Association of Preventive & Social Medicine, 36(4), 275–282. https://doi.org/10.4103/0970-0218.91329
335. Spaniol, L. (2002). Spirituality and connectedness [Editorial]. Psychiatric Rehabilitation Journal, 25(4), 321–322. https://doi.org/10.1037/h0095006
336. https://www.scienceofconnectedness.com/spirituality-definition/
337. Overcoming Barriers to the Provision of Spiritual Care: the place of compassion in clinical practice. Mary Nathan MSc. Reported by Dr Gillian Broster
338. It is astonishing that some governments are now doubting whether people with severe mental illness should be prioritized for COVID-19 vaccination." The Lancet Psychiatry www.thelancet.com/psychiatry Published online February 20, 2020, https://doi. org/10.1016/S2215-0366(20)30048-1
339. Narenji, F., Nahidi, F., Ebadi, A., & Nasiri, M. (2018). Maternal care for spiritual health of unborn child during pregnancy: A qualitative study with content analysis approach. Spirituality in Clinical Practice, 5(4), 251
340. Ryan T. Howell, https://www.psychologytoday.com/ca/blog/cant-buy-happiness/201302/why-be-spiritual-five-benefits-spirituality
341. Park CL, Masters KS, Salsman JM, Wachholtz A, Clements AD, Salmoirago-Blotcher E, Trevino K, Wischenka DM. Advancing our understanding of religion and spirituality in the context of behavioral medicine. J Behav Med. 2017 Feb;40(1):39-51. doi: 10.1007/s10865-016-9755-5. Epub 2016 Jun 24. PMID: 27342616; PMCID: PMC5183527.

342. Zimmer, Z., Jagger, C., Chiu, C. T., Ofstedal, M. B., Rojo, F., & Saito, Y. (2016). Spirituality, religiosity, aging and health in global perspective: A review. *SSM - population health, 2,* 373–381. https://doi.org/10.1016/j.ssmph.2016.04.009
343. Crossley D. Religious experience within mental illness: opening the door on research. Br J Psychiatry. 1995;166:284-286.
344. Rob Whitley,, Religion and mental health-what is the link, Psychology Today 18, Dec 2017 (https://www.psychologytoday.com/gb/blog/talking-about-men/201712/religion-and-mental-health-what-is-the-link)
345. Moreira-almeida a, neto fl, koenig hg. Religiousness and mental health: a review.braz j psychiatry. 2006 sep;28(3):242-50.
346. Weber SR, Pargament KI. The role of religion and spirituality in mental health. Curr Opin Psychiatry. 2014 Sep;27(5):358-63.
347. Applebaum, A. J., Stein, E. M., Lord-Bessen, J., Pessin, H., Rosenfeld, B., & Breitbart, W. (2014). Optimism, social support, and mental health outcomes in patients with advanced cancer. Psycho-oncology, 23(3), 299–306.
348. Scheier MF, Carver CS. Optimism, coping, and health: assessment and implications of generalized outcome expectancies. Journal of Health Psychology. 1985; 4(3):219–247.
349. Scheier MF, Carver CS. Effects of optimism on pychological and physical well-being: Theoretical overview and empirical update. Cognitive Therapy and Research. 1992; 16(2):201–228.
350. Miller DL, Manne SL, Taylor K, Keates J, Dougherty J. Psychological distress and well-being in advanced cancer: The effects of optimism and coping. Journal of Clinical Psychology in Medical Settings. 1996; 3(2):115–130. [PubMed: 24226639].
351. Horney DJ, Smith HE, McGurk M, Weinman J, Herold J, Altman K, et al. Associations between quality of life, coping styles, optimism, and anxiety and depression in pretreatment patients with head and neck cancer. Head & Neck. 2011; 33(1):65–71.
352. Petersen LR, Clark MM, Novotny P, Kung S, Sloan JA, Patten CA, et al. Relationship of optimism-pessimism and health-related quality of life in breast cancer survivors. Journal of Psychosocial Oncology. 2008; 26(4):15–32.
353. Schou I, Ekeberg O, Ruland CM, Sandvik L, Karesen R. Pessimism as a predictor of emotional morbidity one year following breast cancer surgery. Psycho-Oncology. 2004; 13(5):309–320.
354. Brown, J., Hanson, J. E., Schmotzer, B., & Webel, A. R. (2014). Spirituality and optimism: a holistic approach to component-based, self-management treatment for HIV. Journal of religion and health, 53(5), 1317–1328. doi:10.1007/s10943-013-9722-1
355. McCullough ME, Hoyt WT, Larson DB, Koenig HG, Thoresen C. Religious involvement and mortality: A meta-analytic review. Health Psychology. 2000; 19(3):211
356. Foskett, J., A. Roberts, R. Mathews, L. Macmin, P. Cracknell, and V. Nicholls, 2004, From research to practice: The first tentative steps: Mental Health, Religion & Culture, v. 7, no. 1, p. 41-58.
357. Seybold, K. S., and P. C. Hill, 2001, The Role of Religion and Spirituality in Mental and Physical Health: Current Directions in Psychological Science, v. 10, no. 1, p. 21-24.
358. Weaver, A. J., L. T. Flannelly, J. Garbarino, C. R. Figley, and K. J. Flannelly, 2003, A systematic review of research on religion and spirituality in the Journal of Traumatic Stress : 1990-1999: Mental Health, Religion & Culture, v. 6, no. 3, p. 215-228.
359. Gartner, J., 1996, Religious commitment, mental health and proso-cial behaviour: a review of the empirical literature, in EP Shafranske ed., Religion and the clinical practice of psychology: Washington DC, APA, p. 187-214.
360. Rasic DT Belik SL, Elias B, Katz LY, Enns M, Sareen J; Swampy Cree Suicide Prevention Team. Spirituality, religion and suicidal behavior in a nationally representative sample. J Affect Disord. 2009 Apr;114(1-3):32-40
361. Koenig, H. G., D. O. Moberg, and J. N. Kvale, 1988, Religious activi-ties and attitudes of older adults in a geriatric assessment clinic: J.Am. Geriatr.Soc., v. 36, no. 4, p. 362-374.
362. Boscaglia, N. D. M. Clarke, T. W. Jobling, and M. A. Quinn, 2005, The contribution of spirituality and spiritual coping to anxiety and depression in women with a recent diagnosis of gynecological cancer: Int.J.Gynecol.Cancer, v. 15, no. 5, p. 755-761.
363. Naghi, Jesse J., Kiran J. Philip, Anita Phan, Laurent Cleenewerck, and Ernst R. Schwarz. 2012. The effects of spirituality and religion on outcomes in patients with chronic heart failure. Journal of Religion and Health 51: 1124–36

364. Strada, E. Alessandra, Peter Homel, Sharon Tennstedt, J. Andrew Billings, and Russell K. Portenoy. 2013. Spiritual well-being in patients with advanced heart and lung disease. Palliat and Support Care 11: 205–13.
365. Min, J. A., Lee, C. U., & Lee, C. (2013). Mental health promotion and illness prevention: a challenge for psychiatrists. Psychiatry investiga-tion, 10(4), 307–316.
366. Rob Whitley,, Religion and mental health-what is the link, Psychology Today 18, Dec 2017 (https://www.psychologytoday. com/gb/blog/talking-about-men/201712/religion-and-mental-health-what-is-the-link)
367. Moreira-almeida a, neto fl, koenig hg. Religiousness and mental health: a review.braz j psychiatry. 2006 sep;28(3):242-50.
368. Margetic, B., and B. Margetic, 2005, Religiosity and health outcomes: a review of literature: Coll.Antropol., v. 29, no. 1, p. 365-371.
369. REFLECTIONS ON INTEGRATING MIND AND BODY: A CONCEPT RELEVANT TO PSYCHIATRY? Dr Nicki Crowley
370. Zuckerman DM, Kasl SV, Ostfeld AM. Psychosocial predictors of mortality among the elderly poor: the role of religion, well-being, and social contacts. Am J Epidemiol. 1984;119:410–423.
371. Idler EL. Religious involvement and the health of the elderly: some hypotheses and an initial test. Soc Forces. 1987;66:226–238.
372. Miller JF. Assessment of loneliness and spiritual well-being in chronically ill and healthy adults. J Prof Nurs. 1985;2:45–49.
373. Pressman P, Lyons JS, and Larson DB. et al. Religious belief, depression, and ambulation status in elderly women with broken hips. Am J Psychiatry. 1990 147:758–760.
374. MahdiNejad JE1, Azemati H1, Sadeghi Habibabad A2.Religion and Spirituality: Mental Health Arbitrage in the Body of Mosques Architecture. J Relig Health. 2019 Nov 13
375. Rippentrop EA1, Altmaier EM, Chen JJ, Found EM, Keffala VJ.The relationship between religion/spirituality and physical health, mental health, and pain in a chronic pain population. Pain. 2005 Aug;116(3):311-21
376. Waldron-Perrine B1, Rapport LJ, Hanks RA, Lumley M, Meachen SJ, Hubbarth P.Religion and spirituality in rehabilitation outcomes among individuals with traumatic brain injury. Rehabil Psychol. 2011 May;56(2):107-16. doi: 10.1037/a0023552.
377. Mohr S1, Huguelet P.The relationship between schizophrenia and religion and its implications for care. Swiss Med Wkly. 2004 Jun 26;134(25-26):369-76.
378. Mohr S1, Borras L, Gillieron C, Brandt PY, Huguelet P.Spirituality, religious practices and schizophrenia: relevance for the clinician]. Rev Med Suisse. 2006 Sep 20;2(79):2092-4, 2096-8.
379. Li X, Weissman M, Talati A, Svob C, Wickramaratne P, Posner J, Xu D. A diffusion tensor imaging study of brain microstructural changes related to religion and spirituality in families at high risk for depression. Brain Behav. 2019 Feb;9(2):e01209. doi: 10.1002/brb3.1209. Epub 2019 Jan 15.
380. Banquet JP Spectral analysis of the EEG in meditation. Electroencephalogr Clin Neurophysiol. 1973 Aug; 35(2):143-51.
381. Corby JC, Roth WT, Zarcone VP Jr, Kopell BS Psychophysiological correlates of the practice of Tantric Yoga meditation. Arch Gen Psychiatry. 1978 May; 35(5):571-7
382. Sudsuang R, Chentanez V, Veluvan K, Effect of Buddhist meditation on serum cortisol and total protein levels, blood pressure, pulse rate, lung volume and reaction time. Physiol Behav. 1991 Sep; 50(3):543-8.
383. Jevning R, Wallace RK, Beidebach M, The physiology of meditation: a review. A wakeful hypometabolic integrated response.Neurosci Biobehav Rev. 1992 Fall; 16(3):415-24.
384. O'Halloran JP, Jevning R, Wilson AF, Skowsky R, Walsh RN, Alexander C, Hormonal control in a state of decreased activation: potentiation of arginine vasopressin secretionPhysiol Behav. 1985 Oct; 35(4):591-5
385. Walton KG, Pugh ND, Gelderloos P, Macrae P Stress reduction and preventing hypertension: preliminary support for a psychoneuroendocrine mechanism.J Altern Complement Med. 1995 Fall; 1(3):263-83.
386. Lazar SW, Bush G, Gollub RL, Fricchione GL, Khalsa G, Benson H, Functional brain mapping of the relaxation response and meditation.Neuroreport. 2000 May 15; 11(7):1581-5.
387. Wang DJ, Rao H, Korczykowski M, Wintering N, Pluta J, Khalsa DS, Newberg AB, Cerebral blood flow changes associated with different meditation practices and perceived depth of meditation. Psychiatry Res. 2011 Jan 30; 191(1):60-7.
388. Newberg A. B. (2014). The neuroscientific study of spiritual practices. *Frontiers in psychology, 5*, 215. https://doi.org/10.3389/fpsyg.2014.00215

389. Tang YY, Leve LD. A translational neuroscience perspective on mindfulness meditation as a prevention strategy. Transl Behav Med. 2016;6(1):63-72.
390. Fox KC, Dixon ML, Nijeboer S, et al. Functional neuroanatomy of meditation: A review and meta-analysis of 78 functional neuroimaging investigations. Neurosci Biobehav Rev. 2016;65:208-228.
391. Boccia M, Piccardi L, Guariglia P. The Meditative Mind: A Comprehensive Meta-Analysis of MRI Studies. Biomed Res Int. 2015;2015:419808.
392. Tang YY, Holzel BK, Posner MI. The neuroscience of mindfulness meditation. Nat Rev Neurosci. 2015;16(4):213-225.
393. Barnby JM, Bailey NW, Chambers R, Fitzgerald PB. How similar are the changes in neural activity resulting from mindfulness practice in contrast to spiritual practice? Conscious Cogn. 2015;36:219-232.
394. Deborah Cornah , the impact of Spirituality on mental hekath, A review of literature, written for Mental health Foundation and published by Mental health foundation UK, https://www.mentalhealth.org.uk/sites/default/files/impact-spirituality.pdf
395. Thomas, S., Jenkins, R., Burch, T., Calamos Nasir, L., Fisher, B., Giotaki, G., ... Wright, F. (2016). Promoting Mental Health and Preventing Mental Illness in General Practice. *London journal of primary care, 8*(1), 3–9.
396. Verghese A. Spirituality and mental health. Indian J Psychiatry 2008;50:233-7
397. Timble M. Soul in the brain: the cerebral basis of language, art and belief. BJP. 2008;193:175.
398. Margetic, B., and B. Margetic, 2005, Religiosity and health outcomes: a review of literature: Coll.Antropol., v. 29, no. 1, p. 365-371.
399. Mrazek PJ & Haggerty RJ 1994, Reducing the Risks for Mental Disorders: Frontiers for Preventive Intervention Research, National Academy Press, Washington DC.
400. Kodal A, Fjermestad K, Bjelland, Gjestad R, Öst LG, Bjaastad JF, Haugland BSM, Havik OE, Heiervang E, Wergeland GJ. Long-term effectiveness of cognitive behavioral therapy for youth with anxiety disorders.Anxiety Disord. 2018 Jan;53:58-67. doi: 10.1016/j.janxdis.2017.11.003. Epub 2017 Nov 26.
401. Amminger, G. P., Schäfer, M. R., Schlögelhofer, M., Klier, C. M., & McGorry, P. D. (2015). Longer-term outcome in the prevention of psy-chotic disorders by the Vienna omega-3 study. Nature communications, 6, 7934. doi:10.1038/ncomms8934
402. Sussman S[1], Milam J, Arpawong TE, Tsai J, Black DS, Wills TA.Spirituality in addictions treatment: wisdom to know...what it is. Subst Use Misuse. 2013 Sep;48(12):1203-17.
403. Dein S, Cook CC, Koenig H. Religion, spirituality, and mental health: current controversies and future directions. J Nerv Ment Dis. 2012;200(10):852-855. doi:10.1097/NMD.0b013e31826b6dle
404. Daniel LT, Krishnan G, Gupta S. A study to assess the prevalence and pattern of substance use among male adolescents in suburban area of Delhi. Indian J Soc Psychiatry 2017;33:208-12
405. National Academies of Sciences, Engineering, and Medicine; Division of Behavioral and Social Sciences and Education; Board on Children, Youth, and Families; Committee on Supporting the Parents of Young Children; Briner H, Ford M, Gadsden VL, editors. Parenting Matters: Supporting Parents of Children Ages 0-8. Washington (DC): National Academies Press (US); 2016 Nov 21. 2, Parenting Knowledge, Attitudes, and Practices. Available from: https://www.ncbi.nlm.nih.gov/books/NBK402020
406. Dougkas Todd, 'spiritual' university students more successful: Study, Vencouer Sun,2010, https://vancouversun.com/news/staff-blogs/spiritual-university-students-more-successful-study
407. Committee on the Science of Children Birth to Age 8: Deepening and Broadening the Foundation for Success; Board on Children, Youth, and Families; Institute of Medicine; National Research Council; Allen LR, Kelly BB, editors. Transforming the Workforce for Children Birth Through Age 8: A Unifying Foundation. Washington (DC): National Academies Press (US); 2015 Jul 23. 4, Child Development and Early Learning. Available from: https://www.ncbi.nlm.nih.gov/books/NBK310550/
408. Black, M. M., Walker, S. P., Fernald, L., Andersen, C. T., DiGirolamo, A. M., Lu, C., McCoy, D. C., Fink, G., Shawar, Y. R., Shiffman, J., Devercelli, A. E., Wodon, Q. T., Vargas-Barón, E., Grantham-McGregor, S., & Lancet Early Childhood Development Series Steering Committee (2017). Early childhood development coming of age: science through the life course. *Lancet (London, England), 389*(10064), 77–90. https://doi.org/10.1016/S0140-6736(16)31389-7

409. Puchalski C. M. (2001). The role of spirituality in health care. Proceedings (Baylor University. Medical Center), 14(4), 352–357. doi:10.1080/08998280.2001.11927788
410. A National study of college students' search of meaning and purpose The spiritual life of college students , Higher Education Research Institute, The Dallas Morning News, November 29, 2003
411. Jacob, B., White, A., & Shogbon, A. (2017). First-year Student Pharmacists' Spirituality and Perceptions Regarding the Role of Spirituality in Pharmacy Education. American journal of pharmaceutical education, 81(6), 108.
412. The spiritual life of college students , A national study of college students searcg of meaning and purose,Higher education Research Instidtue,University of California. USA https://spirituality.ucla.edu/docs/reports/Spiritual_Life_College_Students_Full_Report.pdf
413. Koenig H. G. (2012). Religion, spirituality, and health: the research and clinical implications. ISRN psychiatry, 2012, 278730. doi:10.5402/2012/278730
414. Saad, M., de Medeiros, R., & Mosini, A. C. (2017). Are We Ready for a True Biopsychosocial-Spiritual Model? The Many Meanings of "Spiritual". *Medicines (Basel, Switzerland),* 4(4), 79. https://doi.org/10.3390/medicines4040079
415. Ross L1.The spiritual dimension: its importance to patients' health, well-being and quality of life and its implications for nursing practice. no J Nurs Stud. 1995 Oct;32(5):457-68.
416. *Drabble, L., Veldhuis, C. B., Riley, B. B., Rostosky, S., & Hughes, T. L. (2018). Relationship Of Religiosity And Spirituality To Hazardous Drinking, Drug Use, And Depression Among Sexual Minority Women. Journal Of Homosexuality, 65(13), 1734–1757.*
417. Zohar, D. and Marshall, I. (2004) *Spiritual Capital: Wealth We Can Live By.* San Francisco: Berrett-Koehler Publishers, Inc.
418. Zohar, D. (1999) *SQ: Spiritual Intelligence, the Ultimate Intelligence.* London: Bloomsbury
419. Publishing PLC.
420. Biswajit Satpathy Spiritual intelligence from the Bhagavad-Gita for conflict resolution *Int. J. Indian Culture and Business Management, Vol. 3, No. 4, 2010* 449
421. Koenig, H. G., McCullough, M., & Larson, D. B. (2000): *The Handbook of Religion and Health.* (NewYork: Oxford University Press, 200)
422. Laird, K. T., Krause, B., Funes, C., & Lavretsky, H. (2019). Psychobiological factors of resilience and depression in late life. *Translational psychiatry, 9*(1), 88. doi:10.1038/s41398-019-0424-7
423. Mosqueiro BP, Fleck MP and Rocha NSd (2019) Increased Levels of Brain-Derived Neurotrophic Factor Are Associated With High Intrinsic Religiosity Among Depressed Inpatients. *Front. Psychiatry* 10:671. doi: 10.3389/fpsyt.2019.00671
424. How to manage and reduce stress (https://www.mentalhealth.org.uk/publications/how-manage-and-reduce-stress)
425. Jonathan Rowson.Revitalising spirituality to address 21st century challenges, Spiritualise December 2014 (https://www.thersa.org/globalassets/pdfs/reports/spiritualise-report.pdf)
426. Wellbeing, The mind, https://www.mind.org.uk/media/2976123/how-to-improve-your-wellbeing-through-physi- cal-activity-and-sport.pdf
427. Fredrickson, B. L., Cohn, M. A., Coffey, K. A., Pek, J., & Finkel, S. M. (2008). Open hearts build lives: Positive emotions, induced through loving-kindness meditation, build consequential personal resources. Journal of personality and social psychology, 95(5), 1045–1062.
428. Mueller PS1, Plevak DJ, Rummans TA. 2001 Religious involvement, spirituality, and medicine: implications for clinical practice. Mayo Clin Proc. Dec;76(12):1225-35.
429. Mizock L, Millner UC, Russinova Z. 2012Spiritual and religious issues in psychotherapy with schizophrenia: cultural implications and implementation. Religions.;3(1):82–98.
430. History of Yoga. https://www.yogabasics.com/learn/history-of-yoga/#:~:text=The%20beginnings%20of%20Yoga%20were,by%20Brahmans%2C%20the%20Vedic%20priests.
431. Awasthi, A (2013) argue that Patanjali belongs to a dualistic philosophical tradition (Sankhya), in which meditation is a spiritual phenomenon, inaccessible to objective research.
432. Bærentsen K. B. (2015). Patanjali and neuroscientific research on meditation. Frontiers in psychology, 6, 915. https://doi.org/10.3389/fpsyg.2015.00915
433. Rao K. R. (2011). Applied yoga psychology: studies of neurophysiology of meditation. J. Conscious. Stud. 18, 161–198.

434. Woods J. H. (1927/2003). The Yoga-Sutra of Patanjali. New York, NY: Dover.
435. Robena Bano, Sanjay Khanna, Pratap Shankar, Dheeraj Kumar Singh, Sachin Tutu, Preet Lakhani Rakesh Kumar Dixit Knowledge, Attitudes, and Practices regarding YOGA in general population World Journal of Pharmaceutical Sciences ISSN (Print): 2321-3310; 2016
436. Rathore, M., & Abraham, J. (2018). The Implication Of Asana, Pranayama And Meditation On Telomere Stability. International Journal Of Yoga, 11(3), 186–193.
437. Magri C, Schridde U, Murayama Y, Panzeri S, Logothetis NK(2012) T he amplitude and timing of the BOLD signal reflects the relationship between local field potential power at different frequencies.J Neurosci.; 32(4):1395-407.
438. Wolfe, U., & Moran, A. (2017). Integrating Brain Science into Health Studies: An Interdisciplinary Course in Contemplative Neuroscience and Yoga. Journal of undergraduate neuroscience education: JUNE: a publication of FUN, Faculty for Undergraduate Neuroscience, 16(1), A77–A82.
439. Ield T., Diego M., Hernandez-Reif M. (2010). Tai chi/yoga effects on anxiety, heart rate, EEG and math computations. Complement. Ther. Clin. Pract. 16 235–238.
440. Coan J, Allen J. (2004) Frontal EEG asymmetry as a moderator and mediator of emotion. Biological Psychology;67:7–49.
441. Liotti M, Mayberg HS.(2001) The role of functional neuroimag-ing in the neuropsychology of depression. Journal of Clinical & Experimental Neuropsychology: Official Journal of the International Neuropsychological Society;23(1):121–136.
442. Revets W, Price J, Furey M.(2008) Brain structural and functional abnor-malities in mood disorders: Implications for neurocircuitry models of depression. Brain Structure and Function. 2008;213:93–118.
443. Walton, K. G., Schneider, R. H., & Nidich, S. (2004). Review of con-trolled research on the transcendental meditation program and cardiovascular disease. Risk factors, morbidity, and mortality. Cardiology in review, 12(5), 262–266
444. Vahia NS, Doongaji DR, Jeste DV, Ravindranath S, Kapoor SN, Ardhapurkar I. (1973) Psychophysiologic therapy based on the concepts of Patanjail. A new approach to the treatment of neurotic and psychosomatic disorders. Am J Psychotherapy;27:557–65. [PubMed : 4761011]
445. Vahia NS.(1969) A therapy based upon some concepts prevalent in India. Indian J Psychiatry;11:7–14.
446. Vahia NS, Doongaji DR, Deshmukh DK, Vinekar SL, Parekh HC, Kapoor SN. A deconditioning therapy based upon concepts of Patanjali. Int J Soc Psychiatry. 1972;18:61–6. [PubMed: 4558096]
447. Satish Chandra P. Yoga and Neurobehavioral Sciences: Indian Perspective. Indian J Psychiatry 2013;55:332-3.
448. Prathikanti, S., Rivera, R., Cochran, A., Tungol, J. G., Fayazmanesh, N., & Weinmann, E. (2017). Treating major depression with yoga: A prospective, randomized, controlled pilot trial. PloS one, 12(3), e0173869. https://doi.org/10.1371/journal.pone.0173869
449. Streeter CC, Gerbarg PL, Whitfield TH, et al.(2017) Treatment of Major Depressive Disorder with Iyengar Yoga and Coherent Breathing: A Randomized Controlled Dosing Study. J Altern Complement Med.;23(3):201-207.
450. Streeter CC, Gerbarg PL, Brown RP, et al. (2020) Thalamic Gamma Aminobutyric Acid Level Changes in Major Depressive Disorder After a 12-Week Iyengar Yoga and Coherent Breathing Intervention. J Altern Complement Med.;26(3):190-197
451. Balasubramaniam, M., Telles, S., & Doraiswamy, P. M. (2013). Yoga on our minds: a systematic review of yoga for neuropsychiatric disorders. Frontiers in psychiatry, 3, 117. https://doi.org/10.3389/fpsyt.2012.00117
452. Rao, N. P., Varambally, S., & Gangadhar, B. N. (2013). Yoga school of thought and psychiatry: Therapeutic potential. Indian journal of psychiatry, 55(Suppl 2), S145–S149. https://doi.org/10.4103/0019-5545.105510
453. Varambally S, Gangadhar BN.(2012) Yoga: a spiritual practice with therapeutic value in psychiatry. Asian J Psychiatr. 2012;5(2):186-189.
454. Jayaram N, Varambally S, Behere RV, et al.(2013) Effect of yoga therapy on plasma oxytocin and facial emotion recognition deficits in patients of schizophrenia. Indian J Psychiatry. 2013;55(Suppl 3):S409-S413
455. Govindaraj R, Naik S, Manjunath NK, Mehta UM, Gangadhar BN, Varambally S.(2018) Add-on Yoga Therapy for Social Cognition in Schizophrenia: A Pilot Study. Int J Yoga.;11(3):242-244.

456. Deshpande, S. N., Bhatia, T., Mohandas, E., & Nimgaonkar, V. L. (2016). Cognitive remediation in schizophrenia-The view from India. Asian journal of psychiatry, 22, 124–128. https://doi.org/10.1016/j.ajp.2016.06.011
457. Cochrane Database Syst Rev. 2017 Sep; 2017(9): CD012052. Published online 2017 Sep 28.
458. Varambally, S., Venkatasubramanian, G., Govindaraj, R., Shivakumar, V., Mullapudi, T., Christopher, R., Debnath, M., Philip, M., Bharath, R. D., & Gangadhar, B. N. (2019). Yoga and schizophrenia-a comprehensive assessment of neuroplasticity: Protocol for a single blind randomized controlled study of yoga in schizophrenia. Medicine, 98(43), e17399.
459. Yang, H., Leaver, A. M., Siddarth, P., Paholpak, P., Ercoli, L., St Cyr, N. M., Eyre, H. A., Narr, K. L., Khalsa, D. S., & Lavretsky, H. (2016). Neurochemical and Neuroanatomical Plasticity Following Memory Training and Yoga Interventions in Older Adults with Mild Cognitive Impairment. Frontiers in aging neuroscience, 8, 277.
460. Gangadhar, B. N., & Porandla, K. (2015). Yoga and mental health services. Indian journal of psychiatry, 57(4), 338–340.
461. Braboszcz, C., Cahn, B. R., Balakrishnan, B., Maturi, R. K., Grandchamp, R., & Delorme, A. (2013). Plasticity of visual attention in Isha yoga meditation practitioners before and after a 3-month retreat. Frontiers in psychology, 4, 914.
462. Schmalzl, L., Powers, C., & Henje Blom, E. (2015). Neurophysiological and neurocognitive mechanisms underlying the effects of yoga-based practices: towards a comprehensive theoretical framework. Frontiers in human neuroscience, 9, 235.
463. STEVEN PINKER, So How Does the Mind Work? Mind & Language, Vol. 20 No. 1 February 2005, pp. 1–24. # BlackwellPublishing Ltd. 2005, 9600 Garsington Road, Oxford, OX4 2DQ, UK and 350Main Street,Malden,MA 02148, USA.
464. Easwaran (1997). The Bhagavad Gita (Easwaran's Classics of Indian Spirituality Book 1) 2nd Edition, Nilgiri Press; 2nd edition (June 1, 2009
465. T.N.Sethumadhavan Srimad Bhagavad Gita Chapter 2, Saankhya Yogah: Yoga of Knowledge Transliterated Sanskrit Text Published In Esamskriti.com & Medhajournal.com Nagpur September 2010
466. Bhagavad Gita The Song of God, Commentary by Swami Mukundananda https://www.holy-bhagavad-gita.org/chapter/6/verse/35 (Last accessed on 16.8.2020)
467. http://stevenpinker.com/files/pinker/files/so_how_does_the_mind_ work.pdf
468. The Bhagavad Gita (Eswaran's Classics of Indian Spirituality Book 1) 2nd Edition, Nilgiris Press; 2nd edition (June 1, 2009)
469. Excerpted from "Srimad Bhagavatam Tenth Canto Part One" by A.C. Bhakti Vedanta Swami Prabhakaran, courtesy of the Bhakti Vedanta Book Trust International, www.krishna.com."
470. Bhatia Scl, Mahabodhi J, Kelli V, Bhatia Sc, Madan V.The Bhagavad Gita, And Contemporary Psychotherapies. Indian J Psychiatry. 2013 Jan;55(Suppl 2): S315-21
471. Awasthi (2013) argue that Patanjali belongs to a dualistic philosophical tradition (Sankhya), in which meditation is a spiritual phenomenon, inaccessible to objective research.
472. T.N.Sethumadhavan Srimad Bhagavad Gita Chapter 2, Saankhya Yogah: Yoga of Knowledge Transliterated Sanskrit Text Published In Esamskriti.com & Medhajournal.com Nagpur September 2010
473. What is the use of the vedas?, https://www.esamskriti.com/e/Spirituality/Bhagavad-Gita/Bhagavad-Gita~-Chapter-2-(Part~4)-Saankhya-Yogah~-Yoga-Of-Knowledge-3.aspx
474. T.N.Sethumadhavan Srimad Bhagavad Gita Chapter 2, Saankhya Yoga: Yoga of Knowledge Transliterated Sanskrit Text Published In Esamskriti.com & Medhajournal.com Nagpur September 2010
475. Broderick J, Crumlish N, Waugh A, Vancampfort D. Yoga versus non-standard care for schizophrenia. Cochrane Database Syst Rev. 2017 Sep 28;9(9):CD012052. doi: 10.1002/14651858.CD012052.pub2. PMID: 28956893; PMCID:
476. Bhagwat Gita in daily life, https://iloveiskcontemple.com/bhagavad-gita-in-daily-life/
477. T.N.Sethumadhavan Srimad Bhagavad Gita Chapter 2, Saankhya Yoga: Yoga of Knowledge Transliterated Sanskrit Text Published In Esamskriti.com & Medhajournal.com Nagpur September 2010
478. T.N.Sethumadhavan Srimad Bhagavad Gita Chapter 2, Saankhya Yoga: Yoga of Knowledge Transliterated Sanskrit Text Published In Esamskriti.com & Medhajournal.com Nagpur September 2010

479. Hamilton Inbadas (2018) Indian philosophical foundations of spirituality at the end of life, Mortality, 23:4, 320-333,
480. Sharma H. (2015). Meditation: Process and effects. *Ayu, 36*(3), 233–237. https://doi.org/10.4103/0974-8520.182756
481. T.N.Sethumadhavan Srimad Bhagavad Gita Chapter 2, Saankhya Yogah: Yoga of Knowledge Transliterated Sanskrit Text Published In Esamskriti.com & Medhajournal.com Nagpur September 2010
482. Hegde S. National seminar on Bhagavad Gita and mental health: Conference proceedings. Asian J Psychiatry. 2009;1:60.
483. Allain, H., Akwa, Y., Lacomblez, L., Lieury, A., & Bentué-Ferrer, D. (2007). Impaired cognition and attention in adults: pharmacological management strategies. Neuropsychiatric disease and treatment, 3(1), 103–116.
484. Amaranath, B., Nagendra, H. R., & Deshpande, S. (2016). Effect of integrated yoga module on the personality of home guards in Bengaluru: A randomized control trial. Journal of Ayurveda and integrative medicine, 7(1), 44–47.
485. Rajesh, S. K., Ilavarasu, J. V., Srinivasan, T. M., & Nagendra, H. R. (2014). Stress and its Expression According to Contemporary Science and Ancient Indian Wisdom: Perseverative Cognition and the Pañca kośas. Men's Sana monographs, 12(1), 139–152
486. Biswajit Satpathy, Spiritual intelligence from the Bhagavad-Gita for conflict resolution Int. J. Indian Culture and Business Management, Vol. 3, No. 4, 2010 449
487. Bhatia Scl, Madabushi J, Kolli V, Bhatia Sk, Madaan V.The Bhagavad Gita, And Contemporary Psychotherapies. Indian J Psychiatry. 2013 Jan;55(Suppl 2): S315-21
488. Kalra, S., Joshi, A., Kalra, B., Shanbhag, V. G., Bhattacharya, R., Verma, K., ... Dalal, K. (2017). Bhagavad Gita for the Physician. Indian journal of endocrinology and metabolism, 21(6), 893–897. doi:10.4103/ijem.IJEM_259_17
489. Pradhan, B., & Derle, S. G. (2012). Comparison of effect of Gayatri Mantra and Poem Chanting on Digit Letter Substitution Task. Ancient science of life, 32(2), 89–92.
490. Susan Thomas1 Shobini L. Rao Effect of Gayatri Mantra Meditation on Meditation Naive Subjects: an EEG and fMRI Pilot Study. The International Journal of Indian Psychology. Volume 3, Issue 2, No.7,
491. Rashi Sharma, To study the effect of Gayatri mantra on Manas Prakruti and stress International Journal of Engineering Development and Research 2018, Volume 6, Issue 2
492. Sushrutha S, Manjunath NK, Bhatta R. Karnataka: 2009. Changes in higher brain functions following recitation of gayatri mantra. M. Sc dissertation Swami Vivekananda Yoga Anushandhan Samsthana, Bangaluru.

ABOUT THE AUTHOR

Amresh Shrivastava,
Professor Emeritus of Psychiatry
MD,DPM.FRCPsych,FRCPC,FAPA
Western University, Canada

Dr. Srivastava is a Professor Emeritus of Psychiatry at the Western University and a Scientist of Mental health at Lawson Health Research Institute, located in London, Ontario, Canada.

Trained from the K.E.M Hospital, University of Mumbai, Dr. Srivastava received his postgraduate degrees and worked in Mumbai for two decades. He holds a Fellowship of the Royal College of Physicians and Surgeons Of Canada (Academic accreditation) FRCPC and a Fellowship of the Royal College of Psychiatry, UK, FRCPsych. He is also a fellow of the American Psychiatric Association (FAPA).

His areas of focus include Suicide prevention, early intervention, and complex mental disorders.

He has served as an editor, reviewer and member of the editorial board of psychiatric journals and published original research reviews, book chapters, academic and non-fiction academic books.

Most notable amongst these is the publication of a reference book series on suicide – "Suicide from a Global Perspective", which encompasses five volumes with contributions from authors from 30 countries.

Dr. Srivastava's professional career spans over 40years in mental health. During this period, he worked in India, the United Kingdom and Canada in the fields of clinical academics, research, and education encompassing Government health services, private practice, universities, and professional organizations.

His areas of focus include Suicide prevention, .

Dr. Srivastava has also had the honour of receiving prestigious research and service awards from professional organizations, hospitals, and University in India, the United States and Canada. The measurement tool for assessing the 'risk of suicide behaviors' called SIS-MAP, developed by Dr. Srivastava, resulted him in being awarded the R.O.Jones award for research from the Canadian Psychiatric Association.

Printed in Great Britain
by Amazon

74036936R00228